Proceedings in Life Sciences

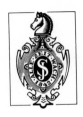

Cerebellar Functions

Edited by
J. R. Bloedel, J. Dichgans, and W. Precht

With 156 Figures

Springer-Verlag
Berlin Heidelberg New York Tokyo 1985

Prof. Dr. James R. Bloedel, Barrow Neurological Institute St. Joseph's
Hospital and Medical Center, 350 West Thomas Rd., Phoenix,
Arizona 85013 USA

Prof. Dr. Johannes Dichgans, Neurologische Klinik der Universität
Tübingen, Liebermeisterstraße 18–20, 7400 Tübingen, FRG

Prof. Dr. Wolfgang Precht, Institut für Hirnforschung, Universität
Zürich, August-Forel-Straße 1, CH-8029 Zürich

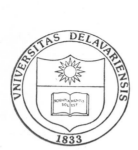

ISBN 3-540-13728-9 Springer-Verlag Berlin Heidelberg New York Tokyo
ISBN 0-387-13728-9 Springer-Verlag New York Heidelberg Berlin Tokyo

Library of Congress Cataloging in Publication Data. Main entry under title: Cerebellar functions. (Proceedings in life sciences) Papers from an international meeting held in Sept. 1983,
sponsored by the Max Planck Society and the Deutsche Forschungsgemeinschaft. Includes
index. 1. Cerebellum–Congresses. I. Bloedel, James R. II. Dichgans, Johannes. III. Precht,
Wolfgang, 1938-. IV. Max-Planck-Gesellschaft zur Förderung der Wissenschaften. V. Deutsche
Forschungsgemeinschaft. VI. Series. [DNLM: 1. Cerebellum–physiology–congresses. WL 320
C4115 1983] QP379.C44 1984 599'.0188 84-14109

© by Springer-Verlag, Berlin Heidelberg 1985.
Printed in Germany.

Typesetting and printing: Beltz, Offsetdruck, Hemsbach/Bergstr.
Bookbinding: Brühlsche Universitätsdruckerei, Giessen
2131-3130-543210

Preface

Over the past few semesters a group of neurologists, neurophysiologists, and brain theorists in various departments of Tübingen University have gathered periodically in an effort to review ideas and evidence on cerebellar functions. At times, general solutions seemed close, when credit was given to various theoretical proposals advanced since the early days of cerebellar physiology, however, it became clear in every case that a large part of the available facts refused to submit to the general ideas.

As believers in the power of scientific discussion, we felt that the time was ripe for posing the problem of the cerebellum once more to a well-articulated group of specialists that would include proponents of every disparate point of view. The sponsorship of the Max Planck Society and of the Deutsche Forschungsgemeinschaft, to whom we express our profound gratitude, made it possible to organize an international meeting in September, 1983. The aim of making new, even extravagant ideas palatable to each other was well accomplished by the participants. We trust that some of the ensuing excitement has been carried over into the printed version. The papers in this book reflect for the most part the talks which were on the program of the meeting. Some of them, the shorter ones, grew out of improvised contributions which we thought fit to be included. Unfortunately, as always happens, one or the other of the invited speakers was unable to attend. Thus we were deprived, for instance, of Masao Ito's presentation . Another participant, O. Oscarsson, whose contribution was a cornerstone of our discussion, was unwilling to put his talk into writing. In spite of this, the papers collected in this volume provide a very timely cross-section of modern cerebellar research.

This field has not yet crystallized into a structure with unambiguous chapter headings. Still, some sort of thread can be followed through the sequence of papers. We start with the contributions describing the main functional contexts in which the cerebellum operates: body posture and locomotion, eye movements, speech, grasping, holding. In the next group of papers some theoretical proposals are collected. Lastly, the hard facts of anatomy and physiology are opposed to the speculative efforts.

October, 1984   J. DICHGANS — V. BRAITENBERG

Contents

How are "Move" and "Hold" Programs Matched?
V. B. Brooks (With 17 Figures) 1

A Cerebellar-dependent Efference Copy Mechanism for Generating
Appropriate Muscle Responses to Limb Perturbations
J. Hore and T. Vilis (With 9 Figures) 24

Motor Programs: Trajectory Versus Stability
W. T. Thach, M. H. Schieber, and R. H. Elble (With 8 Figures) . . 36

Parsimony in Neural Calculations for Postural Movements
G. McCollum, F. B. Horak, and L. M. Nashner (With 10 Figures) . 52

A Synthetic Motor Control System; Possible Parallels With Transformations in Cerebellar Cortex
M. J. Nahvi and M. R. Hashemi (With 2 Figures) 67

Cerebro-Cerebellar Interactions and Organization of a Fast and
Stable Hand Movement: Cerebellar Participation in Voluntary
Movement and Motor Learning
K. Sasaki (With 11 Figures) 70

On the Role of the Subprimate Cerebellar Flocculus in the Optokinetic
Reflex and Visual -Vestibular Interaction
W. Precht, R. H. I. Blanks, P. Strata, and P. Montarolo
(With 13 Figures) 86

The Primate Flocculus in Visual-Vestibular Interactions:
Conceptual, Neurophysiological, and Anatomical Problems
W. Waespe and V. Henn (With 3 Figures) 109

Clinical Evidence for Functional Compartmentalization
of the Cerebellum
J. Dichgans and H. C. Diener (With 8 Figures) 126

Perceptual Analysis of Speech Disorders in Friedreich Disease
and Olivopontocerebellar Atrophy
S. Gilman and K. Kluin (With 6 Figures) 148

Cerebellar Hemispherectomy at Young Ages in Rats
A. Gramsbergen and J. IJkema-Paassen (With 1 Figure). 164

Cerebellar Control of Movement in Fish as Revealed by Small Lesions
    K. Behrend (With 2 Figures) 168

Functional Significance of the Basic Cerebellar Circuit in Motor
    Coordination
    R. Llinás (With 4 Figures) 170

Some Quantitative Aspects of Cerebellar Anatomy as a Guide
    to Speculation on Cerebellar Functions
    M. Fahle and V. Braitenberg (With 13 Figures) 186

Tensorial Brain Theory in Cerebellar Modelling
    A. J. Pellionisz (With 1 Figure) 201

Inferior Olive: Functional Aspects
    P. Strata (With 4 Figures) 230

Climbing Fiber Function: Regulation of Purkinje Cell Responsiveness
    J. R. Bloedel and T. J. Ebner (With 6 Figures) 247

Rhythmic Properties of Climbing Fiber Afferent Responses
    to Peripheral Stimuli
    T. J. Ebner and J. R. Bloedel (With 1 Figures) 260

Cerebellar Climbing Fibers Retrogradely Labeled With
    (^{3}H)-D-Aspartate
    L. Wiklund, G. Toggenburger, and M. Cuenod (With 6 Figures) . . 263

Climbing Fibre Actions of Purkinje Cells — Plateau Potentials and
    Long-Lasting Depression of Parallel Fibre Responses
    C.-F. Ekerot (With 5 Figures) 268

Functional Changes of the Purkinje Cell Following Climbing
    Fiber Deafferentation
    F. Benedetti, P. G. Montarolo, and S. Rabacchi
    (With 1 Figure) 275

Inferior Olive: Its Tonic Inhibitory Effect on the Cerebellar
    Purkinje Cells in the Rat Without Anesthesia
    T. Savio and F. Tempia (With 1 Figure) 278

Tonic Influence of the Climbing Fiber System on the Postural
    Activity
    C. Batini, J. F. Bernard, P. G. Montarolo, and P. Strata
    (With 1 Figure) 280

Sensory Representation of Movement Parameters in the Cerebellar
    Cortex of the Decerebrate Cat
    F. P. Kolb and F. J. Rubia (With 8 Figures) 282

Constraints on Plasticity of Cerebellar Circuitry: Granule
    Cell-Purkinje Cell Synapses
    D. E. Hillman and S. Chen (With 9 Figures) 300

Comparison Between the Developmental Calendars of the Cerebral
    and Cerebellar Cortices in a Precocial and an Altricial Rodent
    A. Schüz and F. M. Hein (With 3 Figures) 318

Three Types of Large Nerve Cells in the Granular Layer of the
    Human Cerebellar Cortex
    E. Braak and H. Braak (With 1 Figure) 322

Local Circuit Neurons in the Cerebellar Dentate Nucleus of Man
    H. Braak and E. Braak (With 1 Figure) 324

Brain Stem Afferents Bilaterally Branching to the Cat Cerebellar
    Hemispheres
    A. Rosina and L. Provini (With 1 Figure) 326

Subject Index 329

Contributors

You will find the adresses at the beginning of the respective contribution

Batini, C 280
Behrend, K. 168
Benedetti, F. 275
Bernard, J. F. 280
Blanks, R. H. I. 86
Bloedel, J.R. 247,260
Braak, E. 322,324
Braak, H. 322,324
Braitenberg, V. 186
Brooks, V. B. 1
Chen, S. 300
Cuenod, M. 263
Dichgans, J. 126
Diener, H. C. 126
Ebner, T. J. 247,260
Ekerot, C. F. 268
Elble, R. H. 36
Fahle, M. 186
Gilman, S. 148
Gramsbergen, A. 164
Hashemi, M. R. 67
Hein, F. M. 318
Henn, V. 109
Hillman, D. E. 300
Horak, F. B. 52

Hore, J. 24
IJkema-Paassen, J. 164
Kluin, K. 148
Kolb, F. P. 282
Llinās, R. 170
McCollum, G. 52
Montarolo, P. 86,275,280
Nahvi, M. J. 67
Nashner, L. M. 52
Pellionisz, A. J. 201
Precht, W. 86
Provini, L. 326
Rabacchi, S. 275
Rosina, A. 326
Rubia, F. J. 282
Sasaki, K. 70
Savio, T. 278
Schieber, M. H. 36
Schüz, A. 318
Strata, P. 86,230,280
Tempia, F. 278
Thach, W. T. 36
Toggenburger, G. 263
Vilis, T. 24
Waespe, W. 109
Wiklund, L. 263

How are "Move" and "Hold" Programs Matched?

V.B. BROOKS[1]

1 Introduction

Motor control is going through a productive "crisis" of concept formation (Holton, 1973; cf. Brooks 1975; Granit, 1981). Research on movements and their neural control control is advancing so rapidly that new concepts have arisen even since the publication of recent "Handbooks" (e.g. Brooks, 1981; Towe and Luschei, 1981; Desmedt, 1983). In this article I adress a question that is implied in Holmes' (1917) description of "decomposition of movements" after cerebellar damage: how does the cerebellum normally assist in the composition of intended movements? How are errors of direction, rate, and range avoided? Since posture and movements merge one into the other, the question is rephrased as: how does the cerebellum match "move" and "hold" programs? (Other functions of the cerebellum, including those with regard to non-programmed movements are not dealt with here, those considerations can be found in broader reviews (e.g. Bloedel and Courville, 1981; Brooks and Thach, 1981; Llinas, 1981).

The point of view put forth in this essay is based on new analyses of multi-joint movements in humans (summarized in Bizzi and Abend, 1983; Jeannerod and Prablanc, 1983), their neural cortical control in monkeys (Georgopoulos et al. 1982), and how single joint movements are learned by monkeys (Brooks et al., 1983). These diverse new findings are woven together by the thought that motor set before and during intended movements depends on cerebellar guidance of precentral responses to internal move commands and to external perturbations. It is proposed that these precentral responses set up and maintain synergic intended postures as well as movements with optimal trajectories, i.e. velocities in relation to the path. The errors of direction, rate, and range of movements during cerebellar dysfunction become parts of a single problem in the concept of trajectory control, which was introduced as a supraspinal control loop for single-joint movements by Cooke (1980). Trajectory control of multi-joint movements was made intelligible by Bizzi's group who showed that the brain governs the trajectory of the object of greatest attention (see Abend et al., 1982; Bizzi and Abend, 1983).

Trajectory control may be most significant as a means to fit simple paths into compound movements that describe patterns. This typically human activity demands scaling of abstract patterns in time or space (Viviani and Terzuolo, 1980). While patterns are the product of the brain's highest level, scaling is done by the middle level of the motor hierarchy which includes the cerebellum and the sensorimotor cortex (c.f. Phillips and Porter, 1977). Trajectory control simplifies the scaling process by combining direc-

---

[1] Dept. of Physiology, The University of Western Ontario London, Ontario, Canada N6A 5C1

Cerebellar Functions
ed. by Bloedel et al.
© Springer-Verlag Berlin Heidelberg 1984

tion, rate, and range into one functional entity: the relation of the directional path to its rate of change. The cerebellum acts like a "clutch" between motor set and motor execution. The precentral "gears" are shifted smoothly only with normal (neo)cerebellar gear-selection. In this sense, the cerebellum conveys the intent of the individual to the machinery of the muscles.

2 Trajectories of Intended Movements

2.1 Description

Intended movements can be recognized by their distinctive "continuous" velocity profile with only one peak. The appearance and moderate speed of these movements is very similar for single-joint ("simple") movements and for the path of the object of greatest attention of multi-joint ("compound") movements. In the case of the arm, for instance, this is usually the path of the hand. The paths of the limb joints that serve to transport the hand are not necessarily continuous, however, since their actions seem to be designed for subsidiary support of the intended handpath (Abend et al., 1982). Bizzi and Abend (1983) have pointed out the hierarchical nature of this arrangement, along the lines postulated by Bernstein (1967). Movements made by monkeys and human subjects seem to follow many of the same rules, allowing us to obtain experimental data from the animal model. Its limitations are set out in Section 3. Figure 1 illustrates the handpath for a multi-joint, free pointing movement in which a human subject uses elbow and wrist, as well as the shoulder to some extent (Jeannerod and Prablanc, 1983). The velocity profile of the handpath is "bell-shaped" (Bizzi's term), i.e., what we have called "continuous".

Descriptions can be made more quantitative when movements are restricted to two joints that operate in the same plane (two degrees of freedom). In Fig. 2A an individual is shown executing a step-tracking task in a horizontal workspace with the immoblized hand by means of an instrumented lever which is moved by the shoulder and elbow. Traces 1-5 of Fig. 2A represent the handpaths of a human subject who has been instructed to move between the targets either in a straight line (1), or in increasingly curved paths (2-5). The velocity profiles, in the row below, grade from single-peaked (1: continuous) to multiple-peaked (5: discontinuous) as the handpaths become more curved and are traversed increasingly in successive, short segments (Abend et al., 1982). Figure 2B illustrates a similar arrangement for a monkey (Georgopoulos et al., 1981). The animal's handpath and velocity profile of a movement like that in Fig. 2A1 closely resemble the human example. The handle method is validated in Fig. 2C which demonstrates that a free reaching movement made by a monkey produces a handpath which is almost identical to those shown in A and B (Gilman et al., 1976. The "decerebellate" example will be considered in Section 3).

Single-joint movements made by human subjects and monkeys resemble each other much in the same way as do multi-joint movements. Figure 3 shows that continuous, bell-shaped velocity profiles indicate use of movement programming as a strategy, but what tactical uses of muscle are actually programmed depends on the circumstances

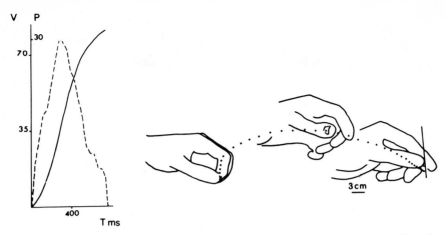

Fig. 1. The handpath of a free pointing movement made with the elbow and wrist as well as the shoulder to some extent has a "bell-shaped", "continuous" velocity profile. Ordinates of graphs on left' Velocity (*V*): mm/s; Position (*P*): mm; abscissa is Time (*T*): ms (Jeannerod and Prablanc, 1983)

and on the muscles used. Examples of continuous elbow movements are illustrated in Fig. 3A and B (Lestienne et al., 1981; Brooks 1983a; Brooks and Watts, 1983 and to be published) which demonstrate how bell-shaped velocity profiles can be achieved with more than just one pattern of muscle activation. The records in column 1 depict relatively slow movements which commence after the braking action of the antagonists is released. The faster movements, in column 2, are propelled by an agonist burst as part of the well known pattern of triphasic agonist-antagonist alternation.

2.2 Functional Purpose of Movement Trajectory

Why do human subjects and monkeys make intended movements with the same kind of bell-shaped, continuous trajectories? An answer is suggested by the way in which monkeys learn to make these movements when they are not constrained to do so in any particular manner. Two naive animals were trained to perform a step-tracking task that required self-paced, accurate elbow movements of any type and speed that they wished to use. (The arrangement is drawn in Figs. 4 and 14). Both animals began with a preponderance of minimally programmed, discontinuous movements and finished with one of maximally programmed, continuous movements (Fig. 4; Brooks et al., 1983; Brooks 1983a).

Two important points emerge, of which the first is especially germane to the argument about velocity profiles. Both animals learned to program their accelerations and decelerations together, right from the very beginning of training. Figure 4B shows that about 90% of all movements with programmed accelerations also have programmed decelerations. That fraction does not change during motor learning. This means that the brain learns to estimate the "move" programs together with, i.e., in relation to, the "hold" programs for arm postures before and after arm movements. Getting set for take-off, making a correct flight, and braking for landing are all learned together. When

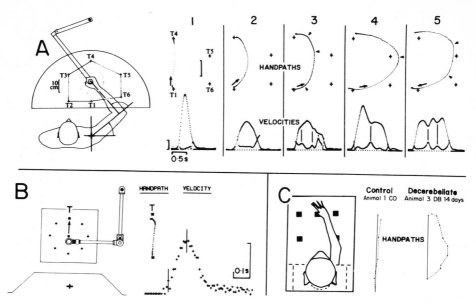

Fig. 2 A-C. Velocity profiles of handpaths of intended, two-joint movements range from "continuos" for human subjects and monkeys. **A,** *left* Human subject performs step-tracking task by moving two-jointed handle between several possible targets (crosses on horizontal workspace), using shoulder and elbow. *Right* Records from one subject, who was told for *1*, only to move the hand to the target, in *2* to *5*, to use a curved path to reach the target. *Arrows* direction of movement, arrowheads point to sharpest curvatures (aligned by vertical lines to curvature plots below velocity traces); **B** Handpaths of intended, two-joint movements made by monkeys resemble those of human subjects. Horizontal workspace for moving a two-jointed handle between targets. Monkey (not shown) is aligned by his shoulder with workspace center, much like human subject in **A**. Traces on the right show the handpath and velocity when handle is moved from workspace center to target equivalent to *T4* in **A**; **C.** Handpaths of free reaching movements resemble those made when turning a two-jointed handle. Monkeys must reach horizontally for food across calibrated workspace. Handpaths are shown (*dotted lines*) for control, and decerebellate monkey when reaching towards food reward (at end of *solid lines*). (**A** Abend et al., 1982; **B** Georgopoulos et al., 1981; **C** Gioman et al., 1976)

these subprograms are matched properly, the velocity profile is bell-shaped, with only minimal discontinuities.

The second point is of more general interest. Use of programmed movements increases rapidly only after the animals give evidence that they have begun to understand the behavioral requirements. These requirements were to flex and extend the elbow alternately from one target to the other without stopping in between, and to hold the hand in the target areas for at least a few seconds before the return move. How understanding opens the gate for successful movement programming is documented in Fig. 4C by the steep increase of the slope of the learning curve after 50% behavioral sureness had been reached (as indicated by the vertical dottet line and the circled area).

Why do animals and human subjects adopt the strategy of using continuous movements when they are not required to do so? Since the need is not imposed upon the subjects, it must be found within the subjects, in the "wisdom of the body" which, after

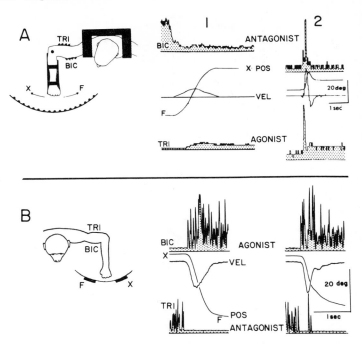

Fig. 3 A, B. Single-joint movements can be programmed for different tactics of muscle use. **A** A human subject performs a step-tracking task with elbow flexions and extensions (monitored by a potentiometer beneath elbow pivot: *black dot*). The seated subject cannot see his arm to which surface EMG leads are attached. Trunk and shoulders are stabilized by a padded block and belts. Targets are 5 deg apart. *Column 1.* Slow, barely continuous, extensions can be started by releasing tonic biceps braking action which holds the arm in flexion posture, and later adding a triceps step which grades over into tonic holding the arm in extension. *Column 2.* Continuous movements with quick (but still moderate) speed require triphasic pattern of pulses for smooth take-off and landing (which has a correction for a small overshoot); **B** Arrangements and movements of a monkey equivalent to **A** (see Fig. 14). The animal (F20) step-tracked targets of 12 deg width, with centers at 16 deg extension *(X)* and 16 deg flexion *(F)*. Records in Columns *1* and *2* depict slow and quick programmed movements, with muscle use roughly equivalent to those in **A**. Both examples are correctly programmed (although there is a correction for a small undershoot in *2*). Samples in *1* and *2* are from monkey F20 when its learning curve (plotted in Fig. 4) had reached 55% behaviorally correct movements. (**A** Lestienne et al., 1981; **B** previously unpublished record from Brooks and Watts, 1983)

all, includes the brain. The need seems to be economy of effort, how to optimize various aspects of the movements to suit them best to the prevailing circumstances. Figure 5 shows how this can be done rather conveniently with this type of velocity profile (Nelson, 1983). Small changes of shape, i.e. of patterns of acceleration and deceleration, permit minimization of acceleration, its rate of change (jerk), energy, or the maintenance of constant stiffness. There is an advantage in easy changes of shape since there likely is need to trade off different kinds of optimization. Figure 3A and B, column 1 would be probable examples for conservation of energy, while the movements in column 2 could minimize any of the other factors in continuous profiles.

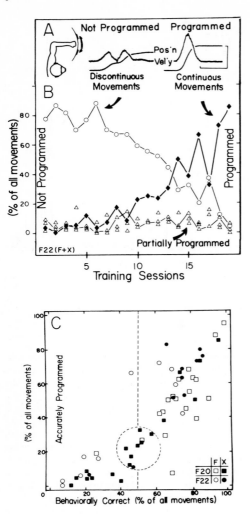

Fig. 4 A-C. Starts and stops are learned together for programmed movements, whose subsequent use depends on understanding of behavioral requirements. *Top row* **A** *far left* monkey performs step-tracking task by turning single-jointed handle with simple elbow flexions and extensions to targets, as in Fig. 14; *right* position and velocity traces of non-programmed, "discontinuous" and programmed, "continuous" movements. Graphs: **B** During motor learning, non-programmed movements (*open circles*) are supplanted by accurately programmed ones (*filled diamonds*). Partial programming did not progress (programmed accelerations but non-programmed decelerations: *open* and *filled triangles*. Graphs represent flexions and extensions of monkey F20: (*F+X*); **C** *Circled area* marks beginning of understanding (50% correct behavior: abscissa) and onset of steeply increasing number of accurate, continuous movements (ordinate). Correct behavior is plotted as moves in the required direction within 2 s of target step for flexions (*F*) and extensions (*X*) of 2 monkeys (F20, F22) for means of 7376 movements for F22 and 3226 for F20. (Brooks et al., 1983)

Fig. 5. Continuous movements can optimize several variables without much adjustment of velocity profile. Comparison of calculated velocity profiles for the same movement time and distance which are optimum with respect to five different objectives: *A* minimum peak acceleration *(solid line); E* minimum energy *(dashed); J* minimum jerk (rate of change of acceleration, *(solid); K* constant stiffness *(dotted). V* which is not a continuous profile, minimizes peak velocity *(solid).* (From Nelson, 1983)

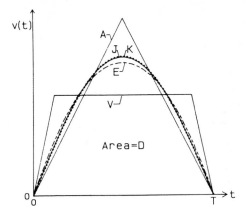

There is a steady gradation between continuous and discontinuous profiles (Brooks, 1974; also see Brooks and Thach, 1981). This is clear in the similar examples for a human subject (Fig. 2A, 1-5) and in those for a monkey (Fig. 6, 1-5). Discontinuous movements become rare after about 10 training sessions (without forcings) as in Fig. 4. They persist longer during learning of relatively difficult movements (c.f. Brooks, 1979). In Fig. 6, movement types 1-4 represent the entire range when the animal had learned to make continuous movements exclusively (of which 90% were made correctly; see abscissa in Fig. 4). They are displayed in decreasing order of peak velocity. Velocities increase with practice by about 1 rad/s, i.e. by about the difference between movements 1 and 2. This form of adaptation is common during work sessions as long as the subject pays attention to the motor performance (see Brooks, 1983a). Movements 3 and 4 still are sill programmed with well-estimated accelerations, but the decelerations represent transitional stages towards frank corrections of the endpoint (also see Fig. 3, B2). The discontinuous movement (Fig. 6, movement 5) was made one year earlier when the animal had already reached that 90% criterion, but when 5% were still discontinuous.

2.3 Maintenance

Once the readiness to make movements with a particular trajectory is set, this "motor set" is maintained against external perturbations by instruction-dependent "long-loop" responses, also called "functional stretch responses". Their successive peaks have been named M1, M2, and M3 (see the review by Lee et al., 1983). M1 is the spinal stretch reflex, M2 the transcortical response to muscle stretch, and M3 grades over into a transcortical "voluntary" response. Motor set has its greatest influence on M1. The point will be made in Section 3 that implementation of motor set is conveyed by the cerebellum, particularly through its influence on transcortical loops that make monosynaptic corticospinal connections. They are more common in man than in monkeys. Long loop responses can be elicited *before* movement onset, when their protective actions reveal the prevailing motor set (Evarts and Tanji, 1974; and see Fig. 12). Motor set enhances useful responses and diminishes unwanted ones which would be counter-productive for

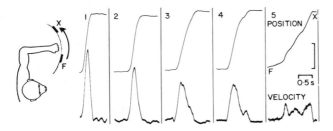

Fig. 6. Velocity profiles of handpaths of intended, single-joint movements range from "continuous" to "discontinuous", much like those for two-joint movements (as in Fig. 2A). The diagram on the *left* describes the arrangement for the step-tracking task executed by a monkey with elbow movements, as in Fig. 15. Extension movements 1-4 are all "programmed", but their decelerations are progressively less well estimated. Extension 5 is discontinuous. Vertical calibration: 16 deg and 120 deg/s. Traces are of individual movements made by monkey F21 between targets of 10 deg width, with their centers at 25 deg extension *(X)* and 12.5 deg flexion *(F)*. (Previously unpublished record from Brooks and Watts, 1983)

the impending movement. Restoration of the handpath and of its velocity by long-loop responses *during* movements was described for perturbed single-joint arm movements of monkeys by Conrad et al. (1974, 1975) and is illustrated in Fig. 10A and 16A and B). Figures 10 and 12 illustrate the use of two practically simultaneous, independent discoveries (made in 1972) of the influence of motor set on long loop responses as measured by precentral and muscular discharges. In both cases, the intention to move the limb in a certain direction was induced by visual cues and was then tested by randomly directed perturbations of the operant arm. In experiments such as those in Fig. 10, the monkeys were instructed to flex or extend the elbow alternately by randomly timed target steps from one position to another. For those in Fig. 12, the instruction to flex or to extend the wrist in random order was conveyed by differently colored lights. The concordant results obtained by Evarts' group and ours have been reviewed with regard to classification of precentral neurons, and to participation of the neocerebellum as demonstrated by dentate unit recording and by dentate cooling respectively (Evarts, 1981; Brooks and Thach, 1981).

The importance of the preservation of the two parameters, directional path and its rate of change, in relation to each other was recognized by Cooke (1980) and is illustrated as trajectory compensation of intended, single-joint movements made by a human subject in Fig. 7. (The divergences of perturbed and non-perturbed trajectories are indicated by arrows). An equivalent plot for monkey movements appears in Fig. 16C.

Motor set also includes braking the moving limb for assumption of another posture. as mentioned in the previous section. A role for long-loop responses in the process of steadying a moving limb such as the arm against sustained perturbations was recognized by Kwan et al. (1979) and is illustrated in Fig. 8 (as the horizontal stippled area denoting the difference between motor set for "resisting" and "yielding" to imposed loads). It is a form of instruction-dependent load compensation which can be thought of as part of trajectory compensation (also see Lacquaniti and Soechting, 1983).

Most people preserve their postural body balance on moving surfaces by long loop responses in synergic patterns of leg muscles (Fig. 9A: ratios of active muscles, a measure

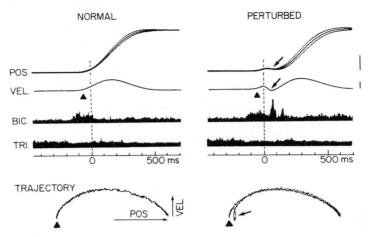

Fig. 7. Long-loop responses assist in "trajectory-compensation" of the arm when a human subject resists perturbations of intended movements. Records of 20 averaged normal and perturbed elbow flexions made (as rapidly as possible) by a normal subject. Movement onset at *filled triangles*, perturbation at *vertical dotted line* (also for reference in the normal record on the *left*). Position traces are enclosed by standard deviations. Trajectory compensation (for the effects of 50 ms torque pulses) is indicated by *arrows* in position, velocity, and trajectory traces. Rectified EMGs show long loop responses of biceps and triceps. Trajectory traces are averaged ("phase-plane") plots of velocity against limb position (calibrations are 30 deg, 50 deg/s, and also apply to position and velocity traces). (Cooke, 1980)

that used to be called "local sign"; Nashner and Grimm, 1978). The important property of response adaptation appears in Fig. 9B, showing how response amplitudes adapt in half a dozen successive trials according to their postural usefulness. Thus, the motor hierarchy implements the intent of the individual by programming long loop responses according to the circumstances of the moment. The responses are also emitted in leg antigravity muscles as part of programs triggered by vestibular gravity receptors when subjects hop on, or fall towards a stable surface (Melvill Jones and Watt, 1971 a, b). The cerebellar deficits depicted in the right column of Fig. 9C and D, will be taken up in Section 3.

In summary of Section 2, we conclude that human subjects and monkeys unconsciously elect to make intended movements with the most advantageous trajectory, in which the object of greatest attention traverses a straight path with a bell-shaped (continuous) velocity profile. This motor set is optimized according to the needs of the moment, and is maintained against perturbations before and during movements by instruction-dependent, "long loop" operated, muscle contractions.

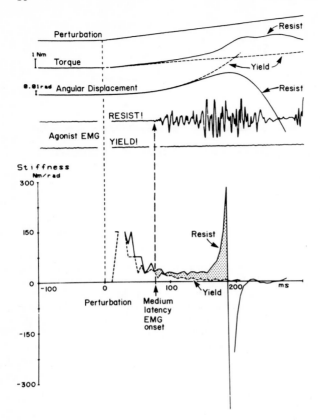

Fig. 8. Limb stabilization is part of trajectory compensation. Long-loop responses precede "load-compensation" of a limb when a human subject resists a perturbation of an intended posture. Stabilization of limb stiffness *(horizontal stippled area)* precedes intended correction of perturbation in order to resist *(solid traces)*. When subject yields *(interrupted traces)*, there is neither a long loop EMG medium latency component nor stiffness stabilization. Traces in upper part of the Figure indicate the perturbation: a rising ramp torque starting at the vertical dotted line at time 0, which alters intended angular displacement *(solid trace)* of the elbow. Agonist *EMG* medium latency component, (starting at *vertical arrow*, increases limb stiffness *(vertical stippled area)* as part of correction of perturbation. (Kwan et al., 1979)

3 Neural Mechanisms for Intended Trajectories

3.1 Motor Cortex

The precentral cortex plays a crucial role in the establishment and maintenance of movement trajectories, although other cortical areas are involved as well (see Fig. 17). Bursts of precentral unit discharge precede and relate to long loop responses of proximal and distal limbs of monkeys (Conrad et al., 1974, 1975; Evarts and Tanji, 1974; Tanji and Evarts, 1976). The task-relation was inferred from the timing of the neural activity (Fig. 10A and B) and has been confirmed by means of precentral spike-triggered averaging of electromyographic activity (Fetz, 1981; Cheney and Fetz, 1984; Fig. 10C and D). These conclusions, drawn from experiments with Cebus and Macaque monkeys, are buttressed by the clinical observation of Marsden et al. (1977) that long loop responses for distal limbs of human subjects are reduced or abolished after lesions of the paths ascending to the sensorimotor cortex (see Fig. 13). Equivalent data for Saimiri monkeys with lesions of forelimb motor cortex (Lenz et al., 1983) show that M2 responses to perturbations of 500 ms duration are decreased for distal but not for proximal muscles. The authors stress this difference, and suggest that it may relate to the degrees of mono-

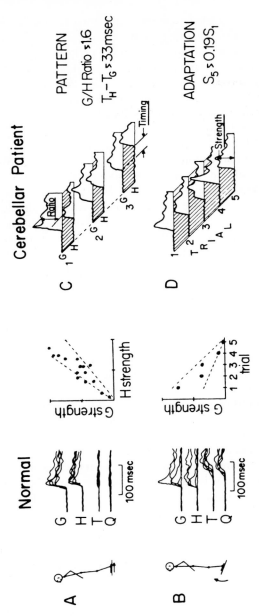

Fig. 9 A-D. Adaptation of human stance requires cerebellar guidance. **A** and **B** Figurines indicate normal stabilization by means of long loop "functional stretch" responses in leg muscles when subjects sway forward in response to backward movement (**A**) or upward tilt (**B**) of platform on which they stand; **C** and **D** Cerebellar deficit is apparent in the abnormal functional stretch responses of muscles in both the functional Pattern data (**C**), and in the adaptation sequence (**D**). These data are plotted in **A** and **B** for the normal cases as ratios and values in successive trials. EMGs are from gastrocnemius *(G)*; hamstrings *(H)*; tibialis anterior *(T)*; quadriceps *(Q)*; minimum criteria for classifying responses as abnormal. (Nashner and Grimm, 1978)

synaptic corticospinal innervation in different primates, man having the greatest which includes such corticomotoneuronal (CM) innervation of proximal as well as distal muscles (see Fig. 10C; see Phillips, 1969; and Phillips and Porter, 1977 for an overall discussion). Cerebral participation may shorten the time needed to detect displacements from an intended path and to generate appropriate, task-related reactions.

The phylogenetic gradation of transcortical synaptic security of responses to perturbations brings out a related point. Evoking long loop responses requires more peripheral input for central summation when CM synapses are sparse. For instance, Vilis ad Cooke (1976) have shown that M2 amplitudes in monkeys' arm muscles depend on perturbations that continue beyond the brief time needed to evoke the segmental M1 response. This fits with the recent demonstration by Hore and Vilis (1984) that torque changes of long durations (at least several hundred ms) are more likely to evoke long loop responses (which can be depressed by neocerebellar dysfunction) than those evoked by brief pulses (10-20 ms). The latter point is illustrated in Fig. 15 (Vilis and Hore, 1977; and see also Tracey et al., 1980; Miller and Brooks, 1981). Furthermore, Hore and Vilis (1984) have suggested that this difference may be related to the greater degree to which set is incorporated into long loop responses to expected perturbations of long, rather than short, durations. This matter will be considered further in Section 3.

How is motor set established for particular movements and for their manner of execution? It may be a reasonable guess that the precentral cortex receives instructions for the sequence of the needed skilled acts through cortico-cortical connections and the basal ganglia, while the details for commands to the spinal cord come from the cerebellum. Some trans-cortical connections perhaps also provide the opportunity for cortical comparison to some integrated form of "intent" of the subject. A diagram of the connections of some of these structures appears in Fig. 17.

Precentral neurons can encode diverse movement properties which depend on the conditions of the task. For instance, in single-joint movements (e.g. as in Figs. 3, 4, 6-10, 13-16) where force, acceleration, or speed are the only controllable parameters besides direction (the path being determined by the structure of the joint), neural codes relate some aspects of directional force to moving or holding the limb. Greater precentral versatility is found when it is required for the task (see reviews by Evarts, 1981; Fetz, 1981). For movements made with two joints (e.g. as in Fig. 1, 2, 11, 12), the direction of the hand path is encoded in the discharge of task-related precentral neurons. Each neuron fires most strongly, although not exclusively, when monkeys make intended movements in a particular direction. This important, recent finding by Georgopoulos et al. (1982, see Fig. 11) implies that the discharges of a population of precentral neurons can encode, i.e., help to establish and maintain, movement trajectories for the object of greatest attention.

3.2 Cerebellum

Evidence that anticipatory subprograms, including those for predictive timing of starts and stops of intended movements, emanate from the neocerebellum has been published by my colleagues and myself since 1968 with increasingly detailed evidence (reviewed in Brooks, 1983a; Brooks and Thach, 1981; Brooks, 1979; and see the important recent work by Hore and Vilis, this Vol.). The generation of precentral start and stop com-

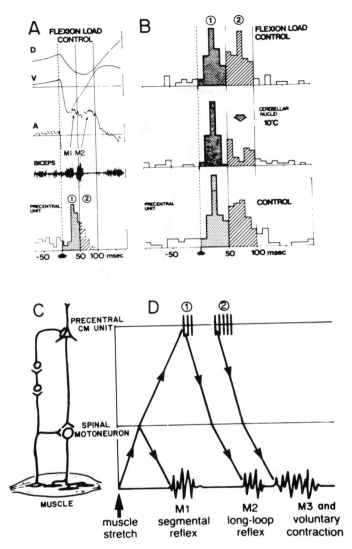

Fig. 10 A-D. Precentral neurons participate in generation of long loop responses which help to compensate perturbations of the path and velocity of monkeys' arm. **A** Movement parameters of a monkey, arranged as in Fig. 14. *D, V,* and *A* are displacement, velocity, acceleration respectively [averages ± SDs *(dotted)* of about 20 trials]; spinal M1 and long loop M2 EMG responses of biceps brachii muscle are also shown. *Arrows* point to resulting changes of acceleration. Lowermost row shows peristimulus time histogram of "early" first *(1)* and second *(2)* responses of a flexion-related precentral neuron following flexion load pulse of monkey's arm (at *arrow* on abscissa); **B** Cerebellar nuclear cooling depresses set-related second *(2)*, but not load reflex-related first *(1)* precentral response to perturbation of monkey's arm from an intended posture (different monkey and unit from A). **C** Diagram of likely neural connections that could generate **D**; **D** The sequence of responses initated by muscle stretch in a subject prepared to make a voluntary contraction of that muscle. Arrows indicate conduction of neural activity over segmental loop (of M1 response) and transcortical (CM) neuron contributing to "voluntary" muscular contraction (A Conrad et al., 1975; B Abter Vilis et al., 1976; C Fetz, 1981)

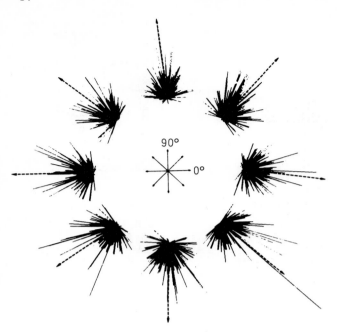

Fig. 11. Direction of the intended handpath can be encoded by a population of precentral neurons. Vector contributions of 241 directionally tuned motor cortical cells of a monkey are drawn for each of 8 movement directions (tested with the arrangement shown in Fig. 2B for two-joint movements). The length of each vector line is proportional to the percent change in cell discharge from the average discharge frequency observed during the 8 movement directions. Notice the spatial congruence between the direction of the vectorial sum (*heavy interrupted lines* in each plot) and the direction of movement (*light interrupted lines* at center). (Georgopoulos et al., 1983)

mands for monkeys' elbow movements is depressed and/or delayed during cerebellar dysfunction, depriving the subject of the programmed phase lead for smooth starts and stops (Meyer-Lohmann et al., 1977; Vilis and Hore, 1980; Miller and Brooks, 1982). "De-programmed" movements faithfully follow degraded precentral discharge (see Fig. 16A and B).

After a cerebellar lesion, the normally straight handpaths of reaching movements are degraded into a series of short segments which correct for the initially wrong direction. Such a degraded, non-programmed movement of a monkey is illustrated in Fig. 2C. It strikingly resembles the sharply curved handpath of a human subject in Fig. 2, A5. It seems a reasonable working hypothesis that cerebellar errors of range, rate and direction arise from cerebellar, failure to modulate the correct assembly of precentral neurons needed to establish the appropriate movement parameters (see Fig. 17; Brooks, 1979; Brooks and Thach, 1981), i.e. the intended trajectory.

Cerebellar patients cannot adapt their stance on shifting ground, because the long loop, functional stretch responses in their leg muscles form neither suitable nor adaptable patterns (Fig. 9C and D). We note, however, that the responses do not drop out, but instead continue, albeit inappropriately. Again, the proposed working hypothesis for this finding is that the diseased cerebellum has failed to prompt the appropriate task-related assembly of precentral neurons for maintenance of the intended motor set. The hypothesis rests largely on the demonstrations by Thach that neocerebellar output neurons in the dentate nucleus can encode motor set (reviewed in Brooks and Thach, 1981) and partly on Strick's evidence that such dentate neurons respond to limb perturbations according to the motor set (Strick, 1983; Fig. 12). Furthermore, some of these dentate responses [and the intercalated ones in the ventral lateral (VL) nucleus of the thalamus] occur early enough in time to influence the instruction-dependent

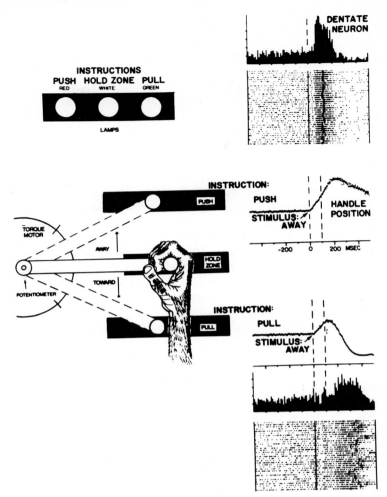

Fig. 12. Influence of motor set on responses of a monkey's dentate neuron to load changes. *Left* Diagram of arm positions of a monkey to pull or push handle from central hold zone. Animals are instructed to do so by a green or red light which comes on in random order 2-5 s before the "move" command. Compare to Fig. 11. The move command consists of a randomly alternating perturbation ("stimulus") produced by the torque motor, and either moves the handle towards or away from the center zone. *Right* Comparison of handle path to the same stimulus which moved the handle away from the monkey (see traces of average handle position) when motor set has been established by prior instruction to either assist or oppose the stimulus (i.e., the "move" command). The traces follow the same displacement for the period between the dashed lines (approximately 90 ms). Response averages and rasters of individual trials of a dentate neuron were recorded when the animal was instructed to prepare to push (*upper records*), and to prepare to pull (*lower records*). Both rasters and response averages show that the same direction of load change evoked an increase in activity when the animal was prepared to push, and a short-latency decrease when the animal was prepared to pull. Each *line* in the rasters represents an individual trial, and each *dot* a single neural discharge. Ordinate scales in impulses/s. (Strick, 1983)

"second early" (2) responses of precentral neurons to limb perturbations (for instance, such as the task-related one in Fig. 10A).

The influence wielded by one structure over another is proved best by concordant results obtained with several methods. Brooks and Thach (1981) have stressed this feature of research on cerebellar and cerebral functions in motor control. Mutually confirmatory results have been obtained from recording of units in the cerebral cortex and in the cerebellar cortex and nuclei of monkeys trained to assume intended arm postures and to make intended arm movements, as well as from "reversible lesions" obtained by cooling of the cerebellar nuclei of similarly trained monkeys while recording in their precentral cortex (cf. Brooks 1983b for a review on use of local brain cooling in research).

Figure 10B provides an example, in that the "second precentral" response to a limb perturbation is depressed by cerebellar nuclear cooling (Vilis et al., 1976). The response latency suggests that it is instruction- (i.e. set-) dependent according to the findings of Tanji and Evarts (1976). Two qualifications apply to the interpretation of Fig. 10B. The effectiveness of evoking long loop responses in proximal muscles of monkeys, and the role of the second precentral responses in this process, depend on the duration of the perturbations (Vilis and Cooke, 1976; Hore and Vilis, 1984). Our working hypothesis, that cerebellar function maintains motor set by activating precentral distributed cell assemblies, predicts that cerebellar dysfunction depresses the long loop, functional stretch responses to unexpected perturbations of intended postures or movements. Cerebellar lesions depress human long loop stretch responses, which are replaced by other responses with delays of about 40-50 ms (Marsden et al., 1977; Fig. 13).

The same delay of about 50 ms is observed for start and stop commands of learned arm movements during cerebellar dysfunction of humans and monkeys (Meyer-Lohmann et al., 1977; Vilis and Hore, 1980). This delay might also account for the difference between the rates of oscillations of normal limbs and those during cerebellar dysfunction, during intended movements or after perturbations from intended postures or movements (see Brooks, 1979). The loss of phase advance by about 50 ms is caused presumably by the inaccessibility of previously learned programs (Brooks, 1979; Vilis and Hore, 1980). Perhaps 50 ms contains a component for central summation time needed to enable central programming. (This could also underlie the recent report by Lee et al. (1983) that human M2/M3 responses of wrist muscles develop fully only when perturbations displace the limb by at least 40-50 ms. This would be a lesser minimal requirement than that of several hundred ms for monkeys, expectedly so in view of their sparser monosynaptic (CM) corticospinal innervation, discussed earlier (also see Wiesendanger and Miles, 1982).

Cerebellar dysfunctions thus degrade execution of programmed movements. The strategy of using programs can be continued, however, as long as the task is well learned (or easy) enough to let the subject succeed. When task performance fails, however, human subjects and monkeys abandon this strategy in favor of using largely non-programmed, discontinuous movements. The handpath of the decerebellate monkey in Fig. 2C is an example. This situation is summarized in Fig. 14, which indicates how cerebellar dysfunction can suspend the results of motor learning, illustrated in Fig. 4. Yet, despite this apparent reversal of the course of learning, we should note that the memory is not lost, but is preserved as mentioned in the Introduction. When reversible lesions are terminated, normal performance returns together with normal local tissue

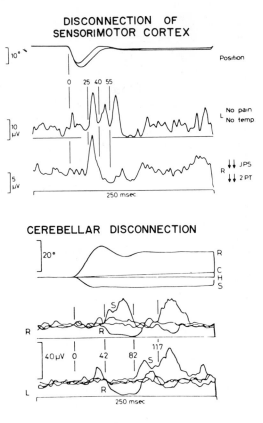

Fig. 13. Disconnections of sensorimotor cortex by lesion in ascending sensory paths (*above*) or of cerebellum (*below*) cause drop-out of long loop responses in human subjects. *Above* Upper traces show displacements of the right and left thumbs from an intended position in a patient with a (stroke) lesion in the right brainstem, who had neither pain nor temperature sensations on the left *(L)* side, and reduced sense of joint position (JPS) and two-point (2PT) tactile discrimination on the right *(R)* side. Lower pair of records show loss of medium- and long-latency responses (after 40 ms and 55 ms) to a fast, brief stretch at time 0 of the right *(R)* long thumb flexor in averages of 24 rectified EMG records. *Below* Responses to sustained stretch (H), halt *(H)*, or release *(R)* of the long thumb flexor in a patient with a left acoustic neuroma caused unilateral left arm ataxia without motor or sensory deficit. The upper traces show, superimposed, the angular position of the right thumb in control *(C)*, *(S)*, *(H)*, or *(R)* trials. Similar records from the left thumb are not shown. The lower pair of records show, superimposed, the rectified EMGs for the 4 conditions for the right and left sides *(R; L* on left margins). The subject flexed the thumb against a standing force of 7 N. At time 0, the thumb was either stretched (by applying a force of 13N for the next 200 ms), released (by decreasing the force to 0.5 N for the next 200 ms), or halted (by arranging for the motor to simulate a stiff spring). Each trace is average of 24 trials which were randomly interspersed. The EMG records from the normal right arm *(R)* show a small spinal monosynaptic response to stretch at about 25 ms, followed by onset of a large long loop response at 42 ms and a voluntary response at 117 ms. Halting also causes a small response with onset at 42 ms, while release silence the muscle at that time. The ataxic left arm *(L)* gives a normal spinal response to stretch, but the long loop response at 42 ms is absent, and another occurs instead at 82 ms. No halt response is evident, but release silences the muscle at the usual latency. (Marsden et al. (*above* 1977, *below* 1978)

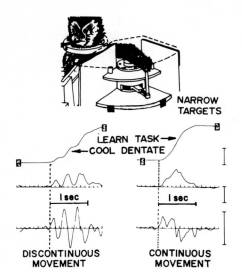

Fig. 14. Opposite changes of movement strategy during motor learning (as in Fig. 4) and during dentate cooling if neocerebellar dysfunction has made performance unsuccessful. *Top row* Diagram of monkey performing relatively difficult (*"narrow targets"*) step-tracking task with single-joint, elbow movements, e.g., as in Figs. 3 and 4. Records are from a normal monkey. (After Brooks et al., 1973; in Brooks and Thach, 1981)

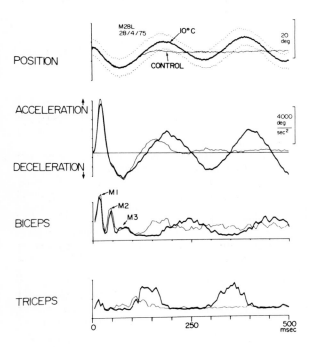

Fig. 15. Cerebellar dysfunction does not alter long loop responses to 10 ms torque pulses of arm muscles in a monkey maintaining an intended arm posture. This figure shows that cooling dentate and interposed nuclei (labelled "10 deg C") had no effect on M1, M2, M3 responses. Traces represent averages of 20 trials ± SDs *(dots)*. *Light line* conctrol; *heavy line* nuclear cooling. (Vilis and Hore, 1977)

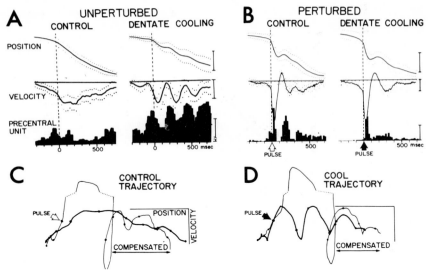

Fig. 16 A-D. Cerebellar dysfunction does not alter trajectory compensation to 10 ms torque pulses of intended arm movements made by a monkey. Control records and those obtained during dentate cooling are compared for unperturbed and perturbed arm extensions (*heavy* and light lines). Unloading perturbations were applied when velocities reached 60 deg/s, indicated for control and cooling records by *open* and *filled arrows*. In all circumstances, discharge of (the two different) precentral neurons remained tightly coupled to movement parameters. C and D compare trajectory compensation for control and during dentate cooling (plotted as in Fig. 7 by matching appropriate records form **A** and**B**). Note 100 ms time intervals marked as dots on trajectory traces. Calibration bars represent 25 deg, 100 deg/s, and 50 deg/s. Traces are averages of about 20 trials (± SDs: dots). Monkey M12, same animal as in Fig. 10A (**A** Conrad et al., 1975; **B** Conrad et al., 1974)

temperatures, with no evidence that the subject had to relearn the task (see Brooks nd Thach, 1981).

When the transcortical route is not the only one for long loop responses, as in the case of monkeys' proximal muscles, the predictions of our working hypothesis depend more strictly on the conditions. Long loop responses are depressed by cerebral or cerebellar disconnections in human subjects (Fig. 13). In contrast, long loop responses of monkeys' proximal muscles to brief perturbations of learned postures and movements are more likely to continue during neocerebellar dysfunction (Fig. 15: Vilis and Hore, 1977; Miller and Brooks, 1981) or precentral dysfunction (Ruegg and Chofflon, 1983). This does not rule out the participation of cerebro-cerebellar guidance in the normal animal, however, any more than in normal human subjects. We are again reminded that task-related, predictive modulation of the motor cortex is more dependent on the duration of the perturbations in subhuman primates than in humans (Hore and Vilis, 1984).

The frequent persistence of monkeys' long loop arm responses to brief perturbations during cerebellar dysfunction (for the reasons set out above) suggests that trajectory compensation should also persist without change. This is indeed the case according to Fig. 16, which is based on the initial papers published about the effects of dentate

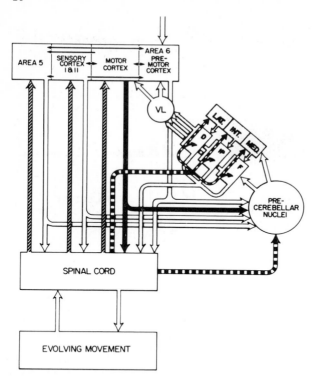

Fig. 17. The "cerebral-cerebellar circuit" drawn as a neural task system to establish and maintain cell assemblies for trajectory control. The diagram is partial and oversimplified, nuclear groups have been combined, connections omitted, and laterality ignored. (Brooks and Thach, 1981, Brooks, 1979)

cooling on monkeys' elbow movements. (Part B is from the very first report, made in association with Mario Wiesendanger who introduced the use of perturbations into our laboratory). The trajectory plots in C and D look different from those in Fig. 7 because larger perturbations were used in relation to the subjects' capability to resist. Both parts A and B document the tightly coupled, faithful relation between abnormal precentral discharge and movements during cerebellar nuclear cooling, referred to in the beginning of this Section.

The cerebellar-cerebral circuit is part of the middle level of the motor hierarchy. It receives instructions from higher levels through the premotor cortex, and issues its own commands to lower levels through the motor cortex and the cerebellum. This circuit is drawn diagrammatically in Fig. 17 to highlight the parallel influences of the cerebellum on the motor cortex and on the brain stem, both of which converge at the lowest level, the spinal "final common path" to the muscles. It is a subject for future research just how this neural task system selects and accesses candidate members of the cell assemblies that will establish and maintain the intended motor set. This line of reasoning follows Bernstein's ideas about the competence of each hierarchical level to determine and adjust its output. One class of outputs of the cerebral-cerebellar circuit are the optimal movement trajectories of the objects of the greatest attention. This example illustrates the workings of hierarchical motor control and how the cerebellum conveys implementation of the subject's intent to the lowest level. Here we glimpse how a neural task system harnesses the machinery of the muscles to serve the mind. How remarkable that this is possible when no parts of the system can read the meaning of the mind!

In summary of Section 3, we conclude that programmed long loop responses of muscles to limb perturbations are generated by instruction-dependent discharges in the motor cortex. These precentral responses are probably triggered by (also programmed) neocerebellar discharges. In human subjects the transcortical route is predominant, but in monkeys parallel subcortical routes contribute, particularly to adjustments of proximal limbs. As a consequence, more central summation appears to be needed for impression of "set" on the cerebral-cerebellar loop. Similar cerebellar and cerebral actions to those following external perturbations may ensue in response to internal commands. The long loop system establishes and maintains motor set for intended postures and movements by trajectory compensation. Cerebro-cerebellar control of trajectories combines direction, rate and range of intended movements into one functional entity.

Acknowledgement. I wish to thank Ms Sherry Watts for composing the illustrations, and Drs. David Cooke, Jon Hore, and Tutis Vilis for helpful discussion of the manuscript.

References

Abend W, Bizzi E, Morasso P (1982) Human arm trajectory formation. Brain 105: 331-348

Bernstein N (1967) The coordination and regulation of movements. Pergamon Press, Oxford New York

Bizzi E, Abend W (1983) Posture control and trajectory formation in single- and multi-joint arm movements. In: Desmedt RE (ed) Motor control mechanism in health and disease, Adv Neurol, vol 39. Raven Press, New York, pp 31-45

Bloedel JR, Courville J (1981) Cerebellar afferent systems. In: Brooks VB (ed) Motor control. Handbook of physiology, sect 1, vol II. Am Physiol Soc (Bethesda), pp 735-829

Brooks VB (1974) Some examples of programmed limb movements. Brain Res 71: 299-308

Brooks VB (1975) Opening remarks for the symposium. Can J Neurol Sci 2: 221-222

Brooks VB (1979) Control of intended limb movements by the lateral and intermediate cerebellum. In: Asanuma H, Wilson VJ (eds) Integration in the nervous system. Igaku Shoin, Tokyo, pp 321-357

Brooks VB (1981) (ed) Motor control, Handbook of physiology, sect 1, vol II. Am Physiol Soc (Bethesda)

Brooks VB (1983a) The cerebellum and adaptive tuning of movements. In: Willis WD, Schmidt RF (eds) Exp Brain Res (Suppl) Springer, Berlin Heidelberg New York (in press)

Brooks VB (1983b) Study of brain function by local, reversible cooling. Rev Physiol Biochem Pharmacol 95: 1-109

Brooks VB, Thach WT (1981) Cerebellar control of posture and movement. In: Brooks VB (ed) Motor control, Handbook of physiology, sect 1, vol II. Am Physiol Soc (Bethesda), pp 877-946

Brooks VB, Watts S (1983) Task-oriented adaptations of cocontraction of opposing muscles ("tuning") depend on the neocerebellum. Soc Neurosci Abstr 9: 606

Brooks VB, Cooke JD, Thomas JS (1973) The continuity of movements. In: Stein RB, Pearson KG, Smith RS, Redford JB (eds) Control of posture and locomotion. Plenum Press, New York, pp 257-272

Brooks VB, Kennedy PR, Ross HG (1983) Movement programming depends on understanding of behavioral requirements. Physiol Behav 31: 561-563

Cheney PD, Fetz EE (1984) Corticomotoneuronal cells contribute to long-latency stretch reflexes in the rhesus monkey. J Physiol 349 (in press)

Conrad B, Matsunami K, Meyer-Lohman J, Wiesendanger M, Brooks VB (1974) Cortical load compensation during voluntary elbow movements. Brain Res 71: 507-514

Conrad B, Meyer-Lohmann J, Matsunami K, Brooks VB (1975) Precentral unit activity following torque pulse injections into elbow movements. Brain Res 94: 219-236

Cooke JD (1980) The role of stretch reflexes during active movements. Brain Res 181: 493-497

Desmedt JE (1983) (ed) Motor control mechanisms in health and disease, advances in neurology, vol 39. Raven Press, New York

Evarts EV (1981) Role of motor cortex in voluntary movements in primates. In: Brooks VB (ed) Motor control, Handbook of physiology, sect 1, vol II. Am Physiol Soc (Bethesda), pp 1083-1120

Evarts EV, Tanji J (1974) Gating of motor cortex reflexes by prior instruction. Brain Res 71: 479-494

Fetz E (1981) Neuronal activity associated with conditioned limb movements. In: Towe AL, Luschei ES (eds) Motor coordination, Handbook of behavioral neurobiology, vol 5. Plenum Press, New York, pp 493-526

Georgopoulos AP, Kalaska JF, Massey JT (1981) Spatial trajectories and reaction times of aimed movements: effects of practice, uncertaintv. and change in target location. J Neurophysiol 46: 725-743

Georgopoulos AP, Kalaska JF, Caminiti R, Massey JT (1982) On the relations between the direction of two-dimensional arm movements and cell discharge in primate motor cortex. J Neurosci 2: 1527-1537

Georgopoulos AP, Caminiti R, Kalaska JF, Massey JT (1983) Spatial coding of movement direction by motor cortical populations. In: Massion J, Paillard J, Schultz W, Wiesendanger M (eds) Neural coding of motor performance, Exp Brain Res (suppl 7). Springer, Berlin Heidelberg New York, pp 327-336

Gilman S, Carr D, Hollenberg J (1976) Kinematic effects of deafferentation and cerebellar ablation. Brain 99: 311-330

Granit R (1981) Comments on history of motor control. In: Brooks VB (ed) Motor control, Handbook of physiology, sect 1, vol II. Am Physiol Soc (Bethesda), pp 1-16

Holmes G (1917) The symptoms of acute cerebellar injuries due to gunshot wounds. Brain 40: 461-535

Holton G (1973) Thematic origins of scientific thought, Kepler to Einstein. Harvard Univ Press, Cambridge

Hore J, Vilis T (1984) Loss of set in muscle responses to limb perturbations during cerebellar dysfunction. J Neurophysiol (in Press)

Jeannerod M, Prablanc C (1983) Visual control of reaching movements. In: Desmedt JE (ed) Motor control mechanisms in health and disease, advances in neurology, vol 39. Raven Press, New York, pp 13-29

Kwan HC, Murphy JT, Repeck MW (1979) Control of stiffness by the medium latency electromyographic response to limb perturbation. Can J Physiol Pharmacol 57: 277-285

Lacquaniti F, Soechting JF (1983) Changes in mechanical impedance and gain of myotatic response during transitions between two motor tasks. In: Massion J, Paillard J, Schultz W, Wiesendanger M (eds) Neural coding of motor performance, Exp Brain Res (Suppl 7). Springer, Verlin Heidelberg New York, pp 135-139

Lee RG, Murphy JT, Tatton WG (1983) Long-latency myotatic reflexes in man' mechanisms, functional significance, and changes in patients with Parkinson' disease or hemiplegia. In: Desmedt JE (ed) Cerebral motor control mechanisms in health and disease, advances in neurology, vol 39. Raven Press, New York, pp 489-508

Lenz FA, Tatton WG, Tasker RR (1983) The effect of cortical lesions on the electromyographic response to joint displacement in the squirrel monkey forelimb. J Neurosci 3: 795-805

Lestienne F, Polit A, Bizzi E (1981) Functional organization of the motor process underlying the transition from movement to posture. Brain Res 230: 121-131

Llinås RR (1981) Cerebellar networks. In: Brooks VB (ed) Motor control, Handbook of physiology, sect 1, vol II. Am Physiol Soc (Bethesda), pp 831-876

Marsden CD, Merton PE, Morton HB, Adam J (1977) The effect of lesions of sensorimotor cortex and the capsular pathways on servo responses from the human long thumb flexor. Brain 100: 503-526

Marsden DC, Merton PE, Morton HB, Adam J (1978) The effect of lesions of the central nervous system on long-latency stretch reflexes in the human thumb. In: Desmedt JE (ed) Cerebral motor control in man: long loop mechanisms. Prog Clin Neurophysiol, vol IV. Karger, Basel, pp 334-341

Melvill Jones G, Watt DGD (1971a) Observations on the control of stepping and hopping movements in man. J Physiol 219: 709-727

Melvill Jones G, Watt DGD (1971b) Muscular control of landing from unexpected falls in man. J Physiol 219: 729-737

Meyer-Lohmann J, Conrad B, Matsunami K, Brooks VB (1975) Effects of dentate cooling on precentral unit activity following torque pulse injections into elbow movements. Brain Res 94: 237-251

Meyer-Lohmann J, Hore J, Brooks VB (1977) Cerebellar participation in generation of prompt arm movements. J Neurophysiol 40: 1038-1050

Miller AD, Brooks VB (1981) Late muscular responses to arm perturbations persist during supraspinal dysfunctions in monkeys. Exp Brain Res 41: 146-158

Miller AD, Brooks VB (1982) Parallel pathways for movement initiation in monkeys. Exp Brain Res 45: 328-332

Nashner LM (1976) Adapting reflexes controlling the human posture. Exp Brain Res 26: 59-72

Nashner LM, Grimm RJ (1978) Analysis of multiloop dyscontrols in standing cerebellar patients. In: Desmedt JE (ed) Cerebral motor control in man: long loop mechanisms. Progr Clin Neurophysiol, vol V. Karger, Basel, pp 300-319

Nelson WL (1983) Physical principles for economics of skilled movements. Biol Cybernet 46: 135-147

Phillips CG (1969) Motor apparatus of the baboon's hand. The Ferrier lacture. Proc R Soc London Ser B 173: 141-174

Phillips CG, Porter R (1977) Corticospinal neurones. Their role in movement. Academic Press, London New York

Ruegg DG, Chofflon M (1983) Peripheral and transcortical loops activated by electrical stimulation of the tibial nerve in the monkey. Exp Brain Res 50: 293-298

Strick PL (1983) The influence of motor preparation on the response of cerebellar neurons to limb displacements. J Neurosci 3: 2007-2020

Tanji J, Evarts EV (1976) Anticipatory activity of motor cortex neurons in relation to direction of an intended movement. J Neurophysiol 39: 1062-1068

Towe AL, Luschei ES (1981) (eds) Motor coordination, Handbook of behavioral neurobiology, vol V. Plenum Press, New York

Tracey DJ, Walmsley B, Brinkman J (1980) "long loop" reflexes can be obtained in spinal monkeys. Neurosci Lett 18: 59-66

Vilis T, Cooke JD (1976) Modulation of the functional stretch reflex by the segmental reflex pathway. Exp Brain Res 25: 247-254

Vilis T, Hore J (1977) Effects of changes in mechanical state of limb on cerebellar intention tremor. J Neurophysiol 40: 1214-1224

Vilis T, Hore J (1980) Central neural mechanisms contributing to cerebellar tremor produced by limb perturbations. J Neurophysiol 43: 279-291

Vilis T, Hore J, Meyer-Lohmann H, Brooks VB (1976) Dual nature of the precentral responses to limb perturbations revealed by cerebellar cooling. Brain Res 177: 336-340

Viviani P, Terzuolo C (1980) Space-time invariance in learned motor skills. In: Stelmach GE, Requin J (eds) Tutorials in motor behavior. Adv Psychol, vol I. North-Holland Publ Co, Amsterdam, pp 525-533

Wiesendanger M, Miles W (1982) Ascending pathway of low-threshold muscle afferents to the cerebral cortex and its possible role in motor control. Physiol Rev 1982, 1234-1270

A Cerebellar-dependent Efference Copy Mechanism for Generating Appropriate Muscle Responses to Limb Perturbations

J. HORE and T. VILIS[1]

1 Introduction

The generation of appropriate muscle responses to a limb or body perturbation requires correct prediction of the nature and consequences of the perturbation. For example, Nashner (1976) demonstrated that the same stretch of the ankle extensors elicited different muscle responses depending on the postural situation in which this stretch occurred. Given a few trials the responses could be altered such that they were appropriate for maintaining postural stability. Thus training can be used to set up stretch reflexes such that they are context-specific. Motor responses can also be altered by prior instruction or intent. Hammond (1956) showed that the muscle response to stretch could be modulated in magnitude depending on whether the subject intended to resist or give way to the stretch. How does motor set, whether mediated by training or prior instruction, modify the muscular response to stretch? One possibility is that set can modulate or gate the synaptic efficacy of stretch reflexes. In the case of Nashner's experiment reflex loops could be modulated or even opened or closed depending on the motor set. Another possibility is that set allows the preprogramming of the appropriate response which then is triggered or released by the initial stretch. This mode is suggested in the experiments of Evarts and Tanji (1976) which dissociated reflex from intended muscle activity. Here set-dependent activity in both muscle and motor cortex was triggered by a perturbation independent of the direction of the initial stretch.

In this paper we will present evidence which suggests that the set-dependent changes in the muscle response to perturbations involves both these mechanisms. In particular the magnitude of the initial muscle responses to stretch that are mediated by segmental and transcortical loops can be modulated by expectation of the nature of the forthcoming perturbation. This expectation or set also affects subsequent components which appear to be preprogrammed in nature. Both set-dependent aspects of the muscular response require the integrity of the cerebellum.

2 Methods

Experiments were performed on five Cebus monkeys. Details of the methods of recording, cerebellar cooling, and the behavioral paradigm have been described fully in

---

[1] Department of Physiology, University of Western Ontario, London, Ontario, Canada

Cerebellar Functions
ed. by Bloedel et al.

recent publications (Vilis and Hore 1980, Hore and Vilis 1984, Flament et al. 1984). In brief the important points of the paradigm were as follows. Monkeys held a handle that was pivoted at the elbow within a target window of 12 deg of horizontal arc. Targets and handle position were displayed on an oscilloscope in front of the monkey. The handle was always held against a constant force that loaded triceps (and assisted the return movement following pulse perturbations). Perturbations were either pulses (20, 40, 60, 80, 100, 140 ms duration) or steps (2000 ms duration). All perturbations initially stretched biceps and resulted in stretch of triceps on the return movement to target. Monkeys were rewarded with fruit juice if they returned the handle to the target region, within 300 ms, after the onset of the perturbation without overshooting. Responses to expected pulses were obtained by averaging responses to about 15 pulses of a particular duration delivered in succession. Responses to unexpected pulses were obtained by delivering a series of 10-20 steps and then randomly interspersing a pulse. This was repeated about 15 times and responses to the pulses were averaged. Cerebellar nuclei were cooled to $10°C$ probe temperature through 2 sheaths that were histologically confirmed to lie lateral and medial to the dentate nucleus.

3 Results

Inherent in preprogramming an appropriate muscular response to a limb disturbance is the ability to predict the nature of the forthcoming disturbance. The possibility for prediction was incorporated into our paradigm by giving the monkey practice trials (usually 15) of a given perturbation type prior to data collection. Two different perturbation types were used: a torque pulse and a torque step. The monkey's EMG response to an expected torque pulse (40 ms duration) is illustrated in Fig. 1A. It consists of a brief response in the agonist biceps (latency 40 ms) whose function is to resist the perturbation and initiate the return movement. This is followed by a phasic burst of activity in the antagonist triceps (latency 60 ms) whose function appears to be to terminate the return movement in the target region. This antagonist response was enhanced if a constant load was placed on the handle which assisted the return movement. An important aspect of this phasic antagonist response is that it could not have been initiated by stretch of the velocity sensitive receptors in the antagonist muscle. The dashed line in Fig. 1A indicates 20 ms after start of stretch of the antagonist, the minimum delay of a spinal stretch reflex. The phasic activity in the antagonist, occurring prior to this, will be referred to as the early antagonist response. In contrast the EMG response to an expected step perturbation (Fig. 1B) consisted of an M2 response followed by a phasic burst in the agonist (M3) and later agonist activity. Thus a phasic burst following M2 occurred in the antagonist when pulses were expected and in the agonist when steps were expected.

What are the characteristics of the early antagonist response to a torque pulse? One possibility is that it is initiated by some receptor that detects the offset of the torque pulse. This possibility was examined by varying the duration of the torque pulse. Practice trials were given for each duration so that the monkey could predict the nature of the forthcoming perturbation. Figure 2 illustrates that the onset of the early antagonist response was not initiated by torque pulse offset. As the torque pulse duration

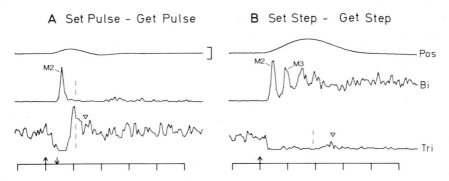

Fig. 1 A, B. EMG responses to expected 40 ms pulses (**A**); and to expected 2000 ms steps (**B**). Traces are averages of the responses to 15 perturbations that initially stretched biceps. A constant force on the handle loaded triceps. *Upward arrows* onset of perturbation; *downward arrow* offset of perturbation. *Dashed line* is drawn 20 ms after velocity reached zero (i.e. at time when stretch of triceps could have produced a stretch reflex). Calibrations: target width 12 deg, time 100 ms/division. *Pos* position; *Bi* biceps; *Tri* triceps; *triangles* peak of return velocity. Monkey Du. (Hore and Vilis 1984)

was increased from 20 to 100 ms the response latency remained fixed. Furthermore for pulse durations of 80 and 100 ms it preceded torque pulse offset. Comparison of the agonist-antagonist responses reveals that they have a reciprocal nature. As the duration of the pulse was increased (see 60 ms response) a second phasic response (M3, latency 70 ms) appeared in the agonist. Simultaneously a trough appeared in the early antagonist response. The magnitude of both agonist peaks (M2 and M3) increased with increasing pulse durations. It is of particular interest that this occurred for the M2 response. Since the magnitude of the torque change was the same for all durations and since the stretch velocity in the initial 40 ms preceding the M2 response was identical for pulse durations of 40 ms or greater, this increase in magnitude can only be attributed to the expectation of longer pulse durations and thus the need for a larger agonist response. In summary the timing of the responses in both the agonist and antagonist muscles appear to be synchronized to torque pulse onset rather than offset. Such a characteristic is consistent with a preprogrammed response that is triggered by initial stretch.

To investigate the preprogrammed nature of the early antagonist response a second test was performed. The monkey was trained to expect a torque step perturbation. A torque pulse was then unexpectedly introduced. The responses to the same pulse perturbations were then compared in two situations: when a pulse was expected (set pulse-get pulse) and when a pulse was unexpected (set step-get pulse). EMG responses for two pulse durations are illustrated in Fig. 3. Figure 3A shows responses in one monkey to 40 ms pulses while Fig. 3B shows responses in another monkey to 100 ms pulses. The first difference between expected and unexpected pairs of responses for both pulse durations is that in the unexpected situation (set step-get pulse) the antagonist EMG response was delayed and followed the start of stretch of the antagonist muscle while in the expected case (set pulse-get pulse) it led it. The second difference is that in the unexpected case a larger agonist response occurred both in terms of M2 size and the

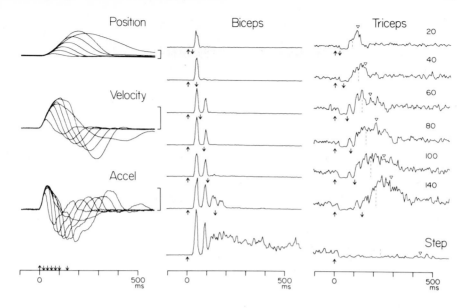

Fig. 2. Movement and EMG traces for perturbations of the same force but different durations. Traces are the average of 15 perturbations that initially stretched biceps. Note that the first peak in the biceps response is an M2. The durations of the perturbations were 20, 40, 60, 80, 100, 140 ms (pulses) and 2000 ms (step). A constant force was applied that loaded triceps. *Arrows, dashed lines* and *triangles* are as in Fig. 1. Calibrations: target – 12 deg; velocity – 200 deg/s; acceleration – 4000 deg/s. Monkey Du. (Hore and Vilis 1984)

presence of subsequent components. It is important to note that the perturbation, the initial movement trajectory, and thus the initial afferent drive is identical for both the expected and unexpected responses for the same pulse duration. The only factor that can account for the difference in the EMG responses in the monkey's different expectation of the forthcoming perturbation. When a step is expected preprogramming appears to direct activity to the agonist even though a pulse is actually received. However afferent feedback also exerts an influence. If it did not the response to an unexpected pulse (set step-get pulse) would be the same as that of an expected step (set step-get step, Fig. 1B) i.e., no antagonist response would be present. The late antagonist activity due to afferent feedback in the set step-get pulse situation however lacks a predictive component as can be seen from the fact that it follows rather than leads the start of stretch of the antagonist.

The next question posed was whether the early antagonist response that occurred when a pulse was correctly predicted was dependent on the integrity of the cerebellum. This was examined by comparing the response to an expected pulse perturbation under normal conditions to the response obtained when the cerebellum was reversibly lesioned by means of cryoprobes placed lateral and medial to the dentate nucleus. The main effect of this cerebellar lesion was a delay in the onset of the antagonist response (Fig. 4). Thus the antagonist response during cooling resembled the unexpected pulse response in that it now followed rather than led the start of stretch of the antagonist. In addition, rather than terminating the return movement it initiated the first cycle of a

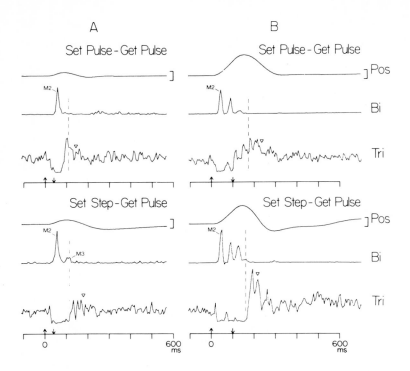

Fig. 3 A, B. Average responses to expected (set pulse-get pulse) and unexpected (set step-get pulse) pulse perturbations of different durations. **A** 40 ms pulse, monkey Bz; **B** 100 ms pulse, monkey Du. Calibration and labels as in Fig. 1

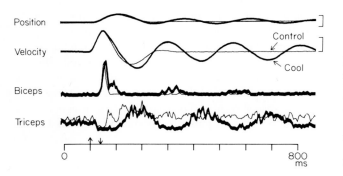

Fig. 4. Averages of EMG responses and movement parameters to 15 expected 40 ms pulse perturbations under normal conditions (control *thin line*) and during cerebellar nuclear cooling (cool *thick line*). Monkey Bz

tremor. During this tremor peak EMG activity in both the agonist and antagonist muscles was aligned to the peak velocity of stretch of the corresponding muscle. This suggests that the EMG responses during cerebellar dysfunction lacked a predictive component and were now driven solely by stretch reflexes.

To verify this we compared the responses to expected pulses of various durations under normal conditions and during cerebellar nuclear cooling. During cerebellar dysfunction both the onset and peak of antagonist activity shifted with pulse duration

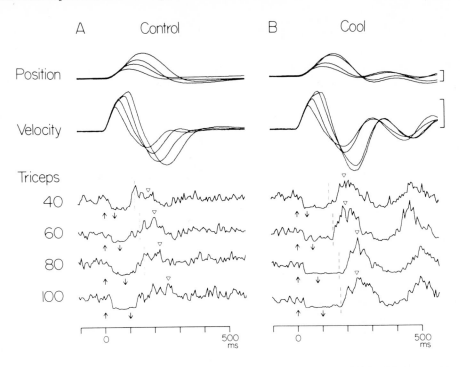

Fig. 5 A, B. Antagonist EMG responses to expected perturbation of different durations. **A** control conditions; **B** during cerebellar nuclear cooling. Each trace is the average of 15 perturbations that initially stretched biceps. Durations of perturbations are indicated on the *left*. *Arrows, dashed lines,* and *triangles* as in Fig. 1. Monkey Mi. (Hore and Vilis 1984)

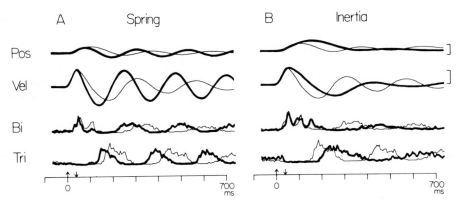

Fig. 6 A, B. Effect of a spring force and increased inertial load on averaged EMG responses to expected limb perturbations during cerebellar nuclear cooling. *Thin line* normal manipulandum (same in **A** and **B**); *thick line* **A** manipulandum acting as a spring. *Thick line* **B** adding mass to manipulandum and increasing force of perturbation so that the same initial peak velocity was achieved. *Arrows* as in Fig. 1. Calibrations: target, 12 deg; velocity, 100 deg/s. Monkey Bz. (Flament et al. 1984)

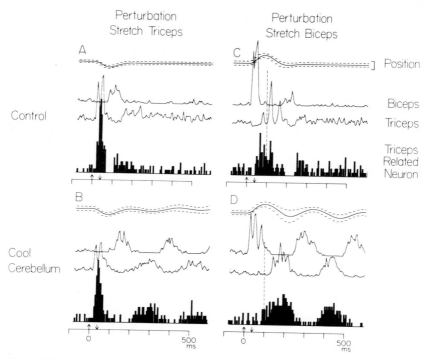

Fig. 7 A-D. Average responses of a triceps-related motor cortex neuron to expected 40 ms pulse limb perturbations that initially stretched triceps under normal conditions (**A**) and during cerebellar nuclear cooling (**B**). In C and D the responses of the same neuron to a perturbation that initially stretched biceps under normal conditions and during cerebellar nuclear cooling are shown. *Dashed line* drawn 100 ms after onset of perturbation. Monkey Bz

(Fig. 5). Thus while under normal conditions onset of the antagonist activity was synchronized to torque pulse onset and led start of stretch of the antagonist muscle, during cerebellar dysfunction the antagonist response lost this preprogrammed quality and now appeared to be driven by stretch reflexes. This aspect of the antagonist response during cerebellar dysfunction is further illustrated when the effect of different mechanical loads on the handle are compared. If a spring load was added to the handle by electronic feedback of a position signal, the tremor increased in frequency (Fig. 6A). At the same time the peak activity in both the agonist and antagonist muscles shifted to again occur at the time of peak stretch velocity. Similarly if the inertia of the handle was increased by the addition of mass to the handle (Fig. 6B), the tremor frequency decreased and the time of peak EMG activity again shifted with the time of peak stretch velocity. Thus the changes observed in both the tremor frequency and the timing of EMG peaks matched the changes one would predict if these EMG responses were mediated by servo-like stretch reflexes.

There is considerable evidence that the normal EMG responses to perturbations are mediated in part by supra-segmental pathways involving a loop through motor cortex (Evarts 1973, Phillips and Porter 1977). In addition the work of Evarts and Tanji (1976) suggests that the components mediating prior instructions or set also traverse the motor cortex. To examine whether the predictive aspect of the early antagonist response was also mediated by the motor cortex and to determine whether this activity in motor cortex was dependent on the integrity of the cerebellum, we compared the responses of units in motor cortex before and after reversible lesions of the cerebellum. Of the various types of units in motor cortex perhaps the most revealing are those that respond reciprocally to both perturbations and voluntary movements and thus most closely resemble the activity of particular muscles involved in the movement. A representative unit of this type is illustrated in Fig. 7. This unit appears to be related to the activity of the triceps muscle. When the perturbation stretched triceps the unit responded with an early excitatory response (latency 20 ms) (Fig. 7A). Thus it could contribute to the M2 response (latency 40 ms) in triceps. When the perturbation stretched biceps the early response was inhibitory and a later excitatory component (latency 40 ms) appeared which preceded the early antagonist response of the triceps muscle (Fig. 7C). During cerebellar cooling no change was observed in the timing of the agonist EMG or the early cortical response (Fig. 7A, B). However when the perturbation initially stretched biceps and the cerebellar nuclei were cooled (Fig. 7D) the activity of the cortical unit was delayed as was activity of triceps. This suggests that the normal early antagonist EMG response, which precedes the start of antagonist stretch, is mediated by motor cortex and is dependent on the integrity of the cerebellum.

4 Discussion

One significance of training is that it enables skilled movements to be performed that are anticipatory or predictive in nature. The results of our experiments suggest that in practised movements this predictive ability is mediated by the cerebellum. In our particular paradigm, that of resisting a perturbation and preventing overshoot of the return movement, the predictive component consists of the early antagonist response. The function of this response is to assist in stabilizing the return movement by generating braking in the antagonist muscle which precedes the start of stretch of the antagonist. Evidence that the early antagonist response is preprogrammed stems from the observation that its onset is synchronized to the onset of the initial perturbation and that its presence is dependent on the correct expectation of the forthcoming perturbation (i.e. a pulse). The reversible lesion studies suggest that this response is mediated by the cerebellum via antagonist related units in motor cortex. Dysfunction of the cerebellum results in loss of this predicitve component and the subsequent reliance on feedback via stretch reflexes. Our results also indicate that in the intact animal the magnitude of these preprogrammed responses can be modulated by afferent feedback. Thus when a perturbation is not what was expected the resulting error in the return trajectory can be minimized by afferent modulation of the magnitude of the EMG responses.

How is the antagonist response preceding the start of antagonist stretch generated? One function of this response is to dissipate the kinetic energy acquired in the inertial components of the limb and handle during the return movement. If this is not dissipated before reaching target position an overshoot will result. Because of the delay inherent between muscle activation and force generation the antagonist must be activated well in advance of reaching final position. One possible mechanism for achieving this is by phase advancing the afferent information by some form of differentiation. A feedforward inhibitory mechanism in the cerebellum has been proposed that may serve this function (Thach 1972). However this does not explain the triggered nature of the antagonist response, i.e. it appears to be synchronized to torque pulse onset rather than offset. An alternate scheme that incorporates both the triggered and the phase advanced nature of this response is an efference-copy mechanism. This mechanism was originally proposed by Helmholtz (1910) to explain why the world does not spin when we move our eyes. In our particular paradigm when the shape of the forthcoming perturbation is correctly anticipated the future velocity of the return movement can be predicted from the agonist command. This is because it is the agonist command that initiates this return movement. Thus the correct antagonist command could, in theory, be computed on the basis of reafference from the agonist command.

Such an **efference-copy** mechanism fits with the known neuroanatomical connections between motor cortex and the cerebellum. Neural discharge from motor cortex is known to project to both the spinal motor neuron pool and by way of collaterals through the pontine nuclei to the cerebellum. Thus as Eccles (1979) observed, the cerebrum cannot begin instituting any action without the cerebellum immediately knowing about it. On the the basis of the collateral or efference-copy the cerebellum can formulate subsequent components of the cerebrum's response. However in order to be effective this formulation must be based on prior experience or learning. Such a concept is consistent with the finding of Evarts and Tanji (1976) that it is not the first but the second, or intended, response in motor cortex that is predominantly affected by prior instruction.

Other schemes for triggering the cerebellum to generate the early antagonist response following a limb perturbation, for example via spino-cerebellar pathways, are not consistent with recent experimental findings. For example Strick (1983) found that it is neurons in dentate and not those in interposed (which receives the bulk of the spino-cerebellar projection) that can be related to set. Furthermore neurons in dentate discharge with a minimum latency of about 30 ms to a limb perturbation which is consistent with them discharging after the first or reflex response in motor cortex (latency about 20 ms).

To illustrate how such an efference-copy mechanism could function in our particular task consider the case when the monkey expects and receives a pulse perturbation (Fig. 8A, set pulse-get pulse). Stretch of the agonist muscle initiates spinal reflexes and activates agonist-related neurons in motor cortex. The motor cortex issues a command to the agonist alpha motor neurons and simultaneously informs the cerebellum of this action. The cerebellum, on the basis of past experience and the expectation of a pulse perturbation, activates antagonist-related motor cortex neurons which in turn generate the early antagonist muscle response (Fig. 1A). Since this response is initiated by the start of agonist muscle stretch it will be synchronized to torque pulse onset. Moreover because its initiation involves a loop of short latency (motor cortex − cerebellum − motor cortex) the onset of antagonist activity can precede the actual stretch of the antagonist muscle.

If instead a step perturbation is expected and received (Fig. 8B, set step-get step) the cerebellum on the basis of this expectation switches the response to the appropriate agonist-related neurons in motor cortex. A reverberatory circuit is formed which contributes to the generation of the M3 and later agonist EMG activity.

Fig. 8 A, B. Schematic diagram
of possible efference-copy
pathways involved in producing agonist and antagonist
EMG responses to expected
pulse perturbations (**A**) and to
expected step perturbations (**B**)

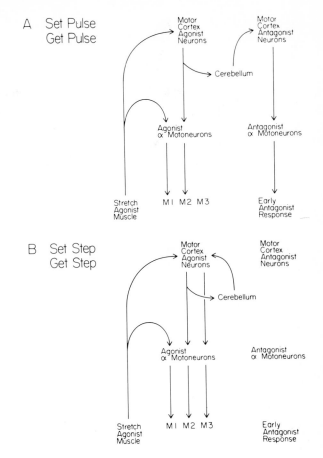

Suppose that a step is expected and instead a pulse is received (Fig. 9A, set step-get
pulse). In this case the cerebellum is not set to program an early antagonist response.
Instead an antagonist response must await the actual stretch of the antagonist muscle.
This results in a delayed or late antagonist response (Fig. 3A, B). The situation for the
antagonist is similar when the cerebellum is lesioned (Fig. 9B). Here the efference-copy
loop is broken and the responses must again await stretch of the antagonist muscle.
Thus the antagonist muscle response is again delayed (Fig. 4, 5) as is the antagonist-
related activity in motor cortex (Fig. 7D).

The significance of the scheme outlined in Figs. 8 and 9 is that a train of preprogrammed responses can be initiated on the basis of a single afferent trigger. In this scheme
the cerebellum acts as more than a switch directing activity to either agonist or antagonist-related units in motor cortex. Rather each command component initiated by
the motor cortex is transformed by the cerebellum into the next of a sequence of
command components. Thus the particular preprogrammed response evolves on the
basis of the transformation set up in the cerebellum by prior experience or instruction.
Possible schemes for how this transformation is realized are considered in detail elsewhere in this volume. The particular paths illustrated in Figs. 8 and 9 are most certainly

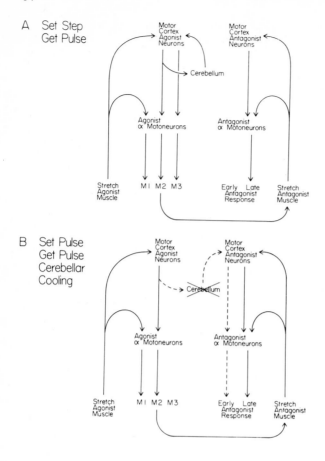

A   Set Step
    Get Pulse

B   Set Pulse
    Get Pulse
    Cerebellar
    Cooling

Fig. 9 A, B. Schematic diagram of possible pathways involved in producing EMG responses to unexpected pulse perturbations (set step-get pulse) (**A**); and to expected pulse perturbations during cerebellar nuclear cooling (**B**)

an oversimplification of the actual situation. For example, it ignores the descending influences of the cerebellum (Bantli and Bloedel, 1976). In addition it omits the role of set in modulating the gain of stretch reflexes. For example, the magnitude of the agonist M2 response is increased as the expected duration of the perturbation is increased (Fig. 2). Decreases in the magnitude of M2 have been observed to step perturbations in patients with cerebellar lesions (Marsden et al. 1977) and in monkeys during cerebellar nuclear cooling (Hore and Vilis 1984). Thus the cerebellum on the basis of set appears to exert a dual role: presetting the gain of stretch reflexes and sequencing preprogrammed responses by means of efference copy.

References

Bantli H, Bloedel JR (1976) Characteristics of the output from the dentate nucleus to spinal neurons via pathways which do not involve the primary sensorimotor cortex. Exp Brain Res 25: 199-220

Eccles JC (1979) Introductory remarks. In: Massion J, Sasaki K (eds) Cerebro-cerebellar interactions. Elsevier/North-Holland, Biomedical Press, Amsterdam

Evarts EV (1973) Motor cortex reflexes associated with learned movement. Science 179: 501-503

Evarts EV, Tanji J (1976) Reflex and intended responses in motor cortex pyramidal tract neurons of monkey. J Neurophysiol 39: 1069-1080

Flament D, Hore J, Vilis T (1984) Dependence of cerebellar tremor on proprioceptive but not visual feedback. Exp Neurol 94: 314-325

Hammond PH (1956) The influence of prior instruction to the subject on an apparently involuntary neuro-muscular response. J Physiol 132: 17P-18P

Helmholtz HV (1910) Handbuch der physilogischen Optik, vol III. Leopold Voss, Hamburg Leipzig

Hore J, Vilis T (1984) Loss of set in muscle responses to limb perturbations during cerebellar dysfunction. J Neurophysiol 51: 1137-1148

Marsden CD, Merton PA, Morton HB, Hallett M, Adam J, Rushton DN (1977) Disorders of movement in cerebellar disease in man. In: Rose F (ed) The physiological aspect of clinical neurology. Blackwell, Oxford, pp 179-199

Nashner LM (1976) Adapting reflexes controlling the human posture. Exp Brain Res 26: 59-72

Phillips CG, Porter R (1977) Corticospinal neurones. Academic Press, London New York

Strick PL (1983) The influence of motor preparation on the response of cerebellar neurons to limb displacements. J Neurosci 3: 2007-2020

Thach WT (1972) Cerebellar output: properties, synthesis and uses. Brain Res 40: 89-97

Vilis T, Hore J (1980) Central neural mechanisms contributing to cerebellar tremor produced by limb perturbations. J Neurophysiol 43: 279-291

Motor Programs: Trajectory Versus Stability

W.T. Thach, M.H. Schieber, and R.H. Elble[1]

1 Introduction

Two subcortical systems converge on motor cortex and brainstem nuclei (Fig. 1). The basal ganglia receive from most or all of cerebral cortex (Kemp and Powell, 1971). Ablation prevents or slows movement, suggesting roles in the initiation and continuation of movement trajectories, and single unit studies have shown relationships to a variety of movement parameters, including direction, velocity/amplitude, pattern and force of muscular activity (Crutcher and Delong, 1984; Delong et al. 1983; Delong and Strick 1974; Georgopoulos et al. 1983a, b). By contrast, the cerebellum receives from a more restricted portion of cerebral cortex, including sensorimotor cortex and parts immediately adjacent in frontal and parietal lobes, and from other portions of the motor apparatus including spinal cord, reticular and vestibular nuclei (Bloedel and Courville 1981; Brodal 1978). Single unit studies had shown that lateral cerebellum fires before movement and even before motor cortex toward which it projects (Thach 1975, 1978), which seems to suggest a role in the programming of the initiation and the direction of trajectory. More medial portions fire later (Strick 1978; Thach 1978) and code for pattern and force of muscular activity (Thach 1978) and movement velocity (Burton and Onoda 1977, 1978; Soechting et al. 1978), which seems to suggest the continuous control of ongoing trajectory (Allen and Tsukahara 1974; Evarts and Thach 1969). Yet cerebellar ablation does not abolish movement trajectory, but instead gives rise to a variety of movement instabilities (Dow and Moruzzi 1958; Holmes 1939). This has suggested specific roles in control of movement and postural stability, possibly acting on reflex pathways (Gilman 1969; Gilman et al. 1971; Granit et al. 1955; Higgins and Glaser 1964; Higgins et al. 1962; Merton 1953; Soechting et al. 1978; Terzuolo et al. 1973; Vilis and Hore 1980; Terzuolo and Viviani 1974). Recent work (Schieber and Thach 1984a, b) on cerebellar unit discharge in monkeys performing trained pursuit tracking movements helps resolve apparent inconsistencies in cerebellar ablation and unit data, and at least in this task, suggests an exclusive role in the control of movement stability.

[1] Department of Anatomy & Neurobiology, Neurology & Neurosurgery, and the McDonnell Center for Higher Brain Functions Washington University School of Medicine St. Louis, Missouri, USA 63110

Cerebellar Functions
ed. by Bloedel et al.
© Springer-Verlag Berlin Heidelberg 1984

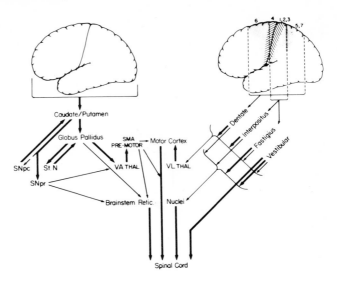

Fig. 1. Connections of basal ganglia and cerebellum: extrapyramidal and prepyramidal. *SMA* Supplementary motor area of cerebral cortex; *PM* Premotor area of cerebral cortex; *VA Thal.* Ventral anterior nuclei of thalamus; *VL Thal.* Ventral lateral nuclei of thalamus; *S.T.N.* Subthalamic nucleus; *SNpc* Substantia nigra pars compacta; *SNpr* Substantia nigra pars reticulata. The basal ganglia receive from the entire cerebral cortex, and project to brainstem nuclei and VA thalamus, which in turn projects indirectly to motor cortex and to brainstem nuclei. The cerebellum receives from sensorimotor cortex (and the immediately adjacent regions) and projects directly to spinal cord, brainstem nuclei, and (via *VL* thalamus) motor cortex

2 Experiments

Monkeys were trained to follow a slowly moving target beam on an oscilloscope with a smooth pursuit tracking movement of the wrist against torque loads (Fig. 1). Parameters were varied such that the target onset was unpredictable in time, the direction either right or left, the total excursion 10-70° of wrist angle, the velocity 8-28°/s, and the torque loads 0-.24 Nm measured at the palm of the hand (aiding or impeding movement, thus dissociating pattern of muscular activity — flexor or extensor — from direction of movement). The tracking window was 10-15° of wrist angle. Once a set of parameter values was selected, identical trials were performed repetitively in blocks. The monkeys could and did anticipate the direction of target movement, and lined up on the leading edge in order not to be left behind when it moved. Even so, a target window of 10° that began to move at 30°/s gave the animal only 330 ms allowed reaction time; he had to be careful not be left behind, or to overshoot the leading edge, or to oscillate excessively once he did get going. The animals had an 11-13 Hz action tremor of 5° or less at the wrist during the ramp tracking.

The principal finding concerns the direction of modulated unit discharge frequency (up or down), and the direction of the wrist movement (right or left). The findings are summarized in Fig. 3. Figure 3A shows the EMG discharge of a long flexor muscle of

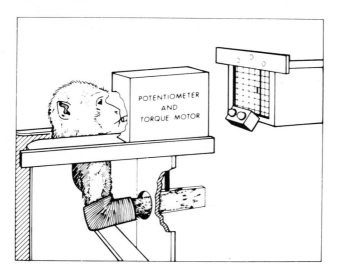

Fig. 2. Sketch of monkey and apparatus used for slow pursuit tracking of a visual stimulus by movement at the wrist. Parameters were varied such that the target onset was unpredictable in time, the direction either right or left, the total excursion 10-70° of wrist angle, the velocity 8-28°/s, the torque loads 0-.24 Nm measured at the palm of the hand, (aiding or impeding movement, thus dissociating pattern of muscular activity – flexor or extensor – from directional movement)

the wrist and the fingers that was located in the forearm averaged over a number of trials. At the top left of Fig. 3A is the stimulus trajectory that the monkey followed during wrist extension, and below it are three graphs showing the muscle EMG during extension. At the top right of Fig. 3A is the target stimulus trajectory that the monkey followed during flexion, and below it are three graphs showing the EMG discharge of the forearm flexor muscle during flexion. The middle two graphs of Fig. 3A show the EMG discharge during extension and flexion under no load, the upper two graphs under flexor load, and the bottom two under extensor load. In flexion under no load (Fig. 3A, middle right graph), the flexor muscle increases discharge as flexion proceeds. When flexing under flexor load (Fig. 3A, right upper graph), the discharge is greatly increased. In flexion under extensor load (Fig. 3A, lower right graph), the flexor muscle is virtually silent as the loaded extensors do all the work even during slow flexor movements. When extending under no load (Fig. 3A, middle left graph), the extensor muscle again does the work, and the flexor muscle is mainly silent. This is true also when extending under extensor load (Fig. 3A, lower left graph). But when extending under flexor load (Fig. 3A, upper left graph), the loaded flexor muscle does the work (the extensor muscles are silent), and the EMG of the flexor muscle slowly lowers to let the load carry the hand and manipulandum in an extensor movement. This is the expected relationship of a muscle's activity for the two directions of movement and for the three different load states, and all the muscles in the forelimb that were used in the task behaved in this way (or the reverse pattern for extensors).

The discharge of a neuron in motor cortex is shown in Fig. 3B. When flexing under no load (Fig. 3B, middle right graph), the discharge frequency increased; the frequency increased even higher when flexion under flexor load (Fig. 3B, upper right graph), but was nil when flexing under extensor load (Fig. 3B, lower right graph). When extending, the neuron was active under flexor load (Fig. 3B, upper left); discharge was slight when extending under no load (Fig. 3B, middle left graph) and nil under extensor load (Fig. 3B, lower left graph). This neuron, therefore, had a discharge pattern during the two directions of movement and the two directions of load similar to that of the flexor

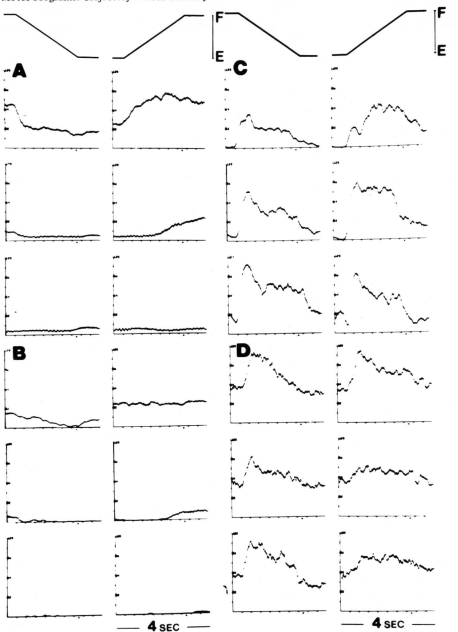

Fig. 3 A-D. Discharge of muscle (EMG) and neurons during slow hold-ramp-hold tracking movements in different directions under different loads. **A** flexor muscle; **B** neuron in precentral cortex; **C** another neuron in precentral cortex; **D** neuron in dentate nucleus of cerebellum. **A** *top left* hold-ramp-hold target trajectory guiding extension; *below* are EMG traces during extension; **A** *top right* stimulus trajectory during flexion; *below* are EMG traces during flexion. On the six graphs, *top row* is under flexor load, the *middle row* under no load, and *bottom row* under extensor load. Conventions are the same for **B-D**. The graphs show that the flexor muscle in **A** and precentral neuron in **B** have patterns that are reciprocal, and that the other precentral neuron in **C** and the dentate neuron in **D** have patterns that are bidirectional

muscle (Fig. 3A). Of all the neurons in motor cortex, half discharged in a pattern that resembled activity in a flexor (like this one) or an extensor muscle. We call this pattern unidirectional or reciprocal.

By contrast, the other half of motor cortex neurons behaved in a distinctly different pattern, an example of which is shown in Fig. 3C. The conventions are the same as in Fig. 3A, B. What is at once apparent is that the pattern of discharge is remarkably similar, regardless of the direction of the movement and the load condition. At the onset of movement there is an abrupt increase of discharge frequency to a peak, which then gradually lowers as the movement progresses. Under conditions which call for marked changes in discharge frequency in muscle (Fig. 3A) and in neurons behaving like muscle (Fig. 3B), the pattern is remarkably constant. We call this pattern of discharge, which is relatively constant for the two directions of movement and the two directions of load, "bidirectional". In the cerebellar nuclei, to our great surprise, *all* of the neurons discharged like that in Fig. 3D: the pattern was bidirectional. Indeed, we did not find any neurons in the cerebellar nuclei that were reciprocal. Because of this, we thought that we had directed the electrode to the wrong parts of the dentate and interposed nuclei — that we were recording from cells that were concerned with parts of the body other than the arm, and that the opposing muscles in these other parts were cocontracting to help keep the rest of the body still (Smith and Bourbonnais 1981; Smith et al. 1983; Frysinger et al. 1984). But this was not the case, for several reasons: (a) the neurons undergoing the greatest changes in discharge frequency (and therefore the most concerned with task performance) were in the middle portion of the interposed and dentate nuclei, and this portion we have shown to contain the greatest numbers of neurons preferentially related to movements of the arm (Asanuma et al. 1983a, b; Thach 1978; Thach et al. 1982); (b) there were no cerebellar neurons in that or other regions that fired in a reciprocal pattern; (c) the bidirectional neurons whose discharge best correlated with performance of this task also correlated well with other movements of the arm — rapid alternating movements, response to flexor and extensor torque pulses, and (d) in all these other movements, the pattern of discharge was reciprocal. Thus, under the conditions of this experiment, all cerebellar neurons (57 in dentate, 45 in interposed) and half the motor cortex neurons that changed activity in relation to movement did so without relation to the trajectory parameters of direction, velocity, position, pattern or force of muscular activity. What movement signal, if any, were they carrying?

Figure 4 shows a single trial of extension. The top trace is position, the middle trace the EMG of a wrist extensor muscle, and the bottom trace the discharge of a neuron in the interposed nuclei. Neurons in interposed (but not those in dentate) and the bidirectional neurons in motor cortex were exquisitely modulated in relation to tremor of the monkey's wrist. The tremor amplitude was as great as 5° and was at a frequency initially of 11-13 cps, though the amplitude increased several fold and the frequency dropped to 5-7 cps after repeated penetrations through the cerebellar nuclei. Peak interposed activity lagged the peak tremor excursion and also the peak EMG (by about 12 ms), which suggested it was carried over the rapidly conducting spinocerebellar pathways known to influence the intermediate cerebellar cortex (and interposed nuclei) but not the lateral (and dentate nucleus) cerebellum. Thus, of all the possible trajectory parameters that cerebellar neurons could conceivably have been coding, the only one detected in this experiment was that relating to tremor — tremor initially physiological

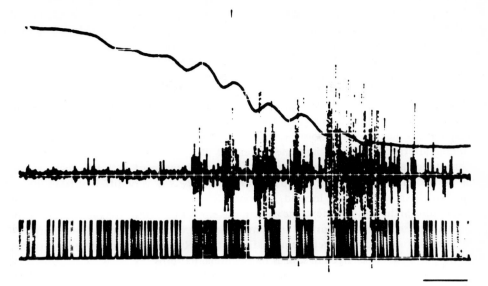

Fig. 4. Cerebellar interpositus neuron and EMG recordings during tremor. Simultaneous position, extensor digitorum EMG (*middle trace*), and extensor related interpositus neuron (*lower trace*) recordings obtained during an extensor ramp maneuver. Scale = 200 ms. By applying extensor and flexor torque pulses to the wrist, 6 of 14 tremor-related interpositus neurons could be classified as excited by stretch of either the extensor or the flexor muscles. The tremor bursts of these interpositus neurons led the peaks in muscle stretch by an average of 51 deg (range 19-86). The interpositus tremor bursts therefore lagged the EMG bursts by an average of 12 s (range 4-22 ms)

(before dropping into a pathological "cerebellar" range), but of sufficient amplitude to jeopardize performance during this demanding task. Under the conditions of this task, cerebellar neurons were concerned with some aspect of the task, or some component of the body, where a premium was set on constancy of pattern, possibly as a carrier frequency to detect tremor and other instabilities of intended and actual movement. We wondered if this could possibly involve the discharge of gamma motor neurons (which the cerebellum is known to control), or the activity of muscle receptors (which are known to influence the cerebellum). This led us to see if we could record from the dorsal root ganglion cells innervating the muscle spindles of the forearm to see if they might also fire in a bidirectional pattern-possibly the cause or the effect (or both) of bidirectional motor cortex and cerebellar activity.

The same monkey in which we had recorded the EMG and the discharge of neurons in motor cortex and cerebellar nuclei was anesthetized, and a standard recording chamber was implanted over the exposed C7-8 dorsal root ganglia (DRG). Single neuron recordings were identified as being those of spindle afferents from forelimb muscles if they had: (a) a receptive field in the muscle belly (and not skin); (b) a spontaneous maintained discharge that (c) could be driven by brief taps to the receptive field; (d) a response to a tuning fork of 128/s frequency applied to the receptive field, with discharge following at 128 or a subharmonic of 64 cps; (e) reciprocal responses to flexor and extensor torque pulses and (f) to rapid alternating movements; and finally (g) a pause in firing when the muscle in which it lay was made to contract by direct electrical shock so as to unload the spindle. One neuron was completely tested and satisfied all of the criteria. Four others were lost before they were completely tested, but satisfied all the criteria tested for. These 5 neurons were identified as muscle spindle afferents. The discharge of one of these is shown in Fig. 5 along with the EMG of the extensor muscle which behaved in a pattern just the opposite of that shown for the extensor muscle in Fig. 3A. Under no load (Fig. 5, middle graphs) the muscle is active during extension (left) and not flexion (right). Under extensor load (Fig. 5, bottom graphs) the muscle is active during both flexion (right) and extension (left); and under flexor load (top graphs) it is inactive during both flexion (right) and extension (left). By contrast, the spindle afferent had much the same pattern of discharge under all the conditions: an abrupt increase in discharge frequency at the onset of movement, with a gradual lowering as the movement progresses. The pattern of discharge was very different from that of the muscle in which it was located, and very different from that of the reciprocal class of neurons in the motor cortex. The pattern was similar to that of the bidirectional class of neurons in the motor cortex, and similar to that of the neurons in the interposed and dentate nuclei of the cerebellum. All five of the DRG cells thus identified as primary spindle afferents discharged in similar bidirectional patterns.

We were led to ask what caused the bidirectional pattern in the spindle afferent discharge, and whether it could be explained by the two conventional means of activating spindle afferents — passive stretch of muscle, and gamma motoneuron drive coactivated with alpha motoneurons. We concluded that it could not for three reasons: (a) the temporal profile of spindle afferent discharge, which abruptly increased at the start of all movements, was not matched by parallel EMG activity in the arm; (b) the constancy of pattern despite varying combinations of passive stretch and gamma coactivation with alpha motoneurons under such diverse conditions, and (c) in the extreme illustrated in Fig. 5, upper left graph, the discharging spindle receptor being located in a muscle that was both passively shortening and electrically silent (the opposite muscle was active under full load and slowly lengthening). The spindle afferent was therefore discharging in a situation quite without either of the two conventional means of activating spindle receptors. Neither can the spindle afferent discharge in Fig. 5 be easily explained as due to the threshold recruitment of the smaller gamma motoneurons before recruitment of any of the larger alpha motoneurons: if this were the case, one might have expected a much greater spindle afferent discharge when the conditions were optimal for driving the spindle afferents by the two conventional means. In Fig. 5, lower right graph, the spindle was in a loaded muscle that was actively lengthening, yet the pattern of spindle afferent discharge was qualitatively and quantitatively similar to that which was observed under the least conventionally favorable conditions in Fig. 5, upper left graph. We must therefore assume that this pattern of constancy of spindle afferent discharge could only have been brought about by changes in gamma drive that were sufficiently dissociated from alpha drive to keep the pattern constant. Figure 7 diagramatically summarizes these findings, emphasizing the variation in the reciprocal EMG (and the inferred alpha motoneuron) discharge as the direction and load vary, and the constancy of the spindle afferent (and inferred gamma motoneuron) discharge across all conditions.

In any event, under the conditions of this task performance, these spindle afferents like all cerebellar neurons and the bidirectional motor cortex neurons did not report on intended or actual trajectory parameters of direction, velocity and position and only

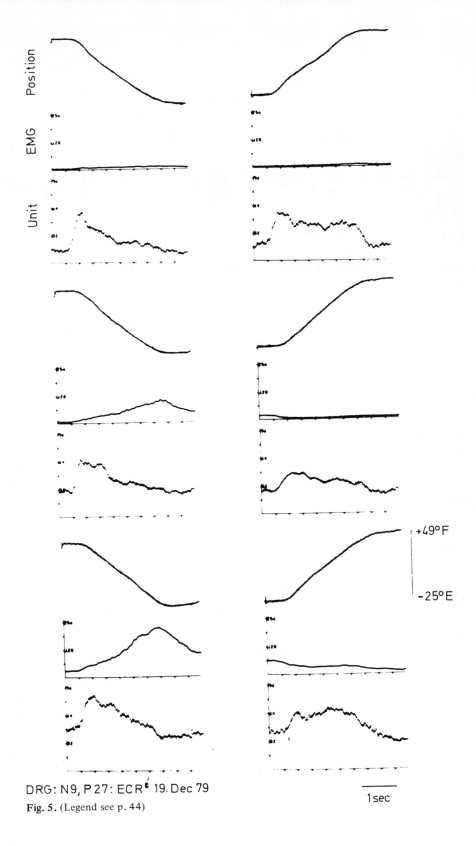

Position

EMG

Unit

+49°F

-25°E

DRG: N9, P27: ECR⁵ 19. Dec 79

Fig. 5. (Legend see p. 44)

1 sec

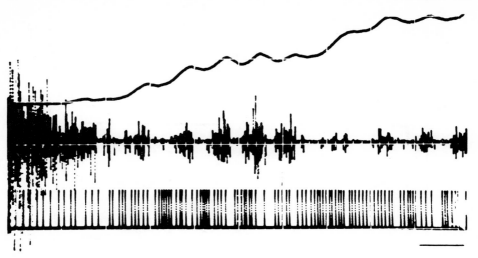

Fig. 6. Spindle afferent and EMG recordings during tremor. Simultaneous position, extensor digitorum EMG (*middle tracing*), and extensor-related muscle spindle (*lower tracing*) recordings obtained
during a flexor ramp maneuver under an extensor torque load. Scale = 200 ms. Two definite (and 3
probable) muscle spindles were studied, one flexor and one extensor. Each was modulated by the
tremor, and their modulations were 180 deg out of phase. Phase analysis was performed, and the
bursts in the spindle afferents led peak muscle stretch by an average of 150 deg (range 133-167).
The EMG bursts therefore followed the spindle bursts by approximately 39 ms (84 deg)

grudgingly on pattern and force of muscle activity. What trajectory parameter did
spindle afferents monitor? Figure 6 shows a single trial of flexion. The upper trace is
position, the middle trace the EMG of a wrist extensor muscle, and the bottom trace
the discharge of a spindle afferent. Like interposed and bidirectional motor cortex
neurons, the spindle afferents discharges exquisitely in relation to tremor.

3 Discussion

Interposed neurons and motor cortex neurons both are influenced by a fast path from
somatosensory afferents — including spindles (Bloedel and Courville 1981; Burton and
Onoda 1977, 1978; Lucier et al. 1975; Mackay and Murphy 1974; Phillips et al. 1971;
Soechting et al. 1978) — at minimum latencies of about 13-15 ms (Thach 1978). Both
sets of neurons discharged (Fig. 4) as did spindle afferents (Fig. 6) in relation to the
tremor and had a phase lag consistent with the possibility that they were driven by
sensory feedback from the tremor. By contrast, the dentate nucleus has no such rapid
somatosensory input, and its activity was not modulated in relation to the tremor, yet
it did have the same pattern of bidirectional discharge. Was it playing a role in generating

Fig. 5. Discharge of spindle afferent (unit) and the EMG of the extensor muscle in which the spindle
was located. Conventions are the same as in Fig. 3. The graphs show that the muscle activity is
reciprocal and the spindle afferent activity is bidirectional

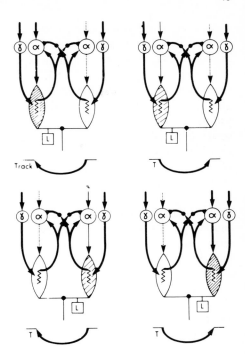

Fig. 7. Diagram summarizing patterns of discharge observed in EMG muscle activity, spindle afferent activity, and presumed activity of alpha and gamma motor neurons and their descending controls during hold-ramp-hold tracking in different directions and under different loads. *Heavy lines* axons that have high discharge frequency; *light lines* those that have lower discharge frequency during the ramp movement. *Dense cross-hatching* of muscle indicates intense EMG activity; *sparse cross-hatching* moderate EMG activity, and *no cross-hatching* little or nor EMG activity during the ramp movement. The diagram shows that the muscle and alpha motor neurons discharge in patterns that are reciprocal and highly varied in oppositely directed movements under different loads, while the spindle afferents and gamma motor neurons have patterns that are bidirectional and relatively symmetric under the different conditions

a similar pattern in gamma motoneurons? Since both ablation (Gilman 1969; Gilman et al. 1971; Higgins and Glaser 1964; Higgins et al. 1962) and stimulation (Granit et al. 1955) studies have shown a path from cerebellar nuclei to gamma motoneurons, this is quite possible.

What would be the purpose of elevated gamma motoneuron and spindle afferent discharge? There has been a recent tendency to regard spindle afferents, and especially the primaries, as preferentially sensitive to length perturbations that are small in amplitude (Matthews 1981). One of the striking observations in the four monkeys that have so far been trained to this task is that they all developed a small (5°) fast (10-13 Hz) tremor, with reciprocal alternating agonist-antagonist EMG discharge during the course of the ramp movements. The tremor does not occur in the holds prior to or following the ramp movement. There is evidence that the normal or "physiological" tremor consists of a natural tendency of the limb to oscillate because of its inertial and the elastic properties of the limb, and that it may be amplified by the action of the segmental stretch reflex (Elble and Randall 1976; Stein and Lee 1981; Young and Hagbarth 1979). Consistent with this view is the fact that the spindle afferents discharge in full-range modulation in relation to the tremor, and were time locked to and we presume the cause of subsequent EMG bursts. The EMG bursts in turn were so timed as to augment (rather than restrain) the tremor (14). Further, the tremor was slowed (as low as 2.5 Hz) with inertial loads, and was eliminated with large viscous loads, suggesting that the tremor was at least in part caused by a peripheral mechanism and was not generated by a central oscillator (Stein and Lee 1981; Young and Hagbarth 1979).

Interposed neurons (and some motor cortex neurons) were exquisitely modulated in relation to tremor: peak activity followed peak EMG activity by 12 ms and peak spindle activity by 50 ms. Was interposed discharge triggered (like EMG) by spindle activity? Did it then act to stop the EMG burst, and thus to restrict the tremor amplitude to within tolerable limits? That this may be so is suggested by the experiments of Vilis and Hore (Vilis and Hore 1980) who cooled deep cerebellar nuclei of monkeys and observed during tremor a prolonged discharge of motor cortex neurons, which was in turn thought to cause the prolonged EMG bursts that resulted in large amplitude, low frequency tremor. In our own monkey, after a number of interposed penetrations without other damage to the animal, the tremor frequency dropped suddenly to 5-7 Hz and increased by fivefold in amplitude. Form these observations we tentatively conclude that interposed nuclei act to limit tremor amplitude, and that they use afferent input to do so. How it does so is unclear: does it act to turn off the alpha motoneuron and the EMG soon after its onset? Does it quicken the response of the motor cortex neurons to stretch and/or inhibit their prolonged discharge? Does it increase the gain or bias of the segmental stretch reflex, and the sensitivity of the spindle, by increasing gamma neuron discharge frequency? How this might work is diagrammed in Figure 8, which emphasizes the symmetry of the sensing and correcting of small perturbations that might result from segmental or higher reflex loop actions. We do not yet know the answers to these questons, yet they would seem to be at the heart of an important aspect of normal cerebellar function.

The discharge of cerebellar neurons under these and, in retrospect, previous (Thach 1975, 1978) testing situations may be viewed as promoting the stability of movement trajectory. This has been seen to include tremor, and may also extend to dysmetria. The physical mechanisms underlying these instabilities are now being explored in greater detail, and would appear to include the neural compensation for the inertial mass, the elastic properties of the moving limb and load, and the damping characteristics needed to control them. Under the conditions of this experiment, these factors would appear to be *all* that the cerebellum is concerned with. This leaves two alternatives as to the interpretation of the results of previous studies in which cerebellar nuclear cell firing was seen to relate to direction (Strick 1978; Thach 1978), velocity (Burton and Onoda 1977, 1978; Soechting et al. 1978) and pattern and force (Thach 1978) of muscular activity. One alternative is that in the one task (a sequential set of prompt fast moves to remembered positions) cerebellar signals code for and control trajectory parameters, and in the present task (visually guided smooth pursuit tracking) they code for and control stability parameters. This seems unlikely: while there are known instances of Purkinje cell discharge relating to a movement parameter and being gated "off" (Frysinger et al. 1984; Smith and Bourbonnais 1981; Lisberger and Fuchs 1974), there seems no precedent for thinking it should shift to an apparently new and different set

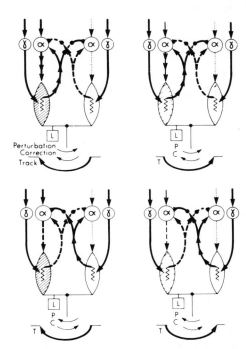

Fig. 8. Diagram of how agonist-antagonist stretch reflex pathways symmetrically activated by γ-motoneurons may correct perturbations entirely through the loaded active agonist muscle. *Top left* during agonist-shortening trajectory, stretch of agonist causes homonymous reflex contraction, while shortening of antagonist removes tonic inhibition from Ia interneuron. *Top right* during agonist-lengthening trajectory, the same perturbation causes a similar correction. *Bottom left* during agonist-shortening trajectory, shortening of agonist removes tonic excitatory Ia input, while stretching antagonist increases inhibition from Ia interneuron. *Bottom right* during agonist lengthening trajectory, the same perturbation causes a similar correction. All corrections are made symmetrically to symmetric tonic spindle afferent discharge in active agonist and silent antagonist which can register lengthenings and shortenings by increasing and decreasing discharge transiently

of controlled variables. A second alternative interpretation is that, in both the task of sequential stepping to remembered positions and the present task of smooth pursuit tracking, the cerebellar neurons were coding for and controlling excitability levels in reflex pathways including gamma motoneurons. Thus, as pointed out previously (Thach 1978), the observed firing relationship to direction, pattern and force of muscluar activity needn't imply cerebellar discharge *controlled* those variables of the trajectory program: it could instead have controlled gamma motoneurons and other neurons which in turn fired in relationship to direction or pattern and force of muscular activity, but whose actual purpose and effect was the control of limb stability as it held positions, resisted perturbations, and made sudden moves successfully without undershoot, overshoot, or oscillation to target positions. While under the circumstances of the present experiment this would appear the more plausible possibility, it must be remembered that the distinction drawn here between trajectory parameters and stability parameters may be rather artificial, since the final trajectory is in fact a composite of both and since the separate origins of the various control signals has yet to be fully disclosed.

Nevertheless, the implication of these experiments is that, at least in slow pursuit tracking, parts of the nervous system other than the cerebellum must be generating the trajectory parameter signals of direction, velocity, pattern and force of muscular activity that are actually used to produce these movements. A first and obvious site to look for these signals in this task performance is the basal ganglia. Reports that basal ganglia neurons fire in relation to direction of limb movement independent of muscle patterns used to make the movement (Crutcher and Delong 1984), amplitude or velocity (or both – Delong et al. 1983; Delong and Strick 1974; Georgopoulos et al. 1983a) of movement, and pattern and force of muscular activity (Crutcher and Delong 1984, in press) would seem to support such a role. Nevertheless, it must be remembered that cerebellar neurons also discharge in relation to trajectory variables in tasks similar to those used for the basal ganglia studies, and only in the present task performance did they lose such a relationship (see also the cocontraction task of Smith and colleagues – Frysinger et al. 1984; Smith and Bourbonnais 1981; Smith et al. 1983). Thus, the present task or some equivalent would appear necessary to adequately dissociate the basal ganglia and the cerebellum in their possibly discrete roles in the control of trajectory and stability, respectively. And, while it is attractive to think that the basal ganglia, because of their connections through to motor cortex and because of their ablation syndromes of akinesia/bradykinesia, may be generating the trajectory parameter signals, some recent evidence suggests this may not be the case. First, there is accumulating evidence that the output of the basal ganglia – the globus pallidus, internal segment, and the substantia nigra, pars reticulata – synthesizes and contains GABA, a putative inhibitory neurotransmitter (Penney and Young 1983), and that basal ganglia output does indeed inhibit target thalamic neurons (Yamamoto et al. 1983). Second, recordings of substantia nigra pars reticulata neurons in relation to visually (and auditorily) targetted saccadic eye movements have shown that neurons uniformly respond with a transient *pause* in the ongoing pattern of high frequency maintained discharge (Hikosaka and Wurtz 1983a, b). These authors show that the substantia nigra pars reticulata neurons project to the superior colliculus (they also project to intralaminar nuclei of the thalamus), which relate to saccade eye movements with bursts of activity that precede and help cause (shown by ablation – Hikosaka and Wurtz 1983a, b) the saccade. While it is possible that substantia nigra pars reticulata neurons may *cause* the saccades by releasing tonic inhibition from collicular and thalamic neurons, these authors suggest that the saccade command signal to colliculus (and to substantia nigra pars reticulata) may originate somewhere else, and that the pars reticulata input is merely a gating signal that allows it to act on the colliculus to generate the saccade. In this scheme, the "ultimate" command for the saccade would then occur in structures other than basal ganglia or colliculus. The authors cite evidence that this could include the frontal eye fields and the parietal lobe of cerebral cortex. Thus it may be the case for limb movement (analogous to eye movement) that the basal ganglia are not the source of an absolute trajectory code to be passed through to premotor, supplementary motor, or motor cortex in a hierarchical fashion. Rather, they may provide a restraint which regulates some one or several of the trajectory variables, such as velocity or amplitude (or both), through an adjustable tonic inhibitory discharge that keeps the system clamped at an inactive level in the absence of movement ("rest"). Such a role would be essentially the same as that proposed for the omni-directional pause cell, a presumed inhibitory pontine neuron that fires at high maintained rates, pausing just prior to (and possibly thereby gating "on") the burst-tonic command neurons that directly initiate the saccade (Zee and Robinson 1979). If these facts and inferences are correct, then the source most nearly approximating an "ultimate" may be frontal and parietal cortex. These are the regions whose ablation gives rise to movement apraxias — highly "conditional" movement disorders, in which movement may occur under some conditions but not others (DeAjuriaguerra and Tissot 1969). Neurons discharging in relation to direction of eye and limb movement have been found in these areas (Georgopoulos et al. 1983a, b, Kalaska et al. 1983, Lynch et al. 1977, Mountcastle et al. 1975, Niki 1974a, b), and while the purity of these signals may still be open to question (as are now similar previous observations on cerebellar relation to direction), they are at least reasonable candidates.

References

Allen GI, Tsukahara N (1974) Cerebrocerebellar communication systems. Physiol Rev 54: 957-1006

Asanuma C, Thach WT, Jones EG (1983a) Distribution of cerebellar terminations and their relation to other afferent terminations in the ventral lateral thalamic region of the monkey. Brain Res Rev 5: 237-265

Asanuma C, Thach WT, Jones EG (1983b) Anatomical evidence for segregated focal groupings of efferent cells and their terminal ramifications in the cerebellothalamic pathway of the monkey. Brain Res Rev 5: 299-322

Bloedel JR, Courville J (1981) Cerebellar afferent systems. In: Brookhart JM, Mountcastle VB, Geiger SR (eds) Handbook of physiology, Sect 1: the nervous system, vol II. Motor control, part 1. Am Physiol Soc (Bethesda), pp 735-829

Brodal P (1978) The corticopontine projection in the rhesus monkey. Origin and principles of organization. Brain 101: 251-283

Burton JE, Onoda N (1977) Interpositus neuron discharge in relation to a voluntary movement. Brain Res 121: 167-172

Burton JE, Onoda N (1978) Dependence of the activity of interpositus and red nucleus neurons on sensory input data generated by movement. Brain Res 152: 41-63

Crutcher MD, Delong MR (1984) Single cell studies of the primate putamen. II. Relations to direction of movement and pattern of muscular activity. (in press)

DeAjuriaguerra J, Tissot R (1969) The apraxias. In: Vinkin PJ, Bruyn GW (eds) Handbook of clinical neurology. North-Holland Publishing Co. Amsterdam, pp 48-66

Delong MR, Strick P (1974) Relations of basal ganglia, cerebellum, and motor cortex units to ramp and ballistic movements. Brain Res 71: 327-355m

Delong MR, Crutcher MD, Georgopoulos AP (1983) Relations between movement and single cell discharge in the substantia nigra of the behaving monkey. J Neurosci 3: 1599-1606

Dow RS, Moruzzi G (1958) The physiology and pathology of the cerebellum. Univ Minnesota Press, Minneapolis

Elble RJ, Randall JE (1976) Motor unit activity responsible for the 8- to 12-Hz component of human physiological finger tremor. J Neurophysiol 39: 370-383

Elble RJ, Schieber MH, Thach WT (1981) Involvement of nucleus interpositus in action tremor. Soc Neurosci Abstr 7: 691

Evarts EV, Thach WT (1969) Motor mechanisms of the CNS: cerebrocerebellar inter-relations. Annu Rev Physiol 31: 451-498

Frysinger RC, Bourbonnais D, Kalaska JR, Smith AM (1984) Cerebellar cortical activity during antagonist cocontraction and reciprocal inhibition of forearm muscles. J Neurophysiol 51: 32-49

Georgopoulos AP, Delong MR, Crutcher MD (1983a) Relations between parameters of step-tracking movements and single cell discharge in the globus pallidus and subthalamic nucleus of the behaving monkey. J Neurosci 3: 1586-1598

Georgopoulos AP, Caminiti R, Kalaska JR, Massey JT (1983b) Spatial coding of movement: a hypothesis concerning the coding of movement direction by motor cortical populations. Exp Brain Res Suppl 7: 327-336

Gilman S (1969) The mechanism of cerebellar hypotonia. An experimental study in the monkey. Brain 92: 621-638

Gilman S, Marco LA, Ebel HC (1971) Effects of medullary pyramidotomy in the monkey. II. Abnormalities of spindle afferent responses. Brain 94: 515-530

Granit R, Holmgren B, Merton PA (1955) The two routes for the excitation of muscle and their subservience to the cerebellum. J Physiol 130: 213-224

Higgins DC, Glaser GH (1964) Stretch responses during chronic cerebellar ablation. A study of reflex instability. J Neurophysiol 27: 49-62

Higgins DC, Partridge LD, Glaser GH (1962) A transient cerebellar influence on stretch responses. J Neurophysiol 25: 684-692

Hikosaka O, Wurtz RH (1983a) Visual and oculomotor functions of monkey substantia nigra pars reticulata. I. Relation of visual and auditory responses to saccades. J Neurophysiol 49: 1230-1253

Hikosaka O, Wurtz RH (1983b) Visual and oculomotor functions of monkey substantia nigra pars reticulata. IV. Relation of substantia nigra to superior colliculus. J Neurophysiol 49: 1285-1301

Holmes G (1939) The cerebellum of man. Brain 62: 1-30

Kalaska JR, Caminiti R, Georgopoulos AP (1983) Cortical mechanism related to the direction of two-dimensional arm movements: relations in parietal area 5 and comparison with motor cortex. Exp Brain Res 51: 247-260

Kemp JM, Powell TPS (1971) The connexions of the striatum and globus pallidus: synthesis and speculation. Philos Trans R Soc London Ser B 262: 441-457

Lisberger SG, Fuchs AF (1974) Responses of flocculus Purkinje cells to adequate vestibular stimulation in the alert monkey: fixation vs. compensatory eye movements. Brain Res 69: 347

Lucier GE, Ruegg DC, Wiesendanger M (1975) Responses of neurones in motor cortex and in area 3a to controlled stretches of forelimb muscles in Cebus monkeys. J Physiol 251: 833-853

Lynch JC, Mountcastle VB, Talbot WH, Yin TC (1977) Parietal lobe mechanisms for directed visual attention. J Neurophysiol 40: 362-389

Mackay WA, Murphy JT (1974) Responses of interpositus neurons to passive muscle stretch. J Neurophysiol 37: 1410-1423

Mattews PBS (1981) Muscles: their messages and their fusimotor supply. In: Brookhart JM, Mountcastle VB, Geiger ST (eds) Handbook of physiology, sect 1: the nervous system, vol II. Motor control. Am Physiol Soc (Bethesda), pp 189-228

Merton PA (1953) Speculations on the servocontrol of movement. In: Malcolm JL, Gray JAB, Wolstenholme GEW (eds) The spinal cord. Little Brown, Boston, pp 183-198

Mountcastle VB, Lynch JC, Georgopoulos A, Sakata H, Acuna C (1975) Posterior parietal association cortex of the monkey: command functions for operations within extrapersonal space. J Neurophysiol 38: 871-908

Niki H (1974a) Prefrontal unit activity during delayed alternation in the monkey. I. Relation to direction of response. Brain Res 68: 185-196

Niki H (1974b) Prefrontal unit activity during delayed alternation in the monkey. II. Relation to absolute versus relative direction of responses. Brain Res 68: 197-204

Penney JB, Young AB (1983) Speculations on the functional anatomy of basal ganglia disorders. Annu Rev Neurosci 6: 73-94

Phillips CG, Powell TPS, Wiesdanger M (1971) Projection from low-threshold muscle afferents of hand and forearm to area 3a of baboon's cortex. J Physiol 217: 419-446

Schieber MH, Thach WT (1984a) Trained slow tracking. I. Muscular production of wrist movement. J Neurophysiol. (in press)

Schieber MH, Thach WT (1984b) Trained slow tracking. II. Bidirectional discharge of spindle afferent, motor cortex, and cerebellar nuclear neurons. J Neurophysiol (in press)

Smith AM, Bourbonnais D (1981) Neuronal activity in cerebellar cortex related to the control of prehensile force. J Neurophysiol 45: 286-303

Smith AM, Kalaska JE, Swetts RW (1983) The activity of dentate and interpositus neurons during maintained isometric prehension. Proc Int Union Physiol Sci 29: 394

Soechting JR, Burton JE, Onoda N (1978) Relationship between sensory input, motor output, and unit activity in interpositus and red nuclei during intentional movement. Brain Res 152: 65-79

Stein RB, Lee RG (1981) Tremor and clonus. In: Brookhart JM, Mountcastle VB, Geiger SR (eds) Handbook of physiology, sect 1: The nervous system, vol II. Motor control, part 1. Am Physiol Soc (Bethesda), pp 325-344

Strick P (1978) Cerebellar involvement in "volitional" responses to load changes. In: Desmedt JE (ed) Progress in clinical neurophysiology. Cerebral motor control in man: long loop mechanisms. Karger, Basel, pp 85-93

Terzuolo CA, Viviani P (1974) Parameters of motion and EMG activities in some simple motor tasks in normal subjects and cerebellar patients. In: Cooper IS, Riklan M, Snider RS (eds) The cerebellum, epilepsy and behavior. Plenum Press, New York, pp 173-213

Terzuolo CA, Soechting JR, Viviani P (1973) Studies on the control of some simple motor tasks. II. On the cerebellar control of movements in relation to the formulation of intentional commands. Brain Res 58: 217-222

Thach WT (1975) Timing of activity in cerebellar dentate nucleus and cerebral motor cortex during prompt volitional movement. Brain Res 88: 233-241

Thach WT (1978) Correlation of neural discharge with pattern and force of muscular activity, joint position, and direction of intended movement in motor cortex and cerebellum. J Neurophysiol 41: 654-676

Thach WT, Perry G, Schieber MH (1982) Cerebellar output: body maps and muscle spindles. In: Palay S, Chan-Palay V (eds) The cerebellum: new vistas. Springer, Berlin Heidelberg New York, pp 440-454

Vilis T, Hore J (1980) Central neural mechanisms contributing to cerebellar tremor produced by limb perturbations. J Neurophysiol 43: 279-291

Yamamoto T, Hassler R, Huber C, Wagner A, Sasaki K (1983) Electrophysiological studies on the pallido- and cerebellothalamic projections in squirrel monkeys (Saimiri sciureus). Exp Brain Res 51: 77-87

Young RR, Hagbarth KE (1979) Participation of the stretch reflex in human physiological tremor. Brain 102: 509-526

Zee DS, Robinson DA (1979) An hypothetical explanation of saccadic oscillations. Ann Neurol 5: 405-414

Parsimony in Neural Calculations for Postural Movements

G. McCollum, F.B. Horak, and L.M. Nashner [1]

1 Introduction

Any movement of the body to maintain or regain erect posture results from a combination of internal, muscular forces with external forces exerted most commonly by the support surface on the foot. That is, erect human posture is characterized by a continuous interaction among the muscular and external forces acting upon the body segments.

The task of erect human stance is to keep the center of mass of the body over the center of foot support. Forward or backward motions are more disequilibrating than lateral perturbations with respect to gravitation; an uncorrected perturbation beyond a confined region of passive stability leads to a fall. There is a continuum (two-dimensional) of ankle, knee, and hip joint angles which satisfy the balance condition in the sagittal plane. In the same way, there is a continuum of ankle, knee, and hip trajectories connecting any two body positions. In particular, from any given posture an equilibrium position can be attained by a continuum of different ankle, knee, and hip joint trajectories.

Taking the properties of the support surface into account further increases the complexity of postural mechanics. A compliant support surface, such as rubber foam, or a surface shorter than the foot is long alters the relations among muscular, gravitational, and support surface reaction forces, necessitating a concomitant redefinition of the limits of equilibrium and of the ankle, knee, and hip joint trajectories by which equilibrium can be attained.

Despite the complexity of postural mechanics, equilibrium is achieved during stance and walking by a rapid, largely automatic process. This led us to suspect that the mechanical calculations performed by the system in directing the change of contractile activity of postural muscles under varying mechanical conditions are also made with economy.

This article is a theoretical exploration, based on experiments by Horak and Nashner (1983), into the organization of mechanical calculations within the sensorimotor system. The focus of this study is a computational system for posture control in which the timing and spatial distribution of muscular contractions required to produce a desired shift in orientation is reduced from an infinite set to a limited number of discrete choices.

---

[1] Neurological Sciences Institute of Good Samaritan Hospital and Medical Center, 1120 N.W. 20th Avenue Portland, Oregon 97209, USA

Cerebellar Functions
ed. by Bloedel et al.

The most fundamental expression of the theme of discreteness is in the firing of muscles in bursts rather than in general, continuous modulation. Bursts, such as occur in postural correction synergies shown later, may vary continuously in magnitude, but always occur in intervals of fairly constant shape. Discreteness is also expressed experimentally in the burst activation of groups of muscles or in particular timing relations termed synergies. The organization of muscle contractions into discrete synergies simplifies the coordination of an action from independently controlling the magnitude and timing of many muscle bursts to controlling the onset time and magnitude of a single synergy. Here we investigate the control and interactions of synergies.

Horak and Nashner found that subjects correcting forward or backward sway perturbations used one of two pure strategies, depending on support surface conditions. When support surface conditions were changed, subjects went through a transition period, during which they used mixtures of the two strategies. A striking finding was the small number of different mixture types.

We consider the transition period between strategies to be a period of search for or calculation of the functionally appropriate strategy. We assume that the calculation being done is this one that we see, a trial by trial testing and discarding of relative amplitude and timing strategies. Thus, the calculation is made with great economy, with minimal use of the nervous system's computational ability; it is reduced to groping in one dimension at a time.

Such parsimony is achieved by recognizing or imposing simplifying constraints. Some are mechanical; the calculation takes into account enduring mechanical properties of the body in question. These mechanical properties determine the strategies to be used in different surface conditions (Nashner and McCollum 1984). Along with gravitation, the mechanical properties of the body determine which parameters must be controlled in each movement and which are already controlled, as described for pure strategies in Section 2.4. In searching for an effective postural control strategy, as in the transitions described by Horak and Nashner (1983), a subject manipulates mechanical parameters of mixed strategies. The set of mechanical parameters modulated must be both adequate to solve the postural problem and also restricted in ways appropriate to allow the subject to modulate only one parameter at a time.

The other aspect of the calculation is how the mechanical parameters are controlled neurally and how movement control is organized neurally to let the subject modulate first one parameter and then another. A control hypothesis consistent with the results of Horak and Nashner is presented. This hypothesis implies exactly the reduction of mechanical variables necessary to perform the transition calculation simply, as a trial by trial search.

Before discussing the transition calculation further, we will describe the individual strategies.

2 Strategies and Synergies

We use the term "muscle synergy" to describe the discrete temporal and spatial patterns of leg and trunk muscle contractions. The term "strategy" refers to the broader context of sensory, motor, and mechanical processes subserving postural movements of a given

A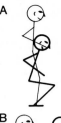

Fig. 1 A-C. The three postural movements most commonly seen in normal subjects responding to perturbations under different support conditions. The three movements form a complete coordinate system for three independent degrees of postural movements in the sagittal plane, one degree of freedom each for ankle, knee, and hip joints. **A** Suspensory strategy; **B** Ankle strategy; **C** Hip strategy

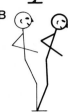

B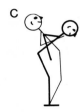

C

pattern. Thus, the ankle and hip strategies include a prescription not only for the ordered contraction of muscles but also for the interpretation of the sensory inputs resulting from the action. In addition, a strategy can be calculated to attain a particular mechanical goal.

The contractions of leg and lower trunk muscles in standing human subjects are organized into three postural synergies, depending upon the direction of perturbation and the support surface conditions (Nashner 1977, Nashner et al. 1979, Horak and Nashner 1983, Nashner and McCollum 1984). The movements effected by these strategies, the suspensory, ankle, and hip strategies, are shown in Fig. 1.

In response to forward and backward displacements of the center of body mass, the ankle strategy (Fig. 1B) is the most efficient in that it effects the greatest center of mass correction in relation to body joint motion. It is the strategy of choice for most normal subjects perturbed while standing on a flat, wide surface. The majority of the work is accomplished by the exertion of torque about the ankles. The hip strategy (Fig. 1C) also moves the center of mass forward and backward. On a surface short in relation to foot length, shear forces on the support surface are generated by hip motions large in comparison to the resulting postural correction. The suspensory strategy (Fig. 1A) moves the center of mass up and down with respect to the support and is the least efficient for returning the center of mass over the foot. This strategy is observed in response to vertical rather than forward and backward perturbations.

The three major strategies shown in Fig. 1 represent three independent degrees of freedom for sagittal plane leg motions, which, if adopted as a coordinate system for sagittal plane motion, would completely specify the mechanics. The motions alone would be sufficient for discussing mechanical changes in postural responses, but we will

Fig. 2 A, B. Ankle synergy EMG patterns: **A** Response to forward sway perturbations, and **B** response to backward sway perturbations. EMG's for six muscles are arranged in antagonist pairs, with the dorsal muscle EMG's pointing up and ventral EMG's down. The lower leg: gastrocnemius (*GAST*) up and tibialis anterior (*TIB*) down. The thigh: hamstrings (*HAM*) up and quadriceps (*QUAD*) down. Torso: paraspinal (*PARA*) up and abdominal (*ABD*) down. (Horak and Nashner 1983)

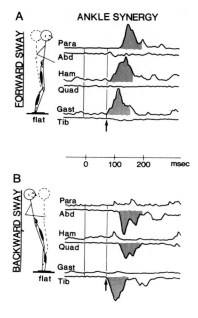

need to study the EMG patterns as well to describe mixtures of synergies and to compare mechanical to neural constraints in the transitions between the ankle and the hip synergies. We will now describe the EMG patterns of the well-practiced ankle and hip synergies.

2.1 Ankle Synergy

Figure 2 shows the EMG patterns associated with the ankle synergy. We have arranged the EMG's in antagonist pairs to make more evident the relation between EMG pattern and mechanical manifestation. For both forward and backward motions, contractions start in ankle joint muscles, radiate to thigh muscles, and then to muscles in the lower trunk. Thus, in response to a forward sway perturbation, muscles on the dorsal aspect of the body fire in turn: gastrocnemius, then hamstrings, then paraspinals. The subject moves the center of mass backward in an approximately rigid rotation about the ankles. In response to a backward sway perturbation, the body rotates forward about the ankle while keeping knee and hip angles fixed by activating the corresponding ventral muscles: tibialis anterior, quadriceps, and then abdominals.

The spatial configuration of muscle responses is important to coordination of ankle and hip joint motions. The time sequence of activations is important to knee stability.

2.2 Hip Synergy

Use of the ankle synergy depends on the support surface affording torque about the ankles. When the support surface is significantly shorter than the foot, the ankle torque that can be exerted is insufficient to rotate the body against inertia and gravitation. The

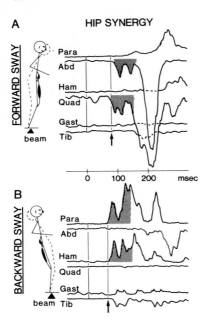

Fig. 3 A, B. Hip synergy EMG patterns: **A** Response to forward sway, and **B** Response to backward sway. EMG's are arranged as in Fig. 2. (Horak and Nashner 1983)

subject must depend upon shear forces. These are best generated by muscles acting about the hip as shown in Fig. 3. In response to a forward sway perturbation, thigh and trunk muscles on the ventral aspect of the body contract in proximal to distal sequence, rather than the dorsal muscles firing in distal to proximal sequence. Similarly, in response to a backward sway perturbation, the dorsal hip muscles are used whereas ventral muscles are used with the ankle synergy.

Note that the muscles on the opposite side and in the opposite sequence are used for the hip synergy. This will be important in the discussion of mechanics, Sections 2.4 and 3.2.

As shown in Fig. 1 and 3, this contractile pattern generates both hip and ankle motions; the hip motion is the direct result of the muscle contractions, while the hip motion causes the ankle motion indirectly through inertia.

As in the case of the ankle strategy, the spatial configuration of muscle responses is important to the coordination of ankle and hip joint motions in the hip strategy. Time sequence is again used to stabilize the knee.

2.3 Trajectories Associated with Ankle and Hip Strategies

By rotating the body about the ankle joints, the ankle strategy can return the body to a fully erect equilibrium position. The hip strategy brings the center of body mass back over the center of support by bending the hips, but it does not return the body to an erect position. While the body is in balance with respect to forward-backward motions, tonic muscle forces are required to maintain the hip-bent position.

Sway trajectories generated by ankle and hip strategy corrections are illustrated in Fig. 4 in two-dimensional position space graphs. The vertical axis is the ankle angle co-

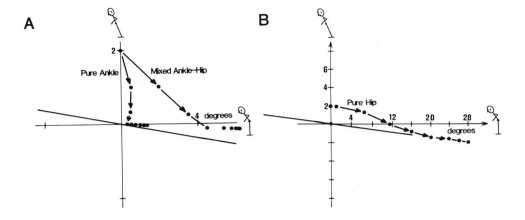

Fig. 4 A, B. Trajectories of a subject reacting to a forward sway perturbation. Erect stance is at the origin, and the coordinates are ankle and hip angles with the foot fixed flat on the floor. (Note that the coordinates are not the strategies shown in Fig. 1, but joint angles). The trajectory ends on the heavy diagonal line across the graph, which is the balance line, the locus of non-erect positions in which the center of mass is over the ankles. The movement starts with the subject leaning forward 2 deg about the ankle joints. Points along the trajectory show position measurements at successive 33 ms intervals. **A** The subject uses a pure ankle synergy and a mixed ankle-hip synergy; **B** The subject uses a pure hip synergy. Note a difference in scale between parts **A** and **B**

ordinate; the horizontal axis, the hip angle coordinate; and the third dimension (pointing out of the page; not shown) the radial distance from the ankle joint to the center of body mass. The heavy diagonal line across the graph, which we call the "balance line", is the locus of all non-erect balanced positions in which the center of body mass is over the ankle joint, while the origin is the erect balanced position.

Figure 4A shows the trajectory followed by a subject using the ankle strategy. The subject starts from a position of forward sway on the ankle rotation axis. The body returns directly to erect stance, the central point on the balance line, following a pathway almost exclusively of ankle joint rotation. The trajectory followed by a subject using a pure hip strategy is shown in Fig. 4B. Starting from the same position of forward sway, the trajectory follows a path initially perpendicular to that of the ankle strategy. It reaches the balance line and then slows. Although this is not an erect position, by placing the center of mass over the ankles, the hip strategy has arrested the perturbation most threatening to biped stance.

2.4 Parameters Controlled

When one of these strategies is performed by a subject standing on the floor, gravitation combines with inherent body mechanics to determine the trajectory followed. Few mechanical parameters are left to be controlled by the subject. In order to understand the mechanical calculation as it unfolds in a transition, we must understand the few controlled parameters.

In the case of the ankle strategy, the trajectory points almost directly towards the origin. Thus, this radially inward pointing corrective action directly opposes the gravi-

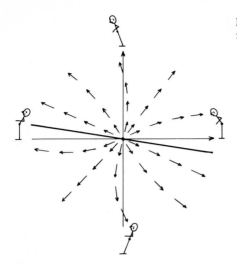

Fig. 5. Lines of fall under gravitation shown schematically in position coordinates as in Fig. 4

tational forces, which tend to accelerate the body radially outward from the origin, as shown in Fig. 5. So unless the trajectory overshoots the origin, its duration of movement toward erect stance is determined by its amplitude.

In the ankle synergy, an ankle torque is first applied in the lower leg, as shown in Fig. 2. This causes a hip torque by inertia. The hip torque is braked shortly thereafter by the action of the proximal muscles. The slight hip motion in some subjects can be seen on videotape, but is stopped within 50-100 ms, as shown in Fig. 2.

When bending at the hips is used as the mode of corrective action, the resulting body motion neither opposes nor follows the direction of gravitational acceleration. Instead, the hip trajectory, as shown in Fig. 4, starts out crossing gravitational lines. When the hip trajectory approaches the locus of non-erect balanced positions later in the movement, it becomes parallel and in the same direction as gravity.

Because later positions of the hip synergy trajectory move in the same direction as gravity, a hip motion will never be stopped by gravity. While hip motions are probably slowed somewhat by muscle viscoelastic forces, a second muscle action is usually needed to stop them. Thus, the duration of a hip movement is determined by the length of time between the original torque and a braking torque. In contrast, because ankle trajectories oppose gravity, a corrective ankle movement has a natural amplitude and duration given by the initial impulse alone, as long as the motion stays on one side of erect stance and does not reverse direction.

The mechanical parameters that need to be controlled, then, for pure ankle and hip postural motions are: for ankle, only amplitude; for hip, both amplitude and duration.

3 Transition and Mixtures

By using mixtures of ankle and hip synergies, subjects generate trajectories intermediate between those generated by pure ankle and pure hip synergies. A corresponding stand-

Fig. 6. A standard EMG pattern for mixing the ankle and hip synergies. EMG's are shown in a format identical to that of Fig. 2

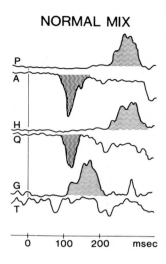

NORMAL MIX

ard mixed EMG pattern is shown in Fig. 6. Subjects pass through such trajectories and mixed patterns in transitions between ankle and hip synergies.

The parameters controlled in the mixed strategies are the same three as in the two pure strategies together. In order to show this and to show how and when control is exerted, we will first consider the nature of mixtures as observed by Horak and Nashner (1983).

3.1 Subjects in Transition

Subjects stood on a surface which varied in front to back length, from longer than the foot to less than half as long. They reacted to abrupt forward or backward translations of the support surface. After a change of surface length, there was a transition period in which the synergy and the postural correction movement changed. Elements of both discreteness and continuity were found in the contractile patterns associated with transitions from one support surface to another. A striking finding was the small number of different mixture types.

When interactions between the two synergies were observed during transition trials, antagonist muscle pairs at a given segment were not normally co-activated, nor did contractions in one segmental muscle inhibit the antagonist. Instead, the overall spatial properties of each synergy were preserved during the interaction, while the timings of bursts within each synergy were adjusted in the following way: The first burst command to arrive at a segment fired the muscle in the usual timing relation, while a subsequent command arriving during the first was delayed until completion of the first.

Synergy mixtures which did not agree with these observations were observed in a population of Parkinsonian patients with stance and gait instability (Horak et al. 1984). However, these abnormal mixtures were also functionally ineffective and accounted for much of the instability problems of the patients.

In order to explain the limited set of normal mixture types, we first hypothesize

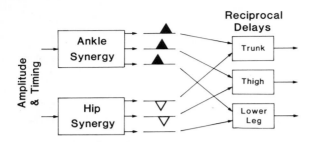

Fig. 7. Separate ankle and hip synergy generators with output converging at the segmental level. The first impulse command arriving at a segment is executed first. The second is delayed until the first is over, and is then executed in full

an independent central generator for each synergy, as shown in Fig. 7. The only parameters determined centrally, outside the generators, are the amplitude and onset of each. A second hypothesis, which leads from these continuous control parameters to a set of discrete choices, is a lower level segment by segment interaction between individual muscle commands, such that the first burst to arrive at a segment delays subsequent bursts. We call it "reciprocal delay".

As shown in Fig. 8, it follows from the above rules for interaction of synergies that there is a limited set of several discrete choices of timing organization for mixtures. The relative amplitudes of the two synergies can also vary, and to the extent that amplitude affects burst durations, relative amplitude may also subtly affect timing. While the onset time of each burst can vary according to our proposed organizational principles, the timings of individual muscle bursts are eliminated as independent variables, because these depend on the relative amplitude and timing relations between the two synergies.

If mixtures are actually produced in the way we have proposed, then two predictions can be made: During forward sway perturbations, the time interval between gastrocnemius and hamstrings onset will have a discrete bimodal distribution (shown in Fig. 9), and the termination time of quadriceps to the subsequent onset of hamstrings will be constant. Both of these predictions are confirmed, but with tentativeness arising from the small number of mixtures produced by each subject.

By hypothesizing independent central generators, central control over relative amplitude and relative onset time, and peripheral interactions among the individual burst commands, we have reduced the control of timing from a large number of independent, continuous onset parameters to several discrete choices. If the relative timing between synergies is fixed, then there is only relative amplitude to vary. Conversely, fixing relative amplitude of synergies leaves relative timing the single variable. This brings us easily down to a one dimensional search alternating between amplitude and timing variables. We assume that ankle torque is maximized early on, so that only relative amplitude remains to vary.

3.2 Mechanics of a Common Mixture Pattern

A standard mixture, generated by interposing the hip synergy muscles between the ankle and thigh components of the ankle synergy sequence of contractions, is shown in Fig. 6. The first muscles to fire in response to a forward sway perturbation are gastrocnemius, quadriceps, and abdominals. In extending the ankles and flexing the

Fig. 8. Variety of possible timing organizations arising from separate synergy generation with reciprocal delay

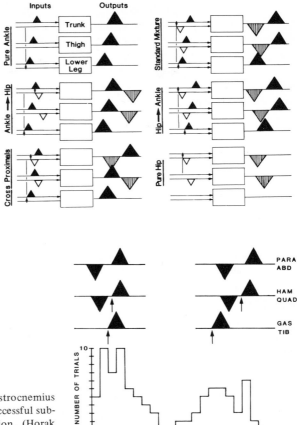

Fig. 9. Histogram of delay from gastrocnemius onset to hamstrings onset for one successful subject, showing a bimodal distribution. (Horak and Nashner, submitted)

hips these three muscles energize the naturally occuring antiphase motions of the ankle and hip joints. The symmetric result is true for a response to a backward sway: the first three muscles to fire, the tibialis anterior, hamstrings, and paraspinals, reinforce antiphase ankle and hip motions in the opposite direction.

As in the case of the pure ankle strategy, the trajectory of the body rotating about the ankle in this mixed strategy is limited in time by its amplitude and by gravitation. Overshoot is not a consideration since the mixture is being used because the ankle torque afforded by the support surface length is insufficient to bring the body to erect stance by means of the ankle strategy. So, again, with respect to the ankle torque produced by the combination of gastrocnemius, quadriceps, and abdominals, only the amplitude need be controlled.

Those three muscles also start a hip motion which moves the center of mass in the desired direction. In the ankle strategy, the antiphase hip motion is braked very soon after it is initiated. Here, since it is an important part of the mechanical strategy, it must be let take its course longer. It is braked, as in the pure ankle strategy, by the hamstrings and paraspinals, but delayed from the usual pure strategy timing. This delay is the control variable of duration for the hip motion.

The two motion amplitudes, hip and ankle, are regulated by the two synergy amplitudes in combination, not one to one. The two amplitude parameters, combinations of the synergy amplitudes, are ankle torque and relative synergy amplitude. These two determine the two motion amplitudes.

Before considering the ways these parameters are actually manipulated by subjects in transitions, we will consider what it means mechanically for the variables to be restricted in this way.

4 Computation

The subject is faced with the mechanical problem of determining the optimal synergy for regaining erect stance given an interaction between the body and the support surface which is a priori unknown. We have described the two pure strategies used by subjects to correct forward-backward trajectories, along with the controls that must be exerted and the trajectories followed. There is an infinity of ways a subject could transition between these trajectories, shown in Fig. 4, if each point of the trajectory is individually controllable. In that case, the nervous system must, at the very simplest, perform the equivalent of a variational calculation or embody a Lagrangian formalism. These would be large calculational steps, consuming either time or neural space, but they would allow the subject to completely change strategy in a single trial.

We assume that the computation performed by the nervous system is much simpler than proposed above, because the observed transitions occurred progressively over many trials and resembled a one dimensional search for the functionally appropriate timing and amplitude parameters mixing ankle and hip strategies. Accordingly, we investigate the transition between synergies as if the whole calculation is manifest in the musculoskeletal mechanics of the system.

This form of reduced dimensional searching is consistent with our idea that the complex skeletomuscular mechanics is simplified by a naturally occurring division of the body position space into distinct regions, each characterized by a minimal set of muscles moving the body in a reduced dimensional plane of position space (Nashner and McCollum 1984). Also, such a search can be implemented using the control system hypothesized in Section 2.5.

If the search is to be one dimensional, the successful subject must reduce the mechanical problem to one dimension or to separable parameters, each of which can be determined independently of the others. In the transition from ankle to hip synergy, for example, the amount of ankle muscle activation might first be reduced to the maximum allowed by the support surface. Then, when the ankle activation is already determined, the hip torque could be increased independently to make up for the lack of corrective thrust.

Greene (1982) has pointed out that in using such variables as amplitude and duration of hip and ankle motions, the nervous system is choosing between naturally occuring musculoskeletal motions rather than constructing each trajectory anew. This reduces the number of controlled variables from infinite to finite. The way the nervous system implements this reduction, for postural responses, is by using discrete muscle bursts and synergies of muscle bursts rather than by continuously varying activation.

Then mechanics determines the relation between burst amplitude, position, and momentum. If the nervous system doesn't need to calculate these relations, it can find functionally appropriate postural responses relatively simply.

In this spirit, the nervous system has three variables to control: ankle torque, relative amplitude of the two synergies, and delay from hip torque exertion to braking. There are various ways, a priori, that the three may be simply used, but combinations of mechanics and neural organization constrain the way control variables are used.

5 Constraints on the Modulation of Amplitude and Timing Organization

Ankle torque is presumably maximized early in the transition between synergies, so the two variables modulated during most of the transition are relative amplitude and timing organization. Amplitude and delay have similar mechanical roles in the standard mixture (Fig. 6): if the relative amplitude is shifted in favor of the hip synergy, then the hip motion will increase, as it will if the delay is lengthened between the firing of the gastrocnemius, quadriceps, and abdominals and the onset of the hamstrings and paraspinals. The important point is that this delay is not an independent variable in the transitions observed by Horak and Nashner (1983).

Under the control organization described in Section 3.1, the only timing variable left is the discrete choice between a limited set of timing organizations. Within each of these timing organizations, amplitude can be gradually modified to give a more effective strategy.

In actual transitions from ankle to hip synergy on the narrow beam, the relative amplitudes of ankle and hip muscles change gradually while the relative ordering of muscle bursts remains the same (See, for example, the later trials in the transition shown in Fig. 10). That is, relative amplitude of ankle and hip synergies is a mechanical variable used by the nervous system in the transition calculation, while relative timing of synergies is held constant over several trials.

However, changes in timing relations also occur; for example, from a crossed proximals timing organization (shown in Fig. 8) during the first through fifth trials of Fig. 10 to the standard mixture pattern during the sixth through sixteenth trials (excluding the ninth).

According to our initial hypothesis for independent generation and peripheral interaction among synergies, the timing organization of a mixed synergy response can be modified by both central and peripheral factors, as schematized in Fig. 7. At the central level, varying the relative onset time of the ankle and hip synergy commands would produce the mixtures in different timing relations.

However, as shown in Fig. 8, only a limited number of timing organizations are possible according to our hypothesis. For example, activation of hip generator simultaneous with or before the ankle generator would produce a prescription of muscle burst commands in which ankle muscles would receive a command from the ankle generator first, while thigh and trunk muscles would receive the hip generator commands first. Due to the reciprocal delay interactions at each segment, this prescription of muscle commands will produce the standard mixture pattern. However, if the hip generator command is progressively delayed in relation to the ankle, then a point is

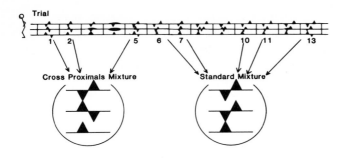

Fig. 10. Transition for one subject from ankle to hip synergy on the narrow beam. The timing organization of actual EMG patterns are presented in abstract form using triangles to represent individual muscle bursts. EMG's are arranged in antagonist pairs as in Fig. 2. *Stick figure* at the left labels the lines by the corresponding mechanical segment of the body. Trials are separated by *light lines*

reached when the ankle generator commands impinge first not only at the ankles but also at the thigh, producing the crossed proximals timing organization observed in Fig. 10. Still later onset of the hip generator command delays hip synergy responses at all segments until after the ankle synergy bursts. Thus, the timing organization of muscle synergies is discrete due to the sequencing of muscle bursts in opposite directions within the ankle and hip synergy generator and to the nature of peripheral interactions, even though the central parameter of relative timing may be continuously variable.

The choice of timing oragnizations is limited further by mechanical considerations; at least one neurally possible combination is functionally ineffective, the one with crossed proximals. This makes the crossed proximal timing organization into a boundary region completely avoided by the most successful subjects, who switch directly across the crossed proximal timing organization from one functionally effective strategy to another. Thus they turn the timing degree of freedom into an even coarser discrete choice.

For all subjects, the reciprocal delay mechanism makes timing organization a discrete choice, used only when the range of amplitude fine tuning is inadequate to reach an effective strategy. This infrequent changing of timing organization, with the resultant inflexibility of the delay time between exertion and braking of hip torque, is a consequence of the organization of the neural control of mixtures.

Mechanically the subject is free to change both duration and amplitude continuously. In order to reduce the mechanical problem of finding the effective strategy to a one dimensional search, one variable must be held fixed. We have seen that timing organization is conveniently frozen into discrete choices by the neural control organization, leaving amplitude to be varied gradually from trial to trial. Thus the requirements for simplifying the mechanical problem are fulfilled by the neural control organization alone; there is no need to invoke a separate control mechanism to make possible the form of strategy search Horak and Nashner observe.

6 Conclusion

We have developed a scheme for understanding how a subject approaches a functionally appropriate synergy. This study is based on another in which subjects were observed to change from one synergy to another. The scheme we have developed has two sides: One is the mechanical description of the problem to be solved and how an equivalent problem can be solved more easily by reducing the number of variables. The other is an hypothesis for the independent central generation of muscle commands and their peripheral interactions, which explains how the number of variables is naturally reduced by the organization of neural commands. Our scheme for movement coordination is the simplest explanation consistent with the experimental data, but is certainly not the only explanation. An assumption inherent to our synthesis is that the subjects' actual behaviors reflect directly the neural processes producing them.

By assuming a scheme of parcellation of muscle activity, first into bursts, then synergies, then discrete choices of timing organization of mixtures, we show that the one by one testing, discarding, and improving of synergies can be the actual calculation method. The stereotypy of the discrete patterns of muscle activity constitutes a set of neural constraints on the calculation. Without constraints, the calculation would be much more complex: firing time and duration. By imposing the constraints and thus simplifying the calculation, the nervous system reduces the amount of neural calculational capacity tied up in routine computations.

Rather than setting absolute constraints, the nervous system retains a measure of flexibility by forcing a choice among a set of discrete timing organizations. Within one timing organization, each pair of antagonist muscles is fired in a particular sequence. Given this sequencing constraint, amplitude variations have a locally linear effect on mechanical performance. Thus, if the nervous system fixes timing organization, it may close in on an effective synergy by amplitude variations.

This is the calculational strategy actually observed: subjects change timing organization rarely, and modulate amplitude within one timing organization. It makes sense that the nervous system could calculate, within one timing organization, whether changes in amplitude could possibly lead to an activation pattern bringing the body to the balance line with maximum afforded ankle torque. But we have no evidence that this is actually done. In any case, since the trajectory of the standard mixture (Figs. 6 and 4A) lies between the hip and ankle trajectories, a subject can find a functionally satisfactory synergy by fixing timing organization and then manipulating amplitude.

We conclude that the data of Horak and Nashner are consistent with the interpretation that the nervous system is simplifying its calculational task for postural adjustments by using stereotyped muscle activation patterns with a structure determined by central synergy generators and local interactions.

Acknowledgements. Lewis M. Nashner and Gin McCollum were supported by Grant NS 12661 from the U.S. Public Health Service and by Grant R-320 from the United Cerebral Palsy Research and Education Foundation. Fay Horak was supported by National Research Service Fellowship NS 06926 from U.S. Public Health Service.

References

Greene Peter H (1982) Why is it easy to control your arms? J Mot Behav 14: 260-286

Horak FB, Nashner LM (1983) Two distinct strategies for stance posture control: Adaptation to altered support surface conditions. Neurosci Abstr 9: 178, and J Physiol (submitted)

Horak FB, Nashner LM, Nutt JGC (1984) Postural instability in Parkinson's disease: motor coordination and sensory organization. Neurose: Abstr 10: 634

Nashner LM (1977) Fixed patterns of rapid postural responses among leg muscles during stance. Exp Brain Res 30: 13-24

Nashner LM, McCollum G (1984) The organization of human postural movements: A formal basis and experimental synthesis. Behav Brain Sci (in press)

Nashner LM, Woollacott M, Tuma G (1979) Organization of rapid responses to postural and locomotor-like perturbations of standing man. Exp Brain Res 36: 463-476

A Synthetic Motor Control System; Possible Parallels With Transformations in Cerebellar Cortex

M.J. NAHVI and M.R. HASHEMI[1]

1 Introduction

In a normal person muscular activity is coordinated so as to take into account the following two factors: (1) information on the pattern of the desired movement and (2) physical constraints such as the dynamics of the moving body, limitations on its input, optimality criteria, etc. The extent of coupling between these two types of factors in producing coordinated muscle activity in the real motor system is not known. However, for the purpose of analysis and modelling one may consider a functional representation as in Fig. 1 in which the command modifier matches the desired movement signal to the dynamics of the system according to given constraints. In this paper we discuss such transformation of a step command in a mechanical system whose output may approximate fast arm movement. Possible parallels with transformations in the neural net of the cerebellar cortex are then mentioned.

2 An Example

Suppose a crane operator wants to move a load suspended from the boom over a certain distance in minimum time. If he suddenly rotates the cab and the boom full range, the load will overshoot its destination and will oscillate before coming to rest (Fig. 2a). To prevent this, he may move the boom to an intermediate position such that at the peak of its swing the load will reach destination. The operator then quickly positions the boom above the load. Since at this time (t = $\frac{T}{2}$ in Fig. 2b) the load has zero velocity it will remain steady. This experiment may be performed using a simple pendulum (e.g. length 1 = 85 cm, T = 2 sec).

The modified input in Fig. 2c can produce the dead beat effect in a shorter time. In fact there exist many classes of inputs which can carry the system from an initial state to a final state within a specified time with a smooth transition. These inputs contain a transition phase, Θ, followed by the final level. The transition phase brings the system to a state such that the arrival at the final level establishes the output steady state immediately. As seen in Fig. 2b this dead beat effect is neither due to approximating the inverse of the system response function nor due to the braking by friction or by a

---

[1]   Sharif University of Technology P.O. Box 3406 Teheran, Iran

Cerebellar Functions
ed. by Bloedel et al.
© Springer-Verlag Berlin Heidelberg 1984

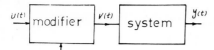

Fig. 1. For explanation see text

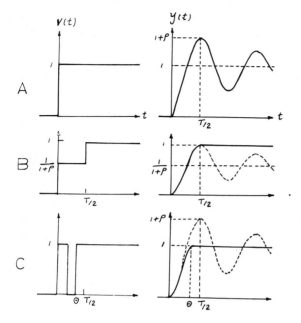

Fig. 2. For explanation see text

reversal of the input. Rather, the modifier may be said to match the input to the system, or to compensate for it, by appropriate use of the system's response to a step. Input modifications may be produced by open loop control, feedback, or combinations. The choice of modified input and the production strategy will depend on input constraints, optimally criteria, system's dynamics, available feedback path, etc.

The above control system has a single dimension and a simple structure. Systems for control of movements are of multilevel structure and deal with several variables or dimensions. They also have many controllers, each of them operating on a separate part of the space under control. Nevertheless extending the above concept of command modification to these systems may facilitate their analysis and modelling.

3 Parallels with Transformations in the Cerebellar Cortex

One of the functions of the cerebellum is to coordinate complex sequences of motor acts so that the total movement is smooth, accurate, and without oscillation. When this function is lost, movement is decomposed into inaccurate, oscillatory, and irregular individual segments. The cerebellar cortex provides part of the transformations and data processing for this coordination.

On may hypothesize that the role of the cerebellar transformations is that of the command modifiers of our previous example, i.e. to match the original command to the physical constraints. Parallels may then be observed. In a rapid but accurate extension of the hand, coordination is achieved by appropriate timing and intensity in the activity pattern of each muscle and between all muscles involved. The EMG of agonist and antagonist muscles contain bursts lasting tens to hundreds of ms, whose duration and relative timing depend on the movement pattern and on the physical constraints. This poses the need for two classes of transformations.

Two basic circuits in the cerebellar cortex can produce two different classes of transformations of potential interest in this respect. One is from mossy fibers to parallel fibers. The Golgi cell feedback plays an important role in this circuit by influencing the spread of activity along the direction of parallel fibers. The other circuit is from parallel fibers to Purkinje cells. In this circuit the inhibition by basket cells produces transformations along the transverse direction. These two circuits extract some input features and on the basis of information from physical constraints produce a multivariable output which participates in the construction of a final modified command for the desired movement.

Cerebro-Cerebellar Interactions and Organization of a Fast and Stable Hand Movement: Cerebellar Participation in Voluntary Movement and Motor Learning

K. SASAKI[1]

1 Cerebro-Cerebellar Interconnections in the Monkey

In higher mammals, especially primates, the hemispherical part of the cerebellum (posterior lobe, neocerebellum) becomes much larger, as the cerebral cortex develops enormously (Dow, 1942; Larsell, 1970). This part is reciprocally connected with the cerebral cortex and is considered important in organizing and controlling voluntary and skilled movements (Evarts and Thach, 1969; Allen and Tsukahara, 1974; Eccles, 1979; Sasaki, 1979; Brooks and Thach, 1981). After mossy and climbing fiber inputs to the cerebellum had been electrophysiologically distinguished (Eccles et al., 1966a, b; 1967), neuronal circuits between the cerebral cortex and the cerebellum of cats and monkeys were electrophysiologically investigated in detail, and those of monkeys were schematically drawn as in Fig. 1 (Sasaki, 1979; cf. Hassler, 1956).

The main features of the diagram in Fig. 1 are: (1) Major inputs to the neocerebellum (lateral part and lateral nucleus) come from the prefrontal (area 9-10), premotor (area 6) and forelimb motor (area 4 L) cortices. The forelimb motor cortex is most powerful in activating the neocerebellum. (2) The output of the neocerebellum (dentate nucleus) goes back contralaterally to those cortical areas that send the major inputs. (3) The cerebello-thalamo-cortical projections onto the forelimb motor and premotor cortices are mediated by superficial thalamo-cortical (T-C) projection neurons originating in the VA-VL region of the thalamus and thus induce surface-negative, depth-positive (s-N, d-P) laminar field potentials in the cortex (see Fig. 2). (4) The projection of the neocerebellum onto the contralateral prefrontal cortex is relayed by deep T-C projection neurons, producing s-P, d-N potentials. (5) The intermediate part and interpositus nucleus of the cerebellum are reciprocally connected with the intermediate part of the contralateral motor cortex (area 4 I) innervating mainly truncal and proximal limb muscles, and also with a part of the premotor cortex. (6) The medial part and medial nucleus of the cerebellum are reciprocally connected with the medial part of the motor cortex bilaterally (area 4 M, hindlimb area) and the bilateral parietal association cortices (area 5). (7) These differential reciprocal interconnections between the cerebral cortex and the cerebellum considerably overlap each other. (8) The projection from the association cortex onto the cerebellum is bilateral, whereas that from the motor cortex is mainly contralateral. The premotor cortex output takes an intermediate role between the association and motor cortices (see Sasaki, 1979).

[1] Department of Physiology, Institute for Brain Research, Faculty of Medicine, Kyoto University, 606 Kyoto, Japan

Cerebellar Functions
ed. by Bloedel et al.
© Springer-Verlag Berlin Heidelberg 1984

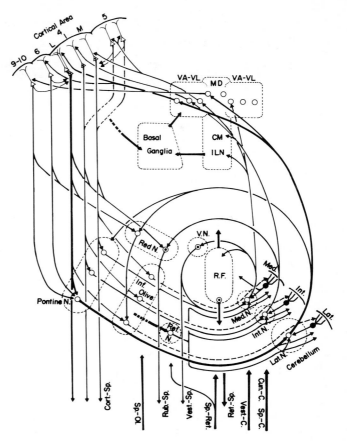

Fig. 1. Neuronal circuit diagram of the cerebro-cerebellar interconnections of the monkey. Several cortical areas are schematically shown in the *upper left* with their numbers. The motor cortex is divided into lateral (forelimb, *4L*), intermediate (truncal and proximal limbs, *4I*), and medial (hindlimb, *4M*) parts. The cerebellum is presented in the lower right with lateral, intermediate, and medial parts, and lateral, interpositus, and medial nuclei. The thalamus is represented by *VA-VL, MD,* and *CM-IL* parts. Pre- and post-cerebellar nuclei are pontine nuclei, inferior olive, reticular nuclei (*Ret. N.*), red nucleus (*Red N.*) and vestibular nuclei (*V.N.*). The brain stem reticular formation (*R.F.*) is also drawn with its descending (*Ret.-Sp.*) and ascending outputs. Corticospinal (*Cort.-Sp.*), rubrospinal (*Rub.-Sp.*) and vestibulospinal (*Vest.-Sp.*) tracts innervate motoneurons together with the reticulospinal tract (*Ret.-Sp.*). Inputs from peripheral sensory organs reach the cerebellum via the cuneo- and spino-cerebellar (*Cun.-C., Sp.-C.*), vestibulo-cerebellar (*Vest.-C.*), spino-reticular (*Sp. Ret.*) and spino-olivary (*Sp.-OI,*) tracts. (After Sasaki, 1979)

The diagram suggests functional significances of the cerebro-cerebellar interactions as summarized below: (1) The prefrontal and premotor cortices activate the neocerebellum which in turn excites the motor cortex via the thalamus. Thus motor commands presumably integrated in the association and premotor cortices are mediated by the neocerebellum, thalamus, and motor cortex before going down to the final common pathway, the motoneurons. (2) The information descending from the motor cortex to motoneurons reaches the cerebellum by collaterals of the pyramidal tract via the pre-

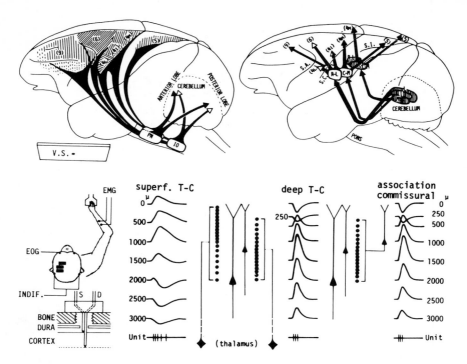

Fig. 2. Schemata of cerebro-cerebellar interconnections in monkeys *(upper diagrams)* and of laminar field potentials of the two thalamo-cortical (superficial and deep *T-C*) and the cortico-cortical (association and commissural) inputs *(lower part)*. Diagram of the methods of chronic experiments on the *lower left*. *Upper diagram* numbers indicate the different cortical areas. *PN* pontine nuclei; *IO* inferior olive; *S.A.* arcuate sulcus; *S.C.* central sulcus; *S.I.* intraparietal sulcus; *M, I, L* medial, interpositus and lateral nuclei of the cerebellum; *R-L, C-M* two nuclear complexes of the thalamus. *Lower diagram* numbers indicate the depth from the cortical surface in μm. Unit: schematical pattern of firing of cortical pyramidal neuron. The presumed excitatory synaptic terminals on apical dendrites of cortical pyramidal neurons in layer *III* and *V* are diagrammatically shown by dots for the three afferent inputs. Laminar field potentials are attributed to electrical dipoles generated in pyramidal neurons by the EPSPs. (After Sasaki, 1979)

cerebellar brain stem nuclei and is modified to recruit different kinds of descending tracts, organizing compound movements with many muscles and joints. In addition, the archi- and paleo-cerebellar parts are certainly centers for feedback control, receiving plenty of informations about the ongoing motor act. They influence motoneurons via several brain stem nuclei (see Sasaki, 1979).

In this paper, experimental data will be presented and discussed about the cerebro-cerebellar interaction upon the initiation of a conditioned (reaction time) hand movement and about motor learning in unanaesthetized behaving monkeys. There will also be speculated about the functional significance of cerebello-prefrontal projections verified electrophysiologically in monkeys. The speculation will take into account the experiences of a patient with an acute cerebellar disorder.

2 Thalamo-Cortical and Cortico-Cortical Responses and Cortical Field Potentials Preceding Visually Initiated Hand Movements

The cerebro-cerebellar and cerebello-cerebral projections in monkeys are schematically illustrated in the upper half of Fig. 2. Laminar field potential analysis in the cerebral cortex after stimulation of various thalamic and cerebellar nuclei revealed two different, elementary cortical responses which are conveyed by two different input systems to the cortex. Superficial thalamo-cortical (T-C) projections produce superficial negativity (active sink) which reverses to positivity (passive source) at about $1500-2000\,\mu$ depth and downwards, presumably due to EPSP currents in the superficial parts of the apical dendrites of pyramidal neurons in the cortex. Deep T-C projections evoke deep negativity which turns to be positive at about $250-500\,\mu$ and more superficially, due to EPSP currents in the deep portion of the apical dendrites and somata of pyramidal neurons. Another major cortical input via cortico-cortical (C-C) projections consisting of association and commissural fibers, elicits superficial positivity and deep negativity which are similar to deep T-C responses (see Sasaki, 1979; Sasaki et al., 1981b). The two different T-C projections of the cerebello-thalamo-cortical pathways are distinguished in Fig. 2 (upper right) by different arrows with open (superficial T-C) and filled (deep T-C) triangle heads. It should be emphasized that dentato-thalamo-forelimb motor cortex projections are mediated exclusively by the superficial T-C projection (4 L).

Based on the analysis of laminar field potentials, studies on premovement activities in various cortical areas were made in behaving monkeys with chronically implanted electrodes on the surface and in the depth of the cortex as shown in the lower left diagram of Fig. 2. Silver needle electrodes ($250\,\mu$ in diameter, insulated except for a pointed tip) were placed on the surface and at 2.5-3.0 mm depth of every locus in about ten different areas of each hemisphere and fixed to the bone by dental cement. Cortical surface and depth potentials were recorded against indifferent electrodes placed in the bone behind the ear on both sides. Potentials were amplified and recorded (with two second time constant) on magnetic tape through a multichannel data recorder. They were averaged after triggering either with the onset of the light stimulus that served as a go-sign to the monkey or the onset of movement. Electrooculogram (EOG), electromyogram (EMG) etc. were also recorded and monitored (see Hashimoto et al., 1979).

Monkeys *(Maccaca fuscata)* were trained to lift a lever by wrist extension in response to a light stimulus delivered in front of the animal by means of a diode emitting green light (V.S.) (see the lower left diagram of Fig. 2). Monkeys had to perform the movement while the light usually lasting about 500 ms was on (at early training stages, 900 or 700 ms). The stimulus was given at random time intervals of 2.5-6.0 s (Gemba et al., 1981).

Figure 3 presents the field potentials generated simultaneously in the prefrontal (A and IPSILATERAL A), premotor (B) and forelimb motor (C) cortices of the same monkey in association with visually initiated hand movements. A-C loci were contralateral to the moving hand. Averaged EMG and reaction time histogram of 100 movements (RT) are given in column C. The averager was triggered by stimulus onset (triangle). After being sufficiently trained, the monkey lifted the lever with reaction times of about 300 ms on the average as seen in RT, in which arrow signs indicate onset and end of the light stimulus. In the part of bilateral prefrontal cortices marked by open circles

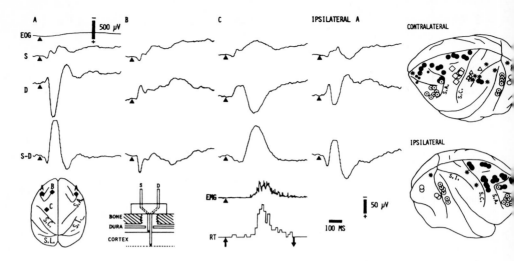

Fig. 3. Cortical field potentials associated with visually initiated hand movements and their distributions in both cortical hemispheres. As shown in the *lower left* diagram, surface *(S)* and depth *(D)* electrodes in four cortical loci *(A-C,* IPSILATERAL *A)* recorded potentials in *S* and *D* rows respectively. Electrical subtraction of *D* from *S* results in the *S-D* potential. Potentials were averaged 100 times, all aligned on the onset *(triangle)* of the stimulus which lasted for 510 ms as illustrated by *arrows* in the *RT* histogram. EOG (electrooculogram) was similarly averaged 100 times and EMG was recorded from wrist extensor muscles by bipolar surface electrodes, rectified, and averaged. Reaction time from the stimulus onset to the movement was plotted as a histogram for the 100 movements in 16 ms bins *(RT)*. Calibration of 500 µV for EOG and 50 µV for cortical potentials. 100 ms time scale for all traces. The recording sites are summarized from 14 monkeys at the well-trained stage and plotted on the dorsolateral aspects of the hemisphere contralateral and ipsilateral to the moving hand on the right. Different symbols represent different kinds of potentials. Loci without marked potentials are indicated by *asterisks.* Some of the electrode sites could not be plotted since they were too crowded in a few areas. (After Sasaki and Gemba, 1982)

with a dot in the center, s-P, d-N potentials appeared at about 40 ms latency after stimulus onset and s-N, d-P potentials followed at about 70 ms. Similar potential sequences emerged in bilateral prestriate cortices as marked by the same symbol. In bilateral premotor cortices, s-P, d-N potentials were recorded at about 40 ms latency as shown in column B and by filled circles in the diagrams on the right. Early s-P, d-N potentials at about 40 ms latency are followed by s-N, d-P ones at about 100-120 ms in the contralateral forelimb motor cortex as exemplified in column C and indicated by open squares in the diagram (CONTRALATERAL), the early component only being observed in the ipsilateral motor cortex (IPSILATERAL). All these potentials preceded the movement as seen in column C.

In these premovement potentials, s-N, d-P components are attributed mainly to superficial T-C responses, whereas s-P, d-N ones are responses either to deep T-C or C-C, or a mixture of both. The s-N, d-P potentials in the forelimb motor cortex contralateral to the moving hand, superficial T-C responses, were presumed to be mediated by the neocerebellum, since the dentate output activates the forelimb motor area through superficial T-C projections (see Sasaki, 1979). This was in fact verified by re-

Fig. 4. Cortical field potentials preceding visually initiated hand movements in the premotor *(A)* and forelimb motor *(B)* cortices contralateral to the moving hand were recorded before *(PREOP., left column)* and four days after *(POSTOP., right column)* unilateral cerebellar hemispherectomy *(shaded* in the *lower inset diagram).* All records were aligned by the stimulus onset pulse. Stimulus duration was 510 ms and 700 ms before and after the operation respectively. Other indications are the same as in Fig. 3. 500 μV for EOG and 50 μV for cortical potentials. 100 ms for all records. The recording sites are shown in the inset diagram with *filled squares.* *S.C.* central sulcus. (Sasaki et al. 1981a)

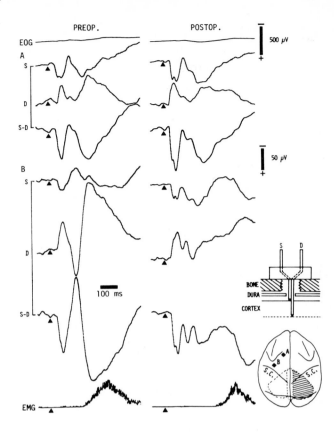

cording after unilateral cerebellar hemispherectomy (Sasaki et al., 1981a; 1982). As shown in Fig. 4, cerebellar hemispherectomy on the side ipsilateral to the moving hand (contralateral to the forelimb motor cortex recorded from) eliminated entirely the s-N, d-P potentials in the forelimb motor cortex and resulted in a prolongation of reaction times by 90-250 ms. These changes lasted for many months, when the hemispherectomy included both the dentate and interpositus nuclei (Sasaki et al., 1982). Premovement potentials in other cortical areas were not reduced in size by cerebellar hemispherectomy (see Gemba and Sasaki, 1984b).

The s-N, d-P premovement potentials in the forelimb motor cortex are directly coupled with the execution of the hand movement, since only these potentials can be eliminated by the substitution experiment in which an examiner lifts the lever for a well trained monkey (Gemba et al., 1981). The early s-P, d-N potentials in the motor cortex and all premovement potentials in other cortical areas remain without much change in the substitution experiment, being more directly involved in sensory and integrative mechanisms rather than execution of the movement on the task (Gemba and Sasaki, 1984a).

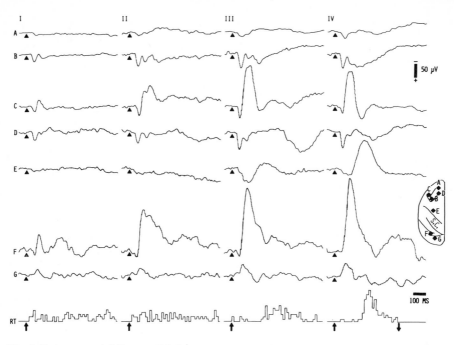

Fig. 5. Premovement *S-D* potentials in seven cortical loci on the left hemisphere of a monkey learn-ing the reaction time movement of the right hand. Columns *I-IV* present four sessions at different stages. *I* was taken in the 2nd session, *II* 21 days after *I, III* 3 days after *II*, and *IV* 36 days after *III*. Potentials were averaged 100 times from every session for respective cortical loci indicated by alphabetical symbols in the inset diagram and each recording. The stimulus was given for 900 ms at stages *I-III* but 510 ms at IV. Only the movements which occurred during the light stimulus were counted in RT histograms and averaged potentials (the later part of 900 ms is curtailed in columns *I-III*). They were aligned by stimulus onset as indicated by *triangle* and upward arrow, the *down-ward arrow* showing the end of 510 ms stimulus. Calibration, 50 µV for all potentials and 100 ms for all traces. *S.C.* central sulcus. (Sasaki and Gemba, 1982)

3 Learning Processes of the Reaction Time Movement and Development of Field Potentials in Different Cortical Areas

Field potentials occurring in association with visually initiated (reaction time) hand movements in the well trained monkey are different from those observed in the early phase of training. Their development and change has been studied. The learning as re-flected in the recorded potentials is exemplified in four stages in Fig. 5. A naive monkey at the beginning of training usually revealed no marked potentials in cortical areas ex-cept the striate cortex in response to the light stimulus. After several training sessions, some evoked potentials were recorded not only from the striate cortex (column I, row G) but also in prefrontal (A-C), premotor (D) and prestriate (F) cortices. Especially C and F loci were remarkable. Potentials in these loci gradually increased in size with successive training sessions as seen in column II (stage II, three weeks after I in this case). At stage I and II, the monkey lifted the lever at its own pace without regard to the light stimulus, as noted in reaction time histograms (RT). However, the monkey may have become more interested in the light stimulus and probably recognized it as "meaning-ful", or at least gazed at the light more eagerly. In any case, for averaging, we took only the records on which the monkey directed its eyes to the light stimulus. One examiner was watching the monkey during every session and cut off records whenever the eyes moved away from the light.

In the next session (3 days later), the monkey suddenly responded to the light stimulus by moving the lever, although movements occurred at longer and more variable latencies than at the well trained stage (compare RT in column III with that in IV). Up to stage III, the stimulus duration was 900 ms instead of 510 ms at stage IV. At stage III, the s-P, d-N followed by s-N, d-P potentials in the association cortices (C and F rows) reached their maximal size and scarcely increased from thereon. The s-P, d-N potentials in the premotor cortex increased a little in size at stage III (D row). Reaction time movements at stage III were preceded by s-P, d-N potentials (ca 40 ms latency) in the forelimb motor cortex but late s-N, d-P potentials were hardly noted (column III, E row). After stage III, repeated trainings for several weeks (3-8 weeks in different monkeys) made reaction times shorter and less variable. The s-N, d-P potentials were gradually manifested and enhanced concomitantly with the improvement of reaction time movements (columns III and IV, E row) (see Fig. 6). After attaining certain fast and stable movements at stage IV, further trainings did not improve the movement any-more and the s-N, d-P potentials in the forelimb motor cortex were saturated in size.

As shown in Fig. 6, another monkey reached stage III as seen in the leftmost col-umn (III) and showed the early s-P, d-N potentials in the premotor (A) and forelimb motor (B) cortices with unstable and long reaction times. The potentials in the contra-lateral motor cortex are aligned 100 times respectively with stimulus (V.S.) and move-ment (L.E.) onset. The latter alignment discloses a small s-N, d-P premovement poten-tial which is hardly seen in the averaging triggered by stimulus onset. These figures reveal that the late s-N, d-P premovement potential gradually increases in size with re-peated trainings from stage III to IV, and that the enhancement of the potential is closely related with faster and less variable reaction times. The wrist movement itself did not change so much, as seen in the averaged EMG records. Individual monkeys took three to eight weeks from stage III to IV. The longest (A) and shortest (B) time courses of the changes in the s-N, d-P potentials and the average reaction times are plotted along stages III to IV for two monkeys in Fig. 7. These appear to imply the time courses of recruitment of cerebro-cerebellar interactions in attaining the fast and stable hand movement.

Fast and accurate timing is undoubtedly one of the most important factors of skill-fulness in movements. It appears likely that cognitive learning of the reaction time movement is associated at least in part with increased activities of the association and premotor cortices, and that attaining fast and accurate reaction time and skillfulness of the movement is intimately related with the recruitment of activities of the cerebro-cerebellar interactions. These interpretations are consistent with the observation in which training was started for the hand movement after cerebellar hemispherectomy ipsilateral to the moving hand (Fig. 8). It took a longer time to train such monkeys than normal monkeys, but the successive appearance of premovement cortical potentials in different areas occurred in the same order and manner as in normal monkeys except for the late s-N, d-P potentials in the contralateral forelimb motor cortex. The hemi-cerebellectomized monkey neither revealed the late s-N, d-P potentials nor attained fast

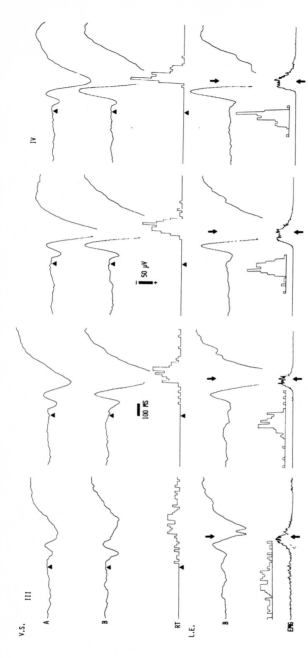

Fig. 6. Premovement *S-D* potentials in the premotor *(A)* and forelimb motor **(B)** cortices are presented in four different sessions at one week interval from stage *III* (leftmost column) to stage *IV* (rightmost column). *V.S.* two rows of the potentials (*A* and *B*) are aligned 100 times by stimulus onset *(triangle)*; *L.E.* row **B** treats the same data as row *B* in *V.S.* but is aligned by movement onset *(arrow)*. Histograms of the onset time of the light stimulus preceding the movement are shown above the EMGs aligned to the onset of movement. The light stimulus lasted for 900 ms in the *leftmost* and *second columns* and 510 ms in the *third* and *rightmost columns*. Calibrations of 50 µV for all cortical potentials and 100 ms for all traces. (Sasaki and Gemba, 1983)

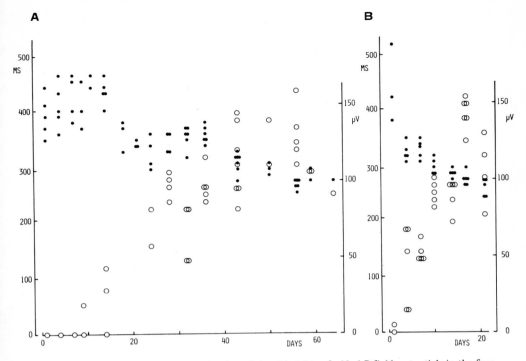

Fig. 7 A, B. Reaction times in ms *(filled circle)* and heights of s-N, d-P field potentials in the fore-limb motor cortex in µV *(open circle)* are plotted against days from stage *III* to *IV (abscissa)*. Examples of two different monkeys are presented in **A** and **B** respectively. The reaction time represents that of the peak in the histogram of 100 samples in every session. For the reaction time and the potential height, several points are given in respective sessions on each day. (Sasaki and Gemba, 1983)

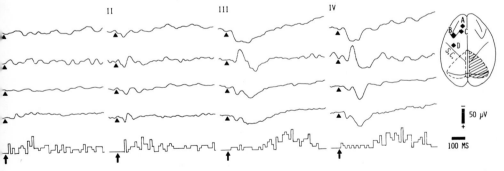

Fig. 8. Premovement S-D potentials in four loci of the left cerebral hemisphere of a monkey whose cerebellar hemisphere on the right side (shaded by *oblique lines*) had been extirpated before training the reaction time movement of the right hand. The potentials were aligned 100 times by the onset of the light stimulus lasting for 900 ms. Their later part is curtailed. Calibration of 50 µV for all potentials and 100 ms for all traces. (Sasaki and Gemba, 1982)

and stable hand movements even with repeated trainings for several months (see Fig. 8). Later histological examination proved that the dentate and interpositus nuclei were largely destroyed by the cerebellar hemispherectomy.

4 Processes of Motor Learning

It is interesting to note in Figs. 5-8 that the latencies of premovement potentials in various cortical areas reveal largely equal values of about 40 ms (35-47 ms) in different loci except the somatosensory cortex which shows a longer latency. The same order of latencies among the striate (primary visual), association (prefrontal and prestriate), premotor and motor cortices suggests that impulses evoked by the visual stimulus arrive at these cortical areas almost simultaneously and in parallel when the motor learning has been accomplished (Fig. 5, stage IV). Also latencies of the potentials in respective cortical areas change little during learning. In every monkey, it was consistently observed that the responsive cortical areas were successively added along the learning process, and that the respective premovement potentials increased in size gradually up to certain levels at different stages without marked changes of their latencies (Fig. 5). These findings appear to imply that visually evoked impulses arrive at the primary visual cortex at the beginning of learning, and simultaneously or several days later at the association and premotor cortices, then several weeks later at the motor cortex and thus let the motor cortex execute the reaction time movement. At the late stage of motor learning, the cerebro-cerebellar neuronal circuits are recruited to activate the motor cortex more efficiently in order to perform the movement in fast and accurate timing skillfully.

The sequential participation of these different cortical areas with much the same latencies suggests that visually evoked impulses are conveyed in a stepwise manner to an increasing number of the different areas involved in a motor program by a kind of "switching" mechanism, i.e., volleys evoked by the visual stimulus are first conveyed only to the primary visual cortex, and then delivered in succession to the association and premotor cortices and later to the motor cortex. Along stages I-III of the learning process, the switching mechanism is supposed to work somewhere in subcortical structures. The early components of premovement potentials recorded at latencies of about 40 ms in these cortical areas were invariably s-P, d-N ones. According to depth profiles in the cortex, they must be either due to deep T-C or C-C responses, or a mixture of both (Sasaki, 1979; Sasaki et al., 1981b). The latencies indicate that the early components are constituted mainly by deep T-C responses rather than by C-C ones. Therefore, the switching mechanism should occur in the thalamus and/or its closely related structures. Thalamic nuclei are candidates for this mechanism, since various paths of information flow, including those from the cerebral cortices, converge onto these nuclei which in turn project divergently onto various cortical areas directly as well as indirectly (Hassler, 1972; Kievit and Kuypers, 1977; Akert and Hartmann-Von Monakow, 1980).

Figure 9 gives two schemata, one for the hypothesized cortico-thalamic interaction distributing visually evoked informations to frontal association plus premotor, posterior association, and motor plus somatosensory cortices during the cognitive learning process (upper diagram, stages I-III), and another for the cerebro-cerebellar interaction initiating

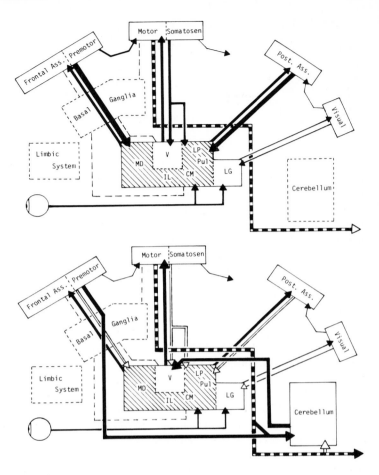

Fig. 9. Two schemata for cortico-thalamic interactions *(upper diagram)* and cerebro-cerebellar inter-actions *(lower diagram)* in motor learning processes. Visual informations come to the visual cortex via LG and also to the prefrontal and premotor cortices as well as the posterior association cortices via extrageniculate and geniculate pathways. These cortices would influence the associational and intralaminar thalamic nuclei(*MD, IL, CM, Pul, LP* etc., shaded by *oblique lines*) and distribute the visual impulses to these cortices themselves and the motor and somatosensory cortices, the latter, especially the motor cortex, send the motor command to motoneurons through the descending tract *(filled* and *open line)* (stage III of the motor learning) *(upper diagram)*. At well trained stage (stage IV), the motor command would start from the prefrontal and premotor cortices, be mediated by the cerebellum and *VA-VL* nuclear complex of the thalamus (V) and activate the motor cortex to execute the movement *(lower diagram)*

fast and accurate reaction time movements at the late skillful learning process (lower diagram, stages III-IV). The associational and intralaminar thalamic nuclei (MD, LP, Pul, CM, IL etc., shaded area) can receive extrageniculate visual inputs and distribute them to the association and premotor cortices, and then eventually to the motor cortex via the VA-VL nuclear region (V). In this distributing and switching mechanism, cortico-thalamic projections might presumably play an important action as illustrated by thick

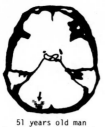

Fig. 10. Drawing after the X-ray computer tomography of a patient with an infarction of left cerebellar hemisphere (posterior lobe). The infarction indicated by *arrow* was localized by enhanced CT 8 days after the onset of the disease

51 years old man
1-cerebellar infarction

lines (upper diagram). After the conditioned (reaction time) movement has just been learned, the motor command should go from the prefrontal association and premotor cortices to the cerebellum which in turn excited the motor cortex via the VA-VL nuclei (lower diagram). This cerebro-cerebellar interaction would gradually be recruited and achieve fast and accurate timing (skilled) movements, and then the cerebro-thalamic interaction might work less than before as illustrated by open lines.

5 Functional Significance of the Cerebello-Prefrontal Projection

A cerebellar projection on the cerebral association cortex was electrophysiologically verified in cats and monkeys (Sasaki et al., 1972a, b, 1979). However, its functional significance has not been clarified so far. In this respect, one may exploit the following observation. The author recently encountered a patient with a cerebellar vascular lesion who claimed very interesting subjective symptoms (Sasaki et al. 1984).

The patient a 51-year-old man, doctor of medicine, suffered from an infarction in the posterior lobe of the cerebellum on the left. On the day after the attack which disturbed his consciousness only for a short time (probably several seconds), he tried the finger-nose test and noted a peculiar experience, i.e., when he moved his left upper limb (lesion side) to point to his nose (or anything else such as eye, ear, navel etc) by his index finger, he felt the nose disappearing from his own body schema, which could clearly be imagined when the upper limb was at rest. The space of several centimeter radius around the target (for instance, the nose) was then imagined as if it were "a sea of clouds". Accordingly he had to point his finger to the "middle of the vague space" and found his finger at his forehead. The trial with the right hand was entirely normal. This subjective symptom lasted only for several days (probably three or four days) after the onset of disease, although dysmetria (hypermetria) endured for about one month or so. X-ray computer tomographic examination revealed the infarction to be localized in about a three centimeter extent in the posterior lobe on the left side, presumably without touching the deep cerebellar nuclei (Fig. 10).

This claim of the patient led me to assume that the cerebello-prefrontal projection transmits the information for personal spatial orientation (Semmes et al., 1963), spatial discrimination based on "egocentric cues" (Pohl, 1973), kinaesthetic discrimination (Mishkin et al., 1977) etc. (see Rosenkilde, 1979). In monkeys, it was shown that the dentate output goes to the dorsal part of dorsolateral prefrontal cortex (area 9) that is just rostral to the premotor cortex (area 6) (Sasaki et al., 1979). In fact, as shown in

Fig. 11 A, B. Deep T-C (*filled squares* in **A**) and superficial T-C (*filled circles* in **B**) responses elicited by stimulation of the contralateral dentate nucleus in monkeys. Averages of response sizes are illustrated by different sizes of the symbols in a relative scale, based on five monkey experiments. *S.a.* arcuate sulcus; *S.cent.* central sulcus; *S.i.* intraparietal sulcus. (After Sasaki et al. 1979)

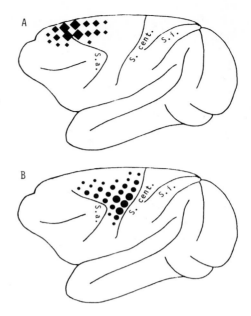

Fig. 11, the prefrontal area receiving the dentate output is continued to the rostral part of premotor cortex. The dentate stimulation induces deep T-C responses in the prefrontal and the rostral part of the premotor cortex, in addition to superficial T-C responses in the premotor and forelimb motor cortices, the rostral part of the premotor cortex being innervated by both deep and superficial T-C projections (Sasaki et al., 1976, 1979).

Thus I hypothesize that the information mediated by the neocerebellum comes back to the dorsal part of the prefrontal cortex in the dynamic state of movement and posture, is compared with information preserved in and around this part of cortex and serves for integrating and perceiving spatial and/or kinaesthetic sensation in the dynamic state. In the resting state, the cerebello-prefrontal projection must not function for such integration and perception as one may have clear personal spatial orientation and body image. But, as soon as the movement starts or the posture is maintained, the proprioceptive information mediated by the neocerebellum should be fed back to the association cortex and should be used for kinaesthetic perception and spatial discrimination. It should be further investigated what part of the neocerebellum is crucial for such integrative functions, the lateral part like crus I and II or the paramedian lobules, the former receiving peripheral informations more indirectly than the latter.

The short duration of the subjective symptom in this patient, which lasted for several days, would suggest powerful compensatory functions of the association cortex and of the neocerebellum. Such a subjective symptom, therefore, can only be found a short time after an acute neocerebellar lesion. Further studies are required to know if the subjective symptom is related to a group of debated cerebellar symptoms, i.e., disturbance in discriminating weight differences, "hefting" a weight (Holmes, 1917; see Fulton, 1949; Dow and Moruzzi, 1957). However, it is interesting to note that everybody who is required to estimate a small difference in weights on both hands invariably moves the hands up and down a little against gravity, obviously utilizing dynamic (probably proprioceptive) information rather than static cutaneous pressures.

Acknowledgement. The author is grateful to Dr. N. Mizuno for help and advice on morphological examinations and Dr. H. Gemba for collaboration throughout chronic experiments. Thanks are also due to Dr. M. Ogawa (Shizuoka Rosai Hospital), Drs. S. Kawaguchi and H. Gemba for collaboration in clinical observation of the patient with cerebellar infarction. Supported by a Grant-in-Aid for Scientific Research from the Ministry of Education, Science and Culture of Japan and by the Japan Society for the Promotion of Science.

References

Akert K, Hartmann-Von Monakow K (1980) Relationships of precentral, premotor and prefrontal cortex to the mediodorsal and intralaminar nuclei of the monkey thalamus. Acta Neurobiol Exp 40: 7-25

Allen GI, Tsukahara N (1974) Cerebrocerebellar communication systems. Physiol Rev 54: 957-1006

Brooks VB, Thach WT (1981) Cerebellar control of posture and movement. In: Brooks VB (ed) Handbook of physiology, sect 1: the nervous system, vol II. Am Physiol Soc (Bethesda), pp 877-956

Dow RS (1942) The evolution and anatomy of the cerebellum. Biol Rev 17: 179-220

Dow RS, Moruzzi G (1958) The physiology and pathology of the cerebellum. Univ Minnesota Press, Minneapolis

Eccles JC (1979) Introductory remarks. In: Massion J, Sasaki K (eds) Cerebro-cerebellar interactions. Elsevier/North-Holland Biomedical Press, Amsterdam, pp 1-18

Eccles JC, Llinas R, Sasaki K (1966a) The excitatory synaptic action of climbing fibres on the Purkinje cells of the cerebellum. J Physiol 182: 268-296

Eccles JC, Llinas R, Sasaki K (1966b) The mossy fibre-granule cell relay in the cerebellum and its inhibition by Golgi cells. Exp Brain Res 1: 82-101

Eccles JC, Sasaki K, Strata P (1967) Interpretation of the potential fields generated in the cerebellar cortex by a mossy fibre volley. Exp Brain Res 3: 58-80

Evarts EV, Thach WT (1969) Motor mechanisms of the CNS: cerebrocerebellar inter-relations. Annu Rev Physiol 31: 451-498

Fulton JF (1949) Physiology of the nervous system. Oxford Univ Press, London New York

Gemba H, Sasaki K (1984a) Studies on cortical field potentials recorded during learning processes of visually initiated hand movements in monkeys. Exp Brain Res 55: 26-32

Gemba H, Sasaki K (1984b) Distribution of potentials preceding visually initiated and self-paced hand movements in various cortical areas of the monkey. Brain Res 306: 207-214

Gemba H, Hashimoto S, Sasaki K (1981) Cortical field potentials preceding visually initiated hand movements in the monkey. Exp Brain Res 42: 435-441

Hashimoto S, Gemba H, Sasaki K (1979) Analysis of slow cortical potentials preceding self-paced hand movement in the monkey. Exp Neurol 65: 218-229

Hassler R (1956) Die extrapyramidalen Rindensysteme und die zentrale Regelung der Motorik. Dtsch Z Nervenheilkd 175: 233-258

Hassler R (1972) Hexapartition of input as a primary role of the thalamus. In: Frigyesi T, Rinvik E, Yahr MD (eds) Corticothalamic projections and sensorimotor activities. Raven Press, New York, pp 551-579

Holmes G (1917) The symptoms of acute cerebellar injuries due to gunshot injuries. Brain 40: 461-535

Kievit J, Kuypers HGJM (1977) Organization of the thalamocortical connexions to the frontal lobe in the rhesus monkey. Exp Brain Res 29: 299-322

Larsell O (1970) The cerebellum from monotremes through apes. Univ Minnesota Press, Minneapolis

Mishkin M, Pohl W, Rosenkilde CE (1977) Kinesthetic discrimination after prefrontal lesions in monkeys. Brain Res 130: 163-168

Pohl W (1973) Dissociation of spatial discrimination deficits following frontal and parietal lesions in monkeys. J Comp Physiol Psychol 82: 227-239

Rosenkilde CE (1979) Functional heterogeneity of the prefrontal cortex in the monkey: A review. Behav Neural Biol 25: 301-345

Sasaki K (1979) Cerebro-cerebellar interconnections in cats and monkeys. In: Massion J, Sasaki K (eds) Cerebro-cerebellar interactions. Elsevier/North-Holland Biomedical Press, Amsterdam, pp 105-124

Sasaki K, Gemba H (1982) Development and change of cortical field potentials during learning processes of visually initiated hand movements in the monkey.Exp Brain Res 48: 429-437

Sasaki K, Gemba H (1983) Learning of fast and stable hand movements and cerebro-cerebellar interactions in the monkey. Brain Res 277: 41-46

Sasaki K, Matsuda Y, Kawaguchi S, Mizuno N (1972b) On the cerebello-thalamo-cerebral pathway for the parietal cortex. Exp Brain Res 16: 89-109

Sasaki K, Kawaguchi S, Matsuda Y, Mizuno N (1972a) Electrophysiological studies on cerebello-cerebral projections in the cat. Exp Brain Res 16: 75-88

Sasaki K, Kawaguchi S, Oka H, Sakai M, Mizuno N (1976) Electrophysiological studies on the cerebello-cerebral projections in monkeys. Exp Brain Res 24: 495-507

Sasaki K, Jinnai K, Gemba H, Hashimoto S, Mizuno N (1979) Projection of the cerebellar dentate nucleus onto the frontal association cortex in monkeys. Exp Brain Res 37: 193-198

Sasaki K, Gemba H, Hashimoto S (1981a) Influences of cerebellar hemispherectomy upon cortical potentials preceding visually initiated hand movements in the monkey. Brain Res 210: 425-430

Sasaki K, Gemba H, Hashimoto S (1981b) Premovement slow cortical potentials on self-paced hand movements and thalamocortical and corticocortical responses in the monkey. Exp Neurol 72: 41-50

Sasaki K, Gemba H, Mizuno N (1982) Cortical field potentials preceding visually initiated hand movements and cerebellar actions in the monkey. Exp Brain Res 46: 29-36

Sasaki K, Kawaguchi S, Gemba H, Ogawa M (1984) On functional significance of the cerebello-prefrontal projection in primates. Neurosci Lett Suppl (in press)

Semmes J, Weinstein S, Ghent L, Teuber H-L (1963) Correlates of impaired orientation in personal and extrapersonal space. Brain 86: 747-772

On the Role of the Subprimate Cerebellar Flocculus in the Optokinetic Reflex and Visual-Vestibular Interaction

W. PRECHT[1], R.H.I. BLANKS[2], P. STRATA[3], and P. MONTAROLO[3]

1 Introduction

1.1 How Did the Interest in the Flocculus Come About? A Brief Review

1.1.2 Relation to the Vestibular System

The flocculus — a part of the vestibulocerebellum or archicerebellum — has long been considered only in conjunction with the vestibular system. Given that this oldest part of the cerebellum develops in close association with the vestibular system (Herrick 1924; Larsell 1934), receives primary and secondary vestibular inputs (cf. ref. Precht 1975, 1978) and projects, via inhibitory Purkinje cell axons, directly to the vestibular nuclei (Fukuda et al. 1972; Baker et al. 1972; cf. ref. Precht 1975, 1978), the vestibular bias in the studies of the flocculus comes as no surprise. Most of the data obtained until about 1975 with anatomical, physiological, and lesion experiments have been summarized elsewhere (Precht 1975) and will not be repeated here. In brief, it has been shown that in all species studied primary and secondary vestibular neurons terminate as mossy fibers in the vestibulocerebellum, and that Purkinje cells of this area project their axons to certain subdivisions of the vestibular nucleus complex thereby exerting monosynaptic inhibition on some of the vestibuloocular relay neurons. Lesions of the flocculus or flocculonodular lobe produced transient nystagmus, positional nystagmus and transient enhancement of postrotatory or caloric nystagmus. In more recent quantitative lesion studies, performed in the cat and primates, the unpredictable nature of the long-term effects of flocculectomy on vestibuloocular reflex (VOR) gain has been stressed (Robinson 1974; Zee et al. 1981). More consistent lesion effects, i.e. a decrease of VOR gain, were obtained in the rabbit (Ito et al. 1982; Nagao 1983). These relatively meager effects of flocculus lesions came as a surprise vis à vis the elaborate interconnections between the vestibulocerebellum and the vestibular nuclei described above. On the other hand, these data emphasize the often subtle nature of cerebellar control on inherently strong brain stem pathways.

1.1.3 Visual and Combined Visual-Vestibular Inputs

The interest in the flocculus was greatly enhanced and expanded by the finding of Maekawa and Simpson (1972, 1973) and Simpson and Alley (1974) that Purkinje cells

[1]   Brain Research Institute, University of Zürich, CH-8029 Zürich, Switzerland
[2]   Departments of Anatomy and Surgery, University of California, Irvine, USA
[3]   Istituto di Fisiologia Umana, Universita di Torino, Torino, Italia

Cerebellar Functions
ed. by Bloedel et al.
© Springer-Verlag Berlin Heidelberg 1984

in the rabbit flocculus receive a direction-selective, retinal slip-coding visual climbing fiber input. The pathway consists of the accessory optic tract and nuclei and the dorsal cap of the inferior olive which projects to the contralateral flocculus. Later it has been shown that optic nerve stimulation also activates a mossy fiber input to the flocculus via the n.reticularis tegmenti pontis (Maekawa et al. 1981). Both mossy and climbing fiber visual pathways can modulate Purkinje cell simple and complex spike activity, respectively, during optokinetic stimulation and they both interact synergistically with vestibular mossy and climbing fiber inputs to the same Purkinje cells (Ghelarducci 1975). It is of interest to briefly note here that in primates visual input to the flocculus is weak (see next paragraph).

The visual input to the flocculus Purkinje cells projecting to VOR neurons was suggested to improve the VOR, an open-loop reflex, by providing the flocculus with a retinal slip "error" signal whenever the VOR was not completely compensatory (Ito et al. 1974). In fact, as pointed out earlier by Meiry (1971), the VOR gain (measured in the dark) could be increased considerably by rotation vis-a-vis a structured background. Is the flocculus responsible for this immediate gain enhancement in the combined visual-vestibular condition? Contrary to previous claims, recent experiments in rabbits (Ito et al. 1982) and cats (Keller and Precht 1979), showed that visual-vestibular interaction in the VOR still occurred after flocculus lesions, provided the velocities of the resulting optokinetic stimuli were not too high. This notion is in agreement with the finding that OKN steady-state velocity in response to high velocity pattern motions was clearly less in flocculectomized as compared to intact cats (Keller and Precht 1979).

Apparently both OKN and visual-vestibular interaction in the VOR require the flocculus only in part of their working range. This point will be taken up again below.

1.1.4 VOR Plasticity and Flocculus

Subsequent to the studies dealing with the importance of the flocculus for immediate visual-vestibular interactions in the VOR, the visual pathway through the cerebellar flocculus was also considered important for inducing the visually guided, plastic and adaptive changes in the VOR (Ito et al. 1974; Gonshor and Melvill-Jones 1976; Ito 1977a, b). This hypothesis appeared attractive also in the light of the Marr (1969) and Albus (1971) hypotheses which postulated that the climbing fiber synapse on Purkinje cells has the capacity to induce long-term changes in the parallel fiber synapses on the same cells. Since the climbing fiber system can signal retinal slip velocity (Simpson and Alley 1974), an error signal being present when the VOR is not compensatory, it was suggested to send such a "teacher's signal" to the Purkinje cells to introduce plastic changes in the parallel fiber synapses activated concurrently by the vestibular stimuli. Ito (1977a, b) showed that Purkinje cells in the horizontal zone of the rabbit flocculus, indeed, underwent some long-term plastic changes in simple spike firing, in parallel with similar changes of the VOR gain. This modification in firing of Purkinje cell simple spikes was considered responsible for the observed changes in the VOR and was accepted as evidence of a learning capacity of the cerebellar cortex. The demonstration that cerebellar floccular lesions strongly impaired long-term VOR adaptation in the rabbit (Ito 1977a, b, Ito et al. 1982, Nagao 1983) and the cat (Robinson 1974) lent further support to this notion. Finally, VOR adaptation was also abolished upon lesions of the visual pathway to the inferior olive while no effects on the plastic adaptive capacity of the VOR was noted when the n.reticularis tegmenti pontis — one of the sources of visual mossy fiber afferents to the flocculus — was destroyed (Miyashita 1981).

Contrary to Ito's hypothesis, postulating the occurrence of learning in the cerebellar cortex, Miles et al. (1980a, b), based on their work in primates, proposed an entirely different hypothesis regarding the functional role of the flocculus in VOR adaptation. Crucial for their hypothesis is the finding (Miles et al. 1980a; Lisberger and Fuchs 1978a, b) that in normal monkeys simple spikes of floccular Purkinje cells carry mainly two independent velocity signals of comparable strength and the same directional preference relating to head and eye velocity. These Purkinje cells were, therefore, classified as gaze velocity cells. Contrary to the rabbit and rat (see Section 2) visual modulation of Purkinje cell simple spikes per se was rare, and only a small percentage of complex spikes responded in the various paradigms applied. Waespe and Henn (1981) studied Purkinje cell activity in response to full-field optokinetic stimulation and concluded that, under certain stimulus conditions, the signal present in Purkinje cell simple spike activity might be equivalent to image slip (see also Waespe et al. this Vol.) Clearly then, eye and head velocity signals appear to dominate Purkinje cell simple spike activity in primates. Thus, gaze velocity Purkinje cells, indeed, show very little or no modulation when the monkey is oscillated in the dark or light when the eyes and head are moving 180° out of phase, and the head and eye velocity signals cancel one another. Modulation of firing is very pronounced, however, when the monkey pursues an object or when he fixates a spot moving with the chair. While in the former case the eye velocity signal dominates the Purkinje cell discharge, it is the head velocity signal in the latter condition. Miles et al. (1980a) propose that the eye velocity signal to Purkinje cells is an efference copy signal to aid — via positive feedback — ocular pursuit. The head velocity signal is part of an inhibitory side path of the VOR pathway which can offset the reduction of eye velocity signals during combined eye-head pursuit.

When Miles et al. (1980b) studied the responses of gaze velocity Purkinje cells in monkeys whose VOR had been modified by magnifying spectacles or left-right reversing prisms they found them to be significantly different from normal monkeys. However, the plastic changes occurring in Purkinje cells cannot explain the adaptive changes observed simultaneously in the VOR and are most likely a consequence rather than the cause of the behavioral changes. The site of the modifiable gain element would then be more likely outside the cerebellum. As pointed out by Miles et al. (1980b) the flocculus may still play a role in the adaptive VOR process providing the brain stem nuclei with information that helps to offset the severe disturbances introduced by the optical devices. The inability to adapt the VOR after vestibulocerebellar lesions also indicates some sort of involvement of the flocculus in the acquisition process. In this context it should be recalled that floccular lesions cause severe disturbances of oculomotricity unrelated to plasticity (see below).

1.1.5 Optokinetic System and Flocculus

Yet another line of research opened a new vista in the understanding of vestibulocerebellar function. Thus, during the past decade several studies have been aimed at a more quantitative description of the optokinetic reflex and its interaction with the VOR in a variety of species (e.g. monkey: Cohen et al. 1977, see also Waespe et al. this Vol.; rabbit: Collewijn 1981; Ito et al. 1982; Batini et al. 1979; cat: Keller and Precht 1979, Maioli and Precht (1984). One of the interesting, and in this context important finding that emerged from these studies is that the optokinetic eye reflex (OKN) of primates and to some extent also of subprimates (Sect. 3) consists of two components that are easily detected when velocity step motions of the surround are used as stimuli: an initial fast rise in slow phase eye velocity brings eye velocity to some species-dependent fraction of final steady-state velocity, and a slowly rising component provides the additional increase of eye velocity to steady-state. When the constant velocity optokinetic stimulation is suddenly terminated, by turning-off the lights, eye velocity quickly falls to a lower level and then continues to decay slowly to zero. This slow decay of eye velocity is known as optokinetic afternystagmus (OKAN). Lesion studies, subsequently performed in primates, have demonstrated that the fast and slow components of OKN can be differentially affected depending on the site of the lesion: removal of the cerebellar flocculus strongly impairs, but not completely abolishes, the fast component of OKN only, and, as a result leads to a prolongation of the time required to reach steady-state velocity (Zee et al. 1981; Waespe et al. 1983); peripheral vestibular lesions affect only the slow build-up of eye velocity during optokinetic stimulation (Cohen et al. 1973).

Flocculus lesions also impaired the steady-state OKN gain at higher stimulus velocities, reduced the gain of the smooth eye tracking of small targets and impaired the ability of the monkey to immediately suppress inappropriate vestibular nystagmus (Takemori and Cohen 1974; Zee et al. 1981; Waespe et al. 1983). It should be added here that visual suppression of vestibular eye movements and OKN deficits at high velocities of stimulation were also seen after nodulus lesions, indicating that we are looking at a vestibulocerebellar rather than a specific floccular lesion symptom (Igarashi et al. 1975).

Single unit studies in the primate flocculus during optokinetic stimulation (Waespe and Henn 1981) are in support of the notion obtained from lesion work, namely that the primate flocculus is involved in supporting rapid changes in eye velocity during OKN and ocular pursuit movements. These findings are extensively discussed in the paper by Waespe et al. (this Vol.).

What is the nature of the pathway leading to the fast optokinetic response? It is of interest to note that, as with flocculus lesions, the fast component is abolished by lesions of the visual cortex (Zee et al. 1982) suggesting that the pathway for the fast OKN component is intimately associated with the geniculo-striate pursuit system which apparently involves the flocculus or, more generally, the vestibulocerebellum, through unknown connections, for optimal performance. Other cerebellar "visual" areas, i.e. the mid-vermis, appear not to be involved in this system (Keller, Precht and Suzuki unpublished). There may exist brainstem pathways which bypass the slow storage network and exert an effect on motoneurons more directly. Evidence for such short latency optomotor connections has been obtained in amphibia (Cochran et al. 1984), but is missing in higher vertebrates at the present time.

The pathway for the slow component of OKN, or the velocity storage network, which the optokinetic system shares with the vestibular system, is apparently not much dependent on the integrity of the cerebellar flocculus, at least in the monkey (Waespe et al. 1983). Given that the tonic peripheral vestibular input is of crucial importance for the velocity storage network and the intimate mutual connections of the vestibular system with the flocculus (cf. ref. Precht 1975), it is surprising to find the slow pathway so little affected by cerebellar lesions. Apparently, in the monkey floccular Purkinje cells, activated conjointly with the fast component of OKN, do not act upon vestibular neurons involved in the VOR and the storage mechanism. That vestibular neurons are not the direct target of gaze velocity Purkinje cells is also apparent from the fact that they continue to be modulated by head velocity in the VOR suppression paradigm (rotation while fixating a point rotating with the platform), in spite of the fact that Purkinje cells are strongly modulated during this task (Miles and Fuller 1975; Lisberger and Fuchs 1978a, b).

Although not directly relevant to the present topic, one other finding, consistently observed after flocculectomy, deserves mention. This deficiency is termed gaze-paretic nystagmus and consists of horizontal centripetal drift of the eyes following a saccade and downbeat nystagmus (Westheimer and Blair 1973; Robinson 1974; Zee et al. 1981). This result implicates involvement of the cerebellar flocculus in the control of the time constant and stability of the velocity-to-position integrator.

1.2 Scope of the Present Paper

In the following we shall concentrate on our own work dealing with the role the cerebellar flocculus may play in controlling the optokinetic reflex and visual-vestibular interaction in subprimate mammals, specifically the rat and cat. While the rat may serve as an example of a lateral-eyed, afoveate species, the cat will serve to exemplify the problem in a frontal-eyed, "foveate" mammal. In addition to comparing these two species we shall refer, whenever appropriate, to work done by others in the rabbit and finally compare subprimate data with those obtained in primates. The latter are extensively treated in the article by Waespe et al. (this volume). Since our studies are still in progress the work is incomplete. Thus, in the rat single unit work and anatomy of the optokinetic system is more advanced than in the cat, while in the latter we have more information on the effects the flocculus may have on eye movements.

2 The Horizontal Optokinetic System and its Relationship with the flocculus in the Rat

2.1 Horizontal Optokinetic Eye Nystagmus

When the head of an alert rat is fixed, and a full-field pattern projected on a cylinder surrounding the animal is rotated or, alternatively, the turntable rotates at constant speed (no vestibular input) vis-à-vis a structured environment, a vigorous optokinetic nystagmus (OKN) results. Its slow phase moves in the direction of pattern rotation, and the quick phases turn the eyes in the opposite direction, often resulting in a net eye position displacement (Schlagfeld shift) into their direction, i.e. opposite to the direction of pattern motion. Provided the animal is fully alert, the steady-state gain of the OKN (eye velocity/pattern velocity) is close to unity up to velocities of 30-60°/s and it is symmetrical in binocular conditions. Thus, as far as the steady-state gain of the OKN of the rat is concerned it functions as a visual field holding reflex over a range very similar to that found in the cat (Maioli and Precht 1984) and is somewhat superior to that found in rabbits (Collewijn 1981). However, all three subprimate species have their high gain range at significantly lower stimulus velocities than the monkey (Cohen et al. 1977). In monocular condition, the rat OKN is dramatically different from that found in cat (Montarolo et al. 1981) and monkey (Pasik and Pasik 1964) in that the effective stimulus direction is almost entirely restricted to the temporonasal one; nasotemporally moving patterns yield weak responses (gain ca. 0.1 or less) at low stimulus velocities and are completely absent at a stimulus velocity of around 50°/s (Fig. 1). Cats and monkeys perform equally well in both directions, even at high velocities, but show a strongly asymmetric OKN, similar to the rat, upon removal of the visual cortex (Montarolo et al. 1981). The fact that the OKN evoked monocularly is highly asymmetric in the rat and apparently little influenced by the cortex makes this animal very suitable to study basic brainstem optokinetic pathways without having to introduce any lesions.

Finally, the initial fast rise in OKN slow phase velocity, often observed in the cat (Maioli and Precht 1984) and monkey (Cohen et al. 1977, see Sect. 1.1), is less frequently observed in rats and, when present, of small amplitude, as described also for the rabbit (Collewijn 1981).

2.2 Optokinetic Pathway Organization

In order to appreciate the various possibilities for the cerebellum to influence and control OKN a brief summary of the horizontal optokinetic pathway organization, as derived from lesion, single unit and anatomical studies, will be given. A more extensive treatment of this topic can be found in Precht (1981, 1982) and Precht et al. (1982). Figure 2 summarizes schematically the essential findings regarding the OKN pathway in the rat. As was found in other species, the pretectum (Pt), more specifically the n. of the optic tract (NOT), is the first central relay station in the rat as well. The evidence is as follows: (1) bilateral lesions abolish OKN and unilateral lesions lead to a disappearance of OKN on stimulation of the contralateral eye (Cazin et al. 1980b); (2) many NOT units (48%) increase their firing rate on temporonasal stimulation of the contralateral eye and give no response to nasotemporal stimuli, while 6% show a change in the opposite direction as well (Fig. 3). These findings are in accordance with OKN behavior (see Sect. 2.1); (3) these directionally specific units code retinal slip velocity, peak at around 1 deg/s slip velocity (Fig. 8) and show no response to vestibular stimulalation, i.e. carry a pure visual sensory signal (Cazin et al. 1980c).

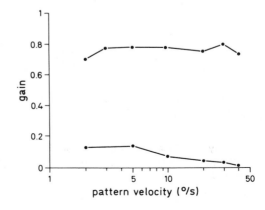

Fig. 1. Steady-state gain of slow phase eye velocity of OKN measured in the rat in monocular temporonasal *(upper)* and nasotemporal *(lower)* directions. Measurements were made with the electromagnetic search coil technique. Gain is defined as the ratio between slow phase eye velocity and stimulus velocity. The stimulus consisted of a random dot pattern projected on a cylindrical screen (unpublished results)

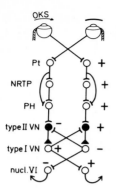

Fig. 2. Schematic diagram of the horizontal optokinetic pathway from the eye through the pretectum *(Pt)*, n.reticularis tegmenti pontis *(NRTP)*, prepositus hypoglossi nucleus *(PH)*, vestibular nuclei *(VN, type I* and *type II* neurons) to the abducens motoneurons *(n.VI)*. On the right-hand side, the response signs, i.e. increase *(+)* and decrease *(-)* in firing, are indicated for an optokinetic stimulus being temporonasal for the left eye (right eye covered). This stimulus causes an OKN with the slow phase to the right, i.e. firing noted in abducens motoneurons is appropriate. On the left-hand side, neuronal groups are identified. *Filled circle* neuron *(type II VN)* is inhibitory in nature. The vestibular commissure is also indicated. Further details, see text

Optokin. response pattern		Ipsil.eye T→N	N→T	Contral.eye T→N	N→T	% of units	Vestib. resp.
Pretectum	Unidirectional*	—	—	↑	—	48	—
	Bidirectional selective	↓	—	↑	—	16	—
		—	—	↑	↓	6	—
		↑	—	↓	—	3	—
NRTP	Unidirectional*	—	—	↑	—	43	Type II
		↑	—	—	—	8	Type I
	Bidirectional selective	↓	—	↑	—	16	Type II
		↑	—	↓	—	33	Type I
PH	Unidirectional*	—	—	↑	—	25	Type II
	Bidirectional selective	↓	—	↑	—	32	Type II
		↑	—	↓	—	37	Type I
VN	Bidirectional selective	↓	(↑)	↑	(↓)	40	Type II
		↑	—	↓	—	60	Type I
Floc	Bidirectional selective	↓	↑	↑*	↓	n=3	Type II
		↑*	↓	↓	↑	n=6	Type I

Fig. 3. Summary of unitary responses to optokinetic stimulation recorded in various pathway nuclei (Abbr. as in Fig. 2). $T \to N$ and $N \to T$ denote temporonasal and nasotemporal pattern motion. *Upward* and *downward arrows* indicate frequency increase or decrease, horizontal lines indicate no response. Unidirectional responses are those which showed an increased firing on temporonasal stimuli of the contralateral eye only and no responses to any other stimulation of either eye. Bidirectional units could either have monocular or binocular inputs. *Asteriks* in the *Floc* (flocculus) responses indicate the strongest responses. Further details, see text

As shown in Figs. 2 and 3, the n.reticularis tegmenti pontis (NRTP), n.prepositus hypoglossi (PH), and the n.vestibularis (VN) are important further links in the optokinetic pathway to ocular motoneurons. All these nuclei contain many neurons that have the same response directionality as Pt neurons, i.e., show a strong increase in firing on temporonasal and little change in discharge on nasotemporal stimulation. In addition, these neurons respond to vestibular stimulation (Fig. 3), i.e. also carry a head and/or eye velocity signal. They all are probably part of the slow build-up or velocity storage network (see 1.1). In summary then, the projections from the Pt to the ocular motoneurons may be as depicted in Fig. 2. There exist direct connections between Pt and NRTP (Teresawa et al. 1979; Cazin et al. 1982; Cazin et al. 1984; Torigoe et al. 1984) and Pt and PH (Cazin et al. 1982, 1984). The NRTP, in turn, projects to the PH (Torigoe et al. 1984; Cazin et al. 1984) and the PH to VN (McCrea et al. 1979). It should be noted that in the rat neither Pt or NRTP have direct projections to VN (Torigoe et al. 1984). While this connectivity has been established anatomically and electrophysiologically it should be emphasized that several other paths may be supplementing this basic circuit. In any event, when a temporonasal stimulus is presented to the left eye (Fig. 2) the Pt,

Fig. 4. Schematic representation of the input and output connections of the flocculus *(Floc)*. Abbr. as in Fig. 2. *Double-headed arrows* mutual connections (see text)

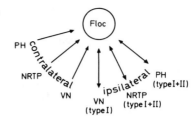

NRTP, PH, type II VN and abducens motoneurons on the right-hand side are excited while on the left the activities are changing in such a way that motoneurons are inhibited. Considering appropriate changes in firing in medial rectus motoneurons, the eyes would move to the right-hand side, i.e. produce a slow OKN phase. Whether motoneurons receive a significant input via pathways not involving the slow build-up path through the VN is not known at the present time but very likely.

This brief review of the existing knowledge on OKN pathway organization in the rat was necessary to illustrate where a motor control system, such as the cerebellum, could potentially interact with the optokinetic reflex. In fact, as schematically illustrated in Fig. 4, there exists anatomical and physiological evidence that the VN (cf. ref. Brodal 1974; Fukuda et al. 1972; Baker et al. 1972), the NRTP (Cazin et al. 1984; Blanks and Precht 1983) and PH (McCrea et al. 1979) project to and receive inputs from the flocculus directly as well as indirectly and are, therefore, all candidates for cerebellar interactions with the optokinetic system. Since all these nuclei are also related to the vestibular system (see above), they may take part in carrying vestibular and combined visual-vestibular signals to and receiving corresponding outputs from the cerebellum. Given the possibility of these multiple interaction sites, the analysis of the role of the cerebellum in optokinetic and visual-vestibular control appears to be rather complicated. As a first step of this analysis we studied the responses of floccular Purkinje cells and other cerebellar neurons to vestibular, optokinetic and combined stimulations (Blanks and Precht 1983) in very much the same conditions we had previously studied the VN (Cazin et al. 1980a), Pt and NRTP (Cazin et al. 1980c) and PH neurons. In the following we shall summarize the main results briefly.

2.3 Responses of Floccular Units to Optokinetic and Vestibular Stimulation

A total of 98 Purkinje cells (P-cells) and 81 non-P-cells in the flocculus were studied during vestibular stimulation, optokinetic stimulation (OKS) in open-loop condition and during a combination of the two. The simple spike activity of 72% of the P-cells responded to both OKS and vestibular stimulation. The remaining P-cells responded only to vestibular stimulation (19%) or to OKS (9%). In many P-cells, activity was often interrupted by bursts or pauses in activity during stimulation. Since the eyes were immobilized, a correlation with these bursts and pauses and eye movements was impossible, although one might assume that they were correlated with quick phases, as shown in the rabbit (Llinas et al. 1976) and monkey (Noda and Suzuki 1979). In the non P-cell group, comprised of those units showing no complex spikes (CS), 73% responded to vestibular stimuli and OKS, 2.5% to vestibular only, and 22% showed only pauses in activity or bursts of spikes which might have been associated with fast eye movements generated in conjunction with vestibular and optokinetic nystagmus.

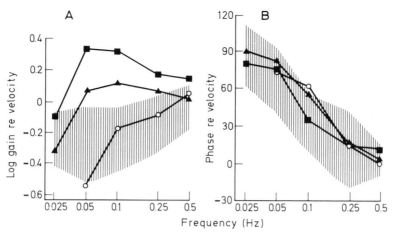

Fig. 5 A, B. Response characteristics of floccular P-cells in the rat during sinusoidal horizontal rotation in the dark. The response gain (**A**) and phase (**B**) relative velocity of three P-cells (two type II cells ■ and ○; one type I P-cell, ▲) are shown in relation to stimulus frequency over the range of 0.025-0.5 Hz. The peak angular velocity was constant (10°/s) at each frequency. *Stippled areas* encompass the mean ± 1 s.d. of the data for all type I and type II P-cells. (Blanks and Precht 1983)

2.3.1 Responses of Cerebellar Units to Vestibular Stimulation

Contrary to the monkey, but similar to the rabbit (see Sect. 1.1), it was relatively easy to detect responses to horizontal rotation in the flocculus. Of those units responding to both vestibular and OKS (n=71) 32 were type I (increase/decrease on ipsilateral/contralateral rotation) and 39 type II (reverse of type I), and the pure vestibular units (n=19) showed all type I responses. It should be mentioned here that the relatively large number of type I responses may in part be due to coexcitation of the vertical canals. In fact, it has recently been shown in the rabbit that with pure horizontal canal stimulation the majority of P-cells shows a type II response (Miyashita 1979; Leonard and Simpson 1983). Since in the rat VN practically all units responded to optokinetic stimulation it is surprising to find ca. 20% of the P-cells that responded only to vestibular stimuli. Presumably these P-cells received a primary vestibular input which is known to show no optokinetic responses (Blanks and Precht 1978).

Responses of P-cells to vestibular stimuli were qualitatively similar to those reported for the vestibular units in the rat (Cazin et al. 1980a), but there were some important quantitative differences that deserve attention. When tested with different amplitudes of oscillations at a given frequency, significant nonlinearities were observed with P-cells but not in non P-cells and VN. Such nonlinearities preclude a linear frequency analysis, given the strong dependence of phase and gain of unitary responses on stimulus amplitude. However, in order to compare P-cell responses with those of the VN, we tested P-cells with frequencies of 0.05-0.5 Hz where the peak amplitude of oscillation was 10 deg/s at each frequency. As shown in Fig. 5, the response phase lead relative to head velocity decreased with increasing frequency, whereas the velocity gain of these units increased with increasing frequency. At low frequencies P-cells had sensitivities very similar to those of VN, but, due to the above mentioned non-linearity, the cerebellar

Fig. 6. Changes in response phase and gain between vestibular only (rotation in dark) and visual-vestibular stimulation (rotation against earth fixed background) for 27 P-cells. The magnitude of the change for each parameter is given by the length of the *arrow* that points in the direction of the phase or gain evoked during combined stimulation. (Blanks and Precht 1983)

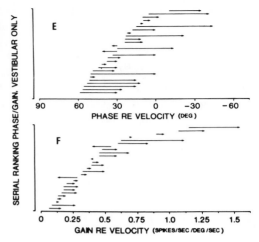

responses were much reduced in relation to VN responses with higher amplitudes at each frequency. Since the VN and non-P-cells did not show this non-linearity, it may be caused by cerebellar circuitry and/or bilateral canal interactions at the level of the cerebellum.

From a comparative point of view it is interesting to emphasize that P-cells in the rat and rabbit show distinct responses during rotation in the dark, while primates don't (see Sect. 1.1). In fact, the sensitivity of rat P-cells, when tested with low amplitudes, is quite similar to that of VN, a finding which again is very different from primates. Do rat P-cells receive different signals compared to primates? As pointed out above (Sect. 1.1) primate gaze velocity P-cells receive a head and eye velocity signal of similar amplitude and preferred directionality, so that when head and eye velocity are equal and opposite, P-cells do not respond to rotation in the dark. If rat P-cells received no or only a weak eye velocity signal, the head velocity signal might dominate and yield the responses seen in the dark. The present experiments in the rat do not allow us to determine the exact signal content of P-cells since the various paradigms used in the primate could so far not be applied in the rat experiments. This point will be taken up again below.

2.3.2 Visual-Vestibular Interaction

In order to examine the interaction between OKS and vestibular stimulation, the phase and sensitivity of cerebellar units in the dark (vestibular only) were compared to values obtained in a lighted, fixed-world environment (OKS and vestibular) at 0.1 Hz ± 15°. As shown in Fig. 6 the presence of the OKS increased sensitivity of the units by ca. 20% and shortened the phase lead (relative velocity) of most P-cells by ca. 25%. Similar changes were seen with non-P-cells (not shown). This visual-vestibular interaction is synergistic and implies that when a unit is activated by rotation to one side in the dark, pattern rotation in the opposite direction likewise causes an increase in firing (see also next section). Only two units showed a non-synergistic interaction, i.e. an increase in phase lead and a decreased sensitivity on combined stimulation. Similar synergistic interaction on combined stimulation has been shown for the rabbit P-cells (Ghelarducci 1975) and vestibular neurons in several species (Dichgans et al. 1973; Allum et al. 1976; Waespe and Henn 1977; Cazin et al. 1980a). The fact that rat and rabbit P-cells show a synergistic interaction very similar to that found in VN may indicate that in these species P-cells more closely reflect the vestibular input. In the monkey (Waespe and Henn 1981), P-cells responded to chair rotation with a frequency increase of SS discharge only during the conflict situation (pattern and chair rotating together so that the VOR needed to be suppressed for image stabilization) when retinal slip was present. They were activated unidirectionally by OKS moving to the same side, i.e. in an apparently "non-synergistic" fashion, probably dictated by the pursuit input. Such type of interaction was very rarely seen in the rat.

2.3.3 Optokinetic Responses of Cerebellar Units

As already pointed out, most cerebellar units showed clear responses to OKS. Fig. 7A illustrates the responses of a type II P-cell to OKS velocity steps of various amplitudes and directions. Note that with ipsilateral OKS firing increases ($+\triangle f$) and partially adapts during continued stimulation, whereas with contralateral OKS firing decreases ($-\triangle f$) and also adapts. On the average, $+\triangle f$ values were larger than $-\triangle f$ values (Fig. 7B). A small number of units showed only unidirectional responses and none were bidirectional, non-selective (increase or decrease in either direction). As already pointed out in Section 2.2.2, primate P-cell SS discharge was increased only to one direction of OKS which was identical to the direction activating the cell in the conflict situation. Also the responses of P-cells to OKS were not maintained except for stimulus velocities exceeding 60°/s. However, the CS of some primate P-cells responded bidirectionally to OKS (Waespe and Henn 1981).

In order to examine the velocity tuning curves for the OKS responses of P-cells, the $\pm\triangle f$ values for flocculus units were examined with velocity steps ranging from 0.25-10°/s. The results indicate that there were some differences in the OKS tuning curves of P-cells compared to non-P-cells. In general, P-cells peaked around 2°/s (Fig. 7B) and non-P-cells achieved their peaks at velocities of ca. 1°/s (Fig. 7D). The values for the tuning curves of non-P-cells and those obtained in Pt, NRTP, PH and VN were similar, while the mean tuning curve of P-cells was shifted towards higher velocities (Fig. 8). The ability of P-cells to fire at higher OKS velocities than other neurons is similar to findings obtained in monkey P-cells (Waespe and Henn 1981 and Waespe et al. this volume). It indicates that they probably receive inputs in addition to those illustrated in Fig. 4 (see below).

Further insights into the responses of floccular units to OKS can be obtained by measuring their response "time constants" (defined as 1/3 the time-to-peak increase or decrease). Some P-cells (10%) showed a slow exponential-like rise or fall in rate with the onset and termination of the OKS step which were governed by time constants of 3-4.5 s (Fig. 9A). This response pattern is similar to that of most VN, PH and NRTP units and seems to indicate an input from the velocity storage network, i.e. that eye velocity and not the visual input is coded in some fashion in these P-cells as well.

Most P-cells (78%), however, showed a faster rise (time constant = 0.5-3.0 s). These cells also were characterized by partial adaptation during OKS and a rapid fall and

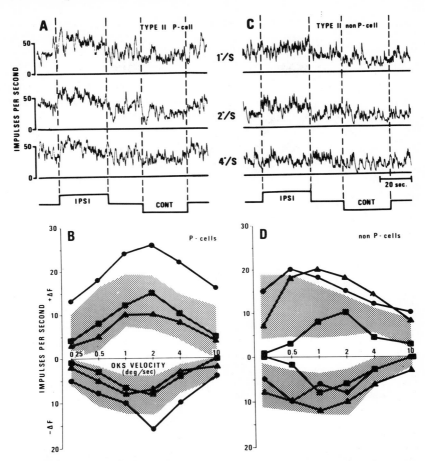

Fig. 7 A-D. The OKS responses of flocculus units are direction-and-speed-selective. Ipsilateral *(IPSI)* OKS increases type II P-cell **(A, B)** and non P-cell **C, D)** activity, whereas contralateral *(CONT)* OKS reduces their discharge rate. In **B** and **D**, response increases (+△f) and decreases (-△f) are plotted for three P-cells **(B)** and non P-cells **(D)**. *Stippled* areas encompass the mean ± 1 s.d. for all type I and II P-cells **(B)** and non P-cells **(D)**. Note that the peak change in firing rate for P-cells occurs with OKS velocities of 1.5-2°/s and 1.0°/s for non P-cells. (Blanks and Precht 1983)

"undershoot" with termination of the stimulus (Fig. 9B). Inputs to these cells may come from the shorter time constant units in NRTP, PH and VN as well as from other brain stem nuclei not yet identified. The optokinetically induced responses in these P-cells probably code retinal slip velocity or some central derivative of it. Activity related to optokinetic afternystagmus appears to be negligible in these units. Eleven percent of the P-cells were unresponsive to vestibular stimulation, but in each case showed a brisk rise and fall (time constant 0.5 s) in rate with the onset and termination of the optokinetic stimulus, respectively (Fig. 9C). In addition, these cells showed only a unidirectional (+△f) response to OKS. The origin of the input to this P-cell type is a problem. Apparently, the signal these cells carry is retinal slip or a central derivative of it, and the input may thus be coming from the Pt. But the Pt (NOT) does not project to the

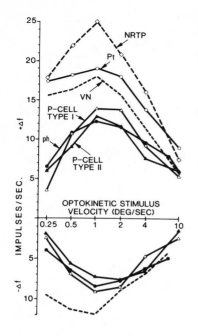

Fig. 8. Summary of the OKS tuning curves in the rat. The average responses of the type I and type II P-cells from the present study are compared to similarly obtained data from neurons of the *NRTP, PT, VN,* and *PH* in the rat. The curves for the *VN* combine the responses of type I and II neurons (Abbreviations *NRTP*, n.reticularis tegmenti pontis; *PT* pretectum; *VN* vestibular nucleus; *PH* prepositus hypoglossi n). (Blanks and Precht 1983)

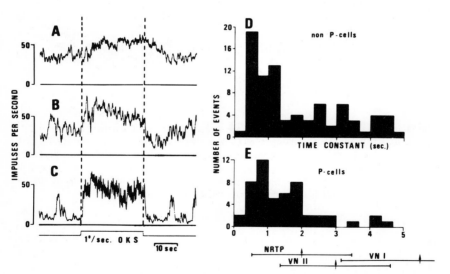

Fig. 9 A-E. Response time constants during constant velocity OKS (stimulus velocity = 1°/s). The neurons in **A** and **B** are type I and type II P-cells, respectively, whereas, the P-cell in **C** was not responsive to horizontal rotation but showed a brisk response to *OKS*. The time constants governing the rise and fall in discharge rate during *OKS* (measured as 1/3 the time to maximum) is shown for non-P-cells **(D)** and for P-cells **(E)**. Note that the *OKS* time constants for P-cells are shorter than those for type I *(VN I)* and type II *(VN II)* vestibular neurons and nucleus reticularis tegmenti pontis *(NRTP)* neurons in the same species. The mean and s.d. for *VN I, VN II,* and *NRTP* are given in **E** by the *arrows* and *horizontal bars.* (Blanks and Precht 1983)

flocculus. The NRTP and PH contain some neurons having very short time constants (Cazin et al. 1980c). However, all these cells also responded to pure vestibular stimuli, and the above P-cells did not. At present, therefore, the origin of the input to these presumed retinal slip coding P-cells is not known. On the basis of our retrograde study of the afferents to the flocculus in the rat (Blanks and Precht 1983) several candidates emerge, e.g. the pontine nuclei. Suzuki and Keller (1982) have, indeed, recorded retinal slip-related activity in the monkey's dorsolateral pontine nuclei. The question also arises of whether these P-cells, having such fast response characteristics, could be involved in the generation of the small initial jump in slow phase velocity of OKN in the rat? At present, however, we do not know whether this initial jump requires the integrity of the flocculus in the rat as it does in the monkey and cat (see Sects. 1.1 and 3).

Responses to Monocular Stimulations. As shown in Fig. 3, the majority of units in the Pt, NRTP and PH responded only to temporonasally directed stimulus motion presented to the contralateral eye, and stimulation of the ipsilateral eye gave no modulation of neural discharge. Some units responded to stimulation of either eye, but with each eye only one stimulus direction was effective. In the VN, however, all units responded to stimulation of both the contra- and ipsilateral eye. It was shown that the responses to stimulations of the ipsilateral eye were mediated by the vestibular commissure connecting the vestibular nuclei on the two sides (Cazin et al. 1980c). While type I VN showed a modulation in firing only with one direction of stimulation of either eye, ca. 10% of the type II units showed not only a strong increase in frequency on temporonasal stimuli (as the remaining 90% of type II units) but decreased firing on nasotemporal stimulation as well (Fig. 3, arrows in parenthesis). It is possible that such bidirectionally selective responses were also present in type I VN but were simply not detected in our sample. Given these response properties of units along the brainstem optokinetic pathway we thought it would be also interesting to study cerebellar units with monocular stimuli. The information derived from such experiments might elucidate further the nature of the nuclei projecting to the flocculus.

Monocular OKS responses of 17 P-cells (13 type I, 4 type II) and 10 non-P-cells (7 type I, 3 type II) were examined by covering first the ipsilateral and then the contralateral eye. Interestingly, the monocular OKS response of most P-cells examined (13/17) was bidirection-selective and of the same polarity regardless of which eye was stimulated, i.e. a type I P-cell in the left flocculus responded with an increase in firing with OKS to the right, independent of which eye was covered. This is in sharp contrast to most of the other nuclei of the optokinetic pathway (see above and Fig. 3).

Even though P-cells could be driven bidirectionally from the ipsi- and contralateral eye, one eye always predominated. Thus, in ca. half the cases, the ipsilateral eye produced the strongest frequency increase, whereas the contralateral eye was most effective in the remaining half. Furthermore, the largest firing increases were produced with temporonasal stimulation of the ipsilateral eye for type I P-cells and with temporonasal stimulation of the contralateral eye for type II. It should be noted that this latter pattern of activation is consistent with the responses of a small portion of type II VN units (the 10% mentioned above).

Examination of the non-P-cells revealed that half showed unidirectional responses to monocular OKS, as the majority of Pt, NRTP, PH and VN, while the remainder responded bidirection-selectively, as did the majority of P-cells.

The binocular responses found in most P-cells are best explained on the basis of convergence of crossed and uncrossed projections from NRTP, PH and VN for which there is ample anatomical (Blanks and Precht 1983) and physiological (Cazin et al. 1984) evidence. Somewhat more difficult to explain are the bidirectional selective responses of P-cells and some non P-cells with monocular OKS, since such a response pattern was not found in the NRTP and PH, and only a small group of VN units showed this response pattern (Fig. 3). Possibly other, not yet identified nuclei, are, in addition to the small VN population, responsible input sources to the cerebellar cortex.

Purkinje Complex Spike Responses to OKS. Up until now, we have considered only the simple spike (SS) responses of P-cells. OKS also modulates CS activity, as has been reported in the rabbit and monkey (see Sect. 1.1). The CS responses were examined in 27 P-cells and in most of them, the OKS responses of the CS were opposite in polarity of those of the SS. In three units, the CS response was bidirectional, but, more typically, there was a unidirectional increase with ipsilateral OKS in type I P-cells and contralateral OKS for type II P-cells. Interestingly, in a few units in the monkey, CS activity in the flocculus showed predominantly bidirectional responses while SS responses were unidirectional (Waespe and Henn 1981). The sensitivity of the CS response in the rat flocculus was low (ca. 1-2 imp/s at 1°/s stimulus velocity) and adapted rapidly. Because of the low sensitivity and limitations of the stimulating system in the low velocity range, the tuning curves for CS activity were not systematically studied. However, the best $+\triangle f$ values were obtained with stimulus velocities below 1°/s. Similar findings have been obtained in the rabbit (cf. ref. Simpson et al. 1979). In conclusion it may be stated that CS activity in the flocculus of subprimates and possibly also primates signals retinal slip, i.e. a visual input per se.

3 The Horizontal Optokinetic System and its Relationship with the Flocculus in the Cat

3.1 Horizontal Optokinetic Eye Nystagmus

As already pointed out in Section 2.1, the OKN in cat and monkey differ from that in the rat in that monocular stimulation yields symmetrical responses of almost identical amplitudes in cat and monkey, while highly asymmetric OKN responses were noted in the rat. Furthermore, the steady-state OKN gain remains high over a wider range of OKS velocities in cat and monkey as compared to the rat. Finally, the initial fast rise in OKN slow phase velocity is readily evoked in the monkey and cat but less frequently seen in rats and, when present, of small amplitude. However, it should be mentioned that the initial fast rise in slow phase velocity, though present in most of the cats studied, appears to be somewhat more difficult to evoke in the cat as compared to the monkey. Thus, in a given experiment it was missing in some trials and present in others, with no obvious relationship to the general state of alertness. If the generation of the fast initial jump is, indeed, largely related to the pursuit system (see Section 1.1) it is not so surprising that the cat — known to have a rather poor pursuit system (Evinger and Fuchs 1978) — shows a poor performance in the OKS paradigm as well. As will be seen below (Section 3.3), the relatively frequent absence of the initial rise of OKN in the cat has some advantage in the interpretation of floccular lesion experiments.

3.2 Optokinetic Pathway Organization

In the cat, the neuronal organization of the optokinetic brainstem pathway is not as well studied as in the rat. However, lesion studies suggest that the Pt and NRTP are — as in the rat — important relay nuclei for horizontal OKN (Precht and Strata 1980). Anatomical studies also support this assumption and, in addition, indicate that the Pt projects to the PH (Magnin et al. 1983) which, in the rat, has been implicated in the optokinetic pathway (see Sect. 2.2). Finally, in the cat the VN readily responds to OKS (Keller and Precht 1979) and projects to the flocculus as do NRTP and PH neurons (cf. ref. Blanks and Precht 1983). It may, therefore, tentatively be assumed that the pathway scheme depicted in Fig. 2, and the connectivity indicated in Fig. 4 for the rat, also applies to the cat.

While the response characteristics of floccular units to optokinetic and vestibular stimuli are not known in the cat, electrical stimulation of the flocculus has been shown to inhibit certain vestibuloocular neurons (Baker et al. 1972). If we assume that some of these neurons are also involved in mediating the signals necessary for the slow build-up of slow phase eye velocity of OKN (see Sect. 1.1) and that floccular P-cells respond to OKS, it will be interesting to examine the responses of VN to OKS with and without the flocculus. Furthermore, the effects of floccular lesions on OKN should be examined. In the next section some preliminary data relating to this topic will be summarized.

3.3 Effects of Flocculus Lesion on OKN and Optokinetic Responses of VN

Selective surgical removal of the flocculus is technically very difficult and has so far not been achieved. Therefore, flocculus lesion in this context implies that the paraflocculus was likewise damaged. When such lesions are performed in the cat (Keller and Precht 1979), the steady-state OKN gain at higher stimulus velocities is clearly lower than that in intact control animals (Fig. 10). Similar results are obtained with total removal of the cerebellum (Fig. 10). As already mentioned in Section 1.1, very similar results were obtained in the rabbit and monkey. The OKN gain deficiency has been explained in the monkey solely by the impairment of the fast initial rise in slow phase OKN velocity by the cerebellar lesion (Waespe et al. 1983). It was claimed that the slow build-up or brainstem pathway was not affected by the lesion in the monkey.

How do floccular lesions affect the initial fast rise in OKN velocity in the cat? Our recent experiments with bilaterally flocculectomized cats revealed that, after such lesions, the initial jump could no longer be detected. Figure 11 shows that the initial jump present prior to the lesion (Fig. 11A) is replaced by a very slow build-up of eye velocity to steady-state even at postoperative time periods as long as 6 weeks after the lesion (Fig. 11B). So it seems that both the gain deficiency as well as the prolonged time to steady-state velocity (Fig. 11) could be — as in primates — explained by the impairment of the fast pathway system.

Is the slow-build up of OKN velocity affected by the lesion? To answer this question the cat is more suitable than the monkey since even in the intact cat the fast rise in velocity is often not present. Thus, if one were to compare the time to steady-state without jump in a control animal with that in a flocculectomized cat, a difference should appear if the lesion affected the slow build-up. The results of one such experiment are shown in Fig. 12. In the control measurement, depicted in Fig. 12B, the slow

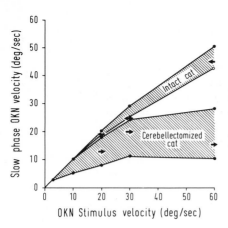

Fig. 10. Steady-state input-output relationship for *OKN* measured in intact and cerebellar lesion cats. The upper crossed hatched area shows the range of data obtained in four intact cats, and the lower region gives the range obtained in three cerebellectomized cats. *Arrows* show individual data points for one cat with a unilateral flocculectomy on the right-hand side. *Arrowheads* to the right *(left)* indicate measurements made for rightward *(leftward)* *OKS* and rightward *(leftward)* slow phase eye movements. (Keller and Precht 1979)

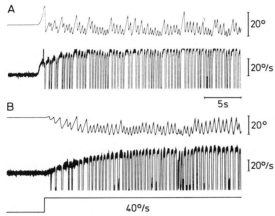

Fig. 11 A, B. Effects of flocculus lesion on the initial fast rise of slow phase OKN velocity in the cat. **A** OKN evoked by a step of surround motion (40°/s) in the intact, and **B** in the flocculectomized cat (4 weeks p.o.). Upper and lower records in **A** and **B** give horizontal eye position and eye velocity, respectively

build-up dominates the time course of OKN velocity and a fast jump is missing in this particular test. After the lesion, the time necessary to reach steady-state (Fig. 12A) is much prolonged compared to those controls showing no initial jump (Fig. 12C, dashed line). It is only in the OKS velocity range below 20 deg/s that the control and lesion measurements are similar. These results suggest that the slow pathway or the velocity storage network is also affected by the cerebellar lesion in the cat and that the lesion results in a significant increase in the time to steady-state. Provided the stimulus velocity is not too large the steady-state gain reached in the lesioned animal may be very similar to that before the lesion.

In support of the findings reported here are the data obtained in a different set of experiments describing the velocity tuning curves of VN units before and after cerebellar lesions (Keller and Precht 1979). As shown in Fig. 13, the mean tuning curves of control and lesion cats differ both in magnitude of responses and peak velocities at which the maximal frequency increase of unit firing is obtained. It appears that flocculus lesion affects the behavior of the nonlinearity, found at all levels of the slow build-up pathway (e.g. Fig. 8). This nonlinearity has been found in various species and in the rabbit occurs already in the retinal ganglion cells (Oyster et al. 1972). It is also subject to

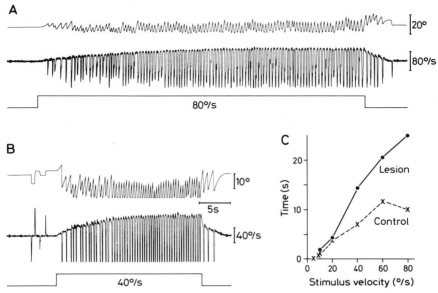

Fig. 12 A-C. Effects of flocculectomy on the time course of the slow build-up of OKN slow phase velocity in the cat. **A** and **B** are recordings taken after and before flocculus lesion. Note that also in the control record **B** the fast rise is missing; **C** comparison of the time to steady-state measured in control records showing no initial rise *(dashed line)* and in flocculectomized condition *(solid line)*. Note that in the latter case, time to steady-state is much prolonged

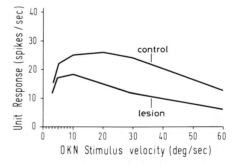

Fig. 13. Effects of cerebellar lesion on the opto-kinetic responses (tuning curves) of vestibular neurons in the cat. Recordings were obtained with the eyes immobilized (open-loop). Note that VN responses after cerebellar lesion peak at lower retinal slip velocities and show an overall reduced response magnitude. (Keller and Precht 1979)

central modification (Collewijn 1975). Since VN seem to play an important role in the slow build-up of OKN velocity, the single unit data of Fig. 13 can, at least in part, explain the prolongation of time to steady-state shown in Fig. 12. It remains to be shown if primates or other subprimates reveal a similar deficiency of the slow build-up when tested under similar conditions.

Unfortunately the rather extensive floccular lesion studies performed in the rabbit (Ito et al. 1982; Nagao 1983) cannot answer this question since the stimulus velocities applied were below those necessary to activate the storage network (Collewijn 1969, 1972), i.e. the authors were testing some sort of a fast pathway which has a maximum amplitude of $2°$ deg/s. The fact, however, that a decrease in OKN gain was observed at these low velocities after the lesion indicates that this small amplitude initial rise is affected by the flocculus lesion. At present the nature of the small initial fast rise in the rabbit is not known. Since the rabbit has no effective pursuit system and OKN is not affected by cortical lesions (Collewijn 1981) it may be an inherent property of brain-stem OKN pathways which, in turn, are under floccular influence. In this context it should be recalled that amphibia are devoid of the slow build-up system and show a fast build-up of OKN slow phase velocity (Dieringer and Precht 1982; Dieringer et al. 1983) which might be, in part produced by the direct input of the relay nucleus in the pre-tectum to ocular motoneurons (Cochran et al. 1984). Similar short-latency paths may likewise exist in higher vertebrates. In fact, flocculectomy in the primate never com-pletely abolished the initial jump in velocity suggesting the existence of extrafloccular pathways, possibly located in the brainstem.

4 Concluding Remarks

After a brief review of the literature concentrating on the importance of the vestibulo-cerebellum for vestibular, visual-vestibular and optokinetic functions, the present paper gave a description of recent work performed in the rat and the cat in regard to floccular function and compared, whenever possible, the subprimate data with those obtained in primates.

In primates, the flocculus is intimately involved in the generation of ocular pursuit and participates in the production of the fast initial rise of slow phase OKN velocity. Its effect on VOR gain is less predictable at least when measured in the subacute post-lesion period. A similar conclusion may tentatively be drawn from studies done in the cat, though more work is needed to substantiate it. While in the monkey the slow build-up system (velocity storage network) is said to be little affected by floccular lesion, changes in the nonlinearity of this system have been noted in the cat after similar le-sions. The latter finding may suggest that floccular P-cells influence vestibular neurons involved in the VOR, while such influence is not evident in the primate.

In afoveate mammals such as the rabbit and rat, having no independent ocular pursuit, the function of the flocculus must obviously be different from that in the monkey and the cat in this respect. Available data suggest that the small and fast initial rise in slow phase OKN velocity, present in these species, is under floccular control, whatever the exact nature of this fast rise may be. Whether the velocity storage system is under floccular control in afoveate species is not known at the present time, though the response properties of P-cells described above make it quite likely. VOR gain, in the rabbit, is consistently decreased after floccular lesions contrary to the unpredictable effects seen in primates and the cat.

Comparing the response properties of floccular P-cells studied during vestibular, optokinetic and combined stimuli in monkey and rat (rabbit) several distinct species differences emerge. In the primate, P-cells receive head and eye velocity signals of similar magnitude and directional preference and little sensory visual input. P-cells of subpri-mates such as the rat and rabbit receive a head velocity signal and probably also a signal related to slow phase eye velocity during OKN and OKAN. However, contrary to pri-mates, P-cell firing in the rat and rabbit is significantly and bidirectionally modulated by vestibular stimulation in the dark implying that cancellation of head and eye velocity signals (if present) is poor.

Another striking difference between primate and rat (rabbit) P-cells is revealed when their responses to OKS are analyzed. In the primate, increases of P-cell discharge on vestibular stimulation (conflict) and OKS have the same directional preference, while in subprimates the OKS and vestibular stimuli have opposite directions to produce the same effect on firing frequency. Since such synergistic interaction is also seen in all vestibular neurons of both primates and subprimates, the P-cells of subprimates much more reflect the properties of brainstem neurons involved in the OKN, whereas in the primate, responses are dominated by the pursuit system. Furthermore, primate P-cells show a maintained firing only during high velocity OKS (when the slow system fails) whereas P-cells of the rat show maintained firing over a large range of velocities, although with a maximal sensitivity at higher velocities (Fig. 8) than the brainstem units. Finally, another major species difference relates to the presence of a strong sensory visual input, both via mossy and climbing fibers, to P-cells in rat and rabbit and the rather weak nature of such an input in the primate.

Acknowledgement. Supported by grants 3.228.82 and 3.403.083 from the Swiss National Science Foundation and the Dr. Eric Slack-Gyr Foundation (W. Precht); Research grants EY03018 and EY00160 from the National Eye Institute (R. Blanks); Twinning Grant of the European Science Foundation to P. Strata, P. Montarolo and W. Precht. The authors would like to thank Mrs E. Hitz, Mrs G. Mack, Mrs E. Schneider, and Mr A. Fäh for excellent technical assistance.

References

Albus JS (1971) A theory of cerebellar function. Math Biosci 10: 25-61

Allum JHJ, Graf W, Dichgans J, Schmidt CL (1976) Visual-vestibular interactions in the vestibular nuclei of the goldfish. Exp Brain Res 26: 463-485

Baker R, Precht W, Llinas R (1972) Cerebellar modulatory action on the vestibulo-trochlear pathway in the cat. Exp Brain Res 15: 364-385

Batini C, Ito M, Kadao RT, Jastreboff PJ, Miyashita Y (1979) Interaction between the horizontal vestibular-ocular reflex and optokinetic response in rabbits. Exp Brain Res 37: 1-15

Blanks RHI, Precht W (1978) Response properties of vestibular afferents in alert cats during optokinetic and vestibular stimulation. Neurosci Lett 10: 225-229

Blanks RHI, Precht W (1983) Responses of units in the rat cerebellar flocculus during optokinetic and vestibular stimulation. Exp Brain Res 53: 1-15

Brodal A (1974) Anatomy of the vestibular nuclei and their connections. In: Kornhuber HH (ed) Handbook of sensory physiology, vol VI/1. Springer, Berlin Heidelberg New York, p 239

Cazin L, Precht W, Lannou J (1980a) Optokinetic responses of vestibular nucleus neurons in the rat. Pflüger's Arch 384: 31-38

Cazin L, Precht W, Lannou J (1980b) Pathways mediating optokinetic responses of vestibular nucleus neurons in the rat. Pflüger's Arch 384: 19-29

Cazin L, Precht W, Lannou J (1980c) Firing characteristics of neurons mediating optokinetic responses to rat's vestibular neurons. Pflüger's Arch 386: 221-230

Cazin L, Magnin M, Lannou J (1982) Non-cerebellar visual afferents to the vestibular nuclei involving the prepositus hypoglossal complex: an autoradiographic study in the rat. Exp Brain Res 48: 309-313

Cazin L, Lannou J, Precht W (1984) An electrophysiological study of pathways mediating optokinetic responses to the vestibular nucleus in the rat. Exp Brain Res 54: 337-348

Cochran SL, Dieringer N, Precht W (1984) Basic optokinetic-ocular reflex pathways in the frog. J Neurosci Vol. 4, No 1, 43-57

Cohen B, Uemura T, Takemori S (1973) Effects of labyrinthectomy on optokinetic nystagmus (OKN) and optokinetic after-nystagmus (OKAN). Equil Res 3: 88-93

Cohen B, Matsuo, Raphan T (1977) Quantitative analysis of the velocity characteristics of optokinetic nystagmus and optokinetic afternystagmus. J Physiol 270: 321-344

Collewijn H (1969) Optokinetic eye movements in the rabbit: input-output relations. Vision Res 9: 117-132

Collewijn H (1972) An analog model of the rabbit's optokinetic system. Brain Res 36: 71-88

Collewijn H (1975) Direction-selective units in the rabbit's nucleus of the optic tract. Brain Res. 100: 489-508

Collewijn H (1981) The oculomotor system of the rabbit and its plasticity. In: Braitenberg V (ed) Studies of brain function, vol V. Springer, Berlin Heidelberg New York, p 240

Dichgans J, Schmidt CL, Graf W (1973) Visual input improves the speedometer function of the vestibular nuclei in the goldfish. Exp Brain Res 18: 319-322

Dieringer N, Precht W (1982) Compensatory head and eye movements in the frog and their contribution to stabilization of gaze. Exp Brain Res 47: 394-406

Dieringer N, Cochran SL, Precht W (1983) Differences in the central organization of gaze stabilizing reflexes between frog and turtle. J Comp Physiol 153: 495-508

Evinger C, Fuchs AR (1978) Saccadic, smooth pursuit and optokinetic eye movements of the trained cat. J Physiol 185: 209-229

Fukuda J, Highstein SM, Ito M (1972) Cerebellar inhibitory control of the vestibulo-ocular reflex investigated in rabbit IIIrd nucleus. Exp Brain Res 14: 511-526

Ghelarducci B (1975) Impulse discharges from flocculus Purkinje cells of alert rabbits during visual stimulation combined with horizontal head rotation. Brain Res 87: 66-72

Gonshor A, Melvill-Jones G (1976) Extreme vestibulo-ocular adaptation induced by prolonged optical reversal of vision. J Physiol 256: 381-414

Herrick CJ (1924) Origin and evolution of the cerebellum. Arch Neurol Psychiat 11: 621-652

Igarashi M, Miyata H, Kato Y, Wright WK, Levy JK (1975) Optokinetic nystagmus after cerebellar uvulonodulectomy in squirrel monkeys. Acta Otolaryngol 80: 180-184

Ito M (1977a) Functional specialization of flocculus Purkinje cells and their differential localization determined in connection with the vestibulo-ocular reflex. In: Baker R, Berthoz A (eds) Control of gaze by brain stem neurons, developments in neuroscience, vol I. Elsevier, Amsterdam, p 514

Ito M (1977b) Neuronal events in the cerebellar flocculus associated with an adaptive modification of the vestibulo-ocular reflex of the rabbit. In: Baker R, Berthoz A (eds) Control of gaze by brain stem neurons, developments in neuroscience, vol I. Elsevier, Amsterdam, p 514

Ito M, Shiida T, Yagi N, Yamamoto M (1974) Visual influence on rabbit's horizontal vestibulo-ocular reflex that presumably is effected via the cerebellar flocculus. Brain Res 65: 170-174

Ito M, Jastreboff PJ, Miyashita Y (1982) Specific effects of unilateral lesions in the flocculus upon eye movements in albino rabbits. Exp Brain Res 45: 233-242

Keller EL, Precht W (1979) Visual-vestibular responses in vestibular nuclear neurons in intact and cerebellectomized, alert cat. Neuroscience 4: 1599-1613

Larsell O (1934) Morphogenesis and evolution of the cerebellum. Arch Neurol Psychiatr 31: 373-395

Leonard CS, Simpson JI (1983) Rotational polarity of Purkinje cell activity in the rabbit flocculus. Soc Neurosci Abstr 9, pt 1: 608

Lisberger SG, Fuchs AF (1978a) Role of primate flocculus during rapid behavioral modification of vestibuloocular reflex. I. Purkinje cell activity during visually guided horizontal smooth-pursuit eye movements and passive head rotation. J Neurophysiol 41: 733-763

Lisberger SG, Fuchs AF (1978b) Role of primate flocculus during rapid behavioral modification of vestibuloocular reflex. II. Mossy fiber firing patterns during horizontal head rotation and eye movement. J Neurophysiol 41: 764-777

Llinas R, Simpson JI, Precht W (1976) Nystagmic modulation of neuronal activity in rabbit cerebellar flocculus. Pflüger's Arch 367: 7-13

Maekawa K, Simpson JI (1972) Climbing fiber activation of Purkinje cell in the flocculus by impulses transferred through the visual pathway. Brain Res 39: 245-251

Maekawa K, Simpson JI (1973) Climbing fiber responses evoked in vestibulocerebellum of rabbit from visual system. J Neurophysiol 36: 649-666

Maekawa K, Takeda T, Kimura M (1981) Neural activity of nucleus reticularis tegmenti pontis. The origin of visual mossy fiber afferents to the cerebellar flocculus of rabbits. Brain Res 210: 17-30

Magnin M, Courjon JH, Flandrin JM (1983) Possible visual pathways to the cat vestibular nuclei involving the nucleus prepositus hypoglossi. Exp Brain Res 51: 298-303

Maioli C, Precht W (1984) The horizontal optokinetic nystagmus in the cat. Exp Brain Res 55: 494-506

Marr D (1969) A theory of cerebellar cortex. J Physiol 202: 437-470

McCrea RA, Baker R, Delgado-Garcia J (1979) Afferent and efferent organization of the prepositus hypoglossi nucleus. Progress in brain research 50. Elsevier/North Holland Biomedical Press, Amsterdam, pp 653-665

Meiry JL (1971) Vestibular and proprioceptive stabilization of eye movements. In: Bach-y-Rita P, Collins CC (eds) The control of eye movements. Academic Press, London New York

Miles FA, Fuller JH (1975) Visual tracking and the primate flocculus. Scinese 189: 1000-1002

Miles FA, Fuller JH, Braitman DJ, Dow BM (1980a) Long-term adaptive changes in primate vestibulo-ocular reflex. III. Electrophysiological observations in flocculus of normal monkeys. J Neurophysiol 43: 1437-1476

Miles FA, Braitman DJ, Dow BM (1980b) Long-term adaptive changes in primate vestibulo-ocular reflex. IV. Electrophysiological observations in flocculus of adapted monkeys. J Neurophysiol 43: 1477-1493

Miyashita Y (1979) Interaction of visual and canal inputs on the oculomotor system via the cerebellar flocculus. In: Granit R, Pompeiano O (eds) Reflex control of posture and movement. Progress in brain research 50. Elsevier/North Holland Biomedical Press, Amsterdam, pp 695-702

Miyashita Y (1981) Differential roles of the climbing and mossy fiber visual pathways in vision-guided modification of the vestibulo-ocular reflex. In: Flohr H, Precht W (eds) Lesion-induced neuronal plasticity in sensorimotor systems. Springer, Berlin Heidelberg New York, pp 305-313

Montarolo PG, Precht W, Strata P (1981) Functional organization of the mechanisms subserving the optokinetic nystagmus in the cat. Neuroscience 6: 231-246

Nagao S (1983) Effects of vestibulocerebellar lesions upon dynamic characteristics and adaptation of vestibulo-ocular and optokinetic responses in pigmented rabbits. Exp Brain Res 53: 36-46

Noda H, Suzuki DA (1979) The role of the flocculus of the monkey in saccadic eye movements. J Physiol 294: 317-334

Oyster CW, Takahashi E, Collewijn H (1972) Direction-selective retinal ganglion cells and control of optokinetic nystagmus in the rabbit. Vision Res 12: 183-193

Pasik T, Pasik P (1964) Optokinetic nystagmus: an unlearned response altered by section of chiasma and corpus callosum in monkeys. Nature (London) 203: 609-611

Precht W (1975) Cerebellar influences on eye movements. In: Lennerstrand G, Bach-Y-Rita P (eds) Basic mechanisms of ocular motility and their clinical implications. Pergamon Press, Oxford New York, pp 261-280

Precht W (1978) Neuronal operations in the vestibular system. In: Braitenberg V (ed) Studies of brain function, vol II. Springer, Verlin Heidelberg New York, p 226

Precht W (1981) Visual-vestibular interaction in vestibular neurons: functional pathway organization. N Y Acad Sci 374: 230-248

Precht W (1982) Anatomical and functional organisation of optokinetic pathways. In: Lennerstrand G (ed) Functional basis of ocular motility disorders. Pergamon Press, Oxford New York, pp 291-302

Precht W, Strata P (1980) On the pathway mediating optokinetic responses in vestibular nuclear neurons. Neuroscience 5: 777-787

Precht W, Cazin L, Blanks RHI, Lannou J (1982) Anatomy and physiology of the optokinetic pathways to the vestibular nuclei in the rat. In: Roucoux A, Crommelinck M (eds) Physiological and pathological aspects of eye movements. Junk, The Hague Boston London, pp 153-172

Robinson DA (1974) The effect of cerebellectomy on the cat's vestibulo-ocular integrator. Brain Res 71: 195-207

Simpson JI, Alley KE (1974) Visual climbing fiber input to rabbit vestibulo-cerebellum: a source of direction-specific information. Brain Res 82: 302-308

Simpson JI, Soodak RE, Hess R (1979) The accessory optic system and its relation to the vestibulo-cerebellum. In: Granit R, Pompeiano O (eds) Reflex control of posture and movement. Progress in brain research 50. Elsevier/North Holland Biomedical Press, Amsterdam, pp 715-724

Suzuki DA, Keller EL (1982) Visuo-oculomotor interactions in dorsolateral pontine nucleus of alert monkey. Soc Neurosci Abstr 291

Takemori S, Cohen B (1974) Loss of visual suppression of vestibular nystagmus after flocculus lesions. Brain Res 72: 213-224

Teresawa K, Otani K, Yamada J (1979) Descending pathways of the nucleus of the optic tract in the rat. Brain Res 173: 405-417

Torigoe Y, Blanks RHI, Precht W (1984) Anatomical studies on the nucleus reticularis tegmenti pontis in the pigmented rat: II. Subcortical afferents (demonstrated by the retrograde transport of horseradish peroxidase). (submitted)

Waespe W, Henn V (1977) Neuronal activity in the vestibular nuclei of the alert monkey during vestibular and optokinetic stimulation. Exp Brain Res 27: 523-538

Waespe W, Henn V (1981) Visual-vestibular interaction in the flocculus of alert monkey. II. Purkinje cell activity. Exp Brain Res 43: 349-360

Waespe W, Cohen B, Raphan T (1983) Role of the flocculus and paraflocculus in optokinetic nystagmus and visual-vestibular interactions: effects of lesions. Exp Brain Res 50: 9-33

Westheimer G, Blair M (1973) Oculomotor defects in cerebellectomized monkeys. Investig Opthal 12: 618-621

Zee DS, Yamazaki A, Butler PH, Gücer G (1981) Effects of ablation of flocculus and paraflocculus on eye movements in primate. J Neurophysiol 46: 878-899

Zee DS, Butler PH, Optican LM, Tusa RJ, Gücer G (1982) Effects of bilateral occipital lobectomies on eye movements in monkeys: preliminary observations. In: Roucoux A, Crommelinck M (eds) Physiological and pathological aspects of eye movements. Junk, The Hague Boston London, pp 225-232

The Primate Flocculus in Visual-vestibular Interactions: Conceptual, Neurophysiological, and Anatomical Problems

W. Waespe and V. Henn [1]

1 Introduction

Unblurred vision is mandatory for the orderly processing of visual information during eye and head movements; image slip on the retina of only a few degrees per second diminishes visual acuity (Westheimer and McKee, 1975). Several mechanisms have developed to generate slow eye movements which are aimed at preventing blurring of images on the retina during movements. Head movements induce in all mammals slow eye movements, i.e. compensatory eye movements, into the direction opposite to the head movement via the *vestibulo-ocular reflex arc* (VOR). Movements of large parts of the visual surround or of single objects induce slow eye movements into the direction of the moving pattern. Continuous rotation of the visual surround induces in foveate and afoveate animals a typical repetitive sequence of eye movements, *optokinetic nystagmus* (OKN). In foveate animals movement of a single target object can elicit *smooth pursuit* eye movements.

There are situations of visual-vestibular interaction in which movements induced by the VOR increase image slip and blurred vision instead of reducing it. During head movements within a head-stationary visual surround, or during tracking of a moving object with the head, the slow eye movements elicited by the VOR are directed opposite to the moving scene or object. These eye movements must be cancelled, otherwise they would take the eyes off the target. It is therefore necessary that signals inducing the different types of slow eye movements interact within the central nervous system. This was recognized already by Mowrer (1937) who suggested that the interaction between vestibular and visual (optokinetic) information takes place in the vestibular nuclei. Ito's hypothesis in 1972 that the flocculus might play a crucial role in such interaction because of its varied and multisensory inputs renewed the interest in the vestibulo-cerebellum. Ito further suggested that the analysis of flocculus activity during visual-vestibular interaction might also furnish hypotheses about principles of cerebellar function in general (Ito, 1982).

The three-neuronal vestibulo-ocular reflex arc is composed of primary vestibular neurons, secondary neurons in the vestibular nuclei and oculomotor neurons (Lorente de Nó, 1933; Fig. 1). The VOR is an open-loop reflex as its output does not influence the input, i.e. its performance does not feed back on the labyrinth. The advantage of an open-loop system is its speed (latency for the VOR is in the order of 10-20 ms). The disadvantage is its susceptability to internal disturbances by lesions. Insufficiencies

---

[1]   Department of Neurology, University Hospital, 8091 Zürich, Switzerland

Cerebellar Functions
ed. by Bloedel et al.
© Springer-Verlag Berlin Heidelberg 1984

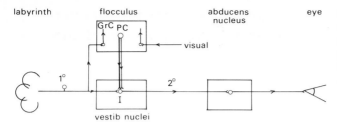

Fig. 1. Scheme of the main connections important in the generation and visual suppression of the VOR in the rabbit. (Ito, 1972, 1976, 1982)

in the VOR with its main function of stabilizing vision could, however, readily be corrected by visual information. Ito suggested that the flocculus is an essential part in the immediate and adaptive (by parametric changes) readjustment of the VOR by visual feedback. The flocculus would be suited for this task (Fig. 1) as it is reported to receive vestibular information directly from primary vestibular fibers as a mossy fiber (MF) input (cat: Brodal and Høivik, 1964; monkey: Carpenter et al. 1972; rabbit: Alley, 1977) and visual information via MFs and climbing fibers (Maekawa and Takeda, 1976). Furthermore, floccular Purkinje cells (P-cells) project to the vestibular nuclei (cat: Angaut and Brodal, 1967; monkey: Dow, 1938; Haines, 1977; rabbit: Alley, 1977) and in the rabbit secondary vestibular neurons are inhibited by stimulation in the flocculus (Fukuda et al., 1972). Ito (1972, 1976, 1982) − based on data in the rabbit − has therefore assumed that floccular P-cells modulate the VOR in relation to visual inputs either on a short-term or long-term basis by directly modulating the activity of secondary vestibular neurons (Fig. 1).

During recent years experimental data accumulated by employing behavioral paradigms and correlating single unit activity to eye movements and a variety of stimuli in alert animals. This permits a test of Ito's floccular hypothesis in the monkey. In the following we will concentrate on the immediate visual-vestibular interactions in the alert monkey and we will mention the visually induced plastic (adaptive) changes of the VOR only briefly (Miles and Lisberger, 1981; Gonshor and Melvill Jones, 1976; Lisberger et al. 1981; Ito, 1982). Also in the following we compare the results obtained in both species, the monkey and the rabbit (see Precht et al., this vol, for a more complete discussion of data from subprimates).

2 Results

2.1 Vestibular and Visually Induced Slow Eye Movements

The gain of the horizontal *vestibular nystagmus* (VN) in the monkey (defined as the ratio of eye velocity to head velocity) is close to 1.0 (Zee et al. 1981; Lisberger et al. 1981). The dominant time constant (T_c) determined by impulses of accelerations or calculated from the response to sinusoidal stimulation, ranges between 10 and 40 s or greater (Raphan et al. 1979; Waespe et al. 1980), and is longer than that found in the activity of eighth nerve fibers which is 5-6 s (Goldberg and Fernandez, 1981; Büttner and Waespe, 1981). By comparison, in the rabbit the gain of the VOR is 0.3-0.5 (Batini et al. 1979; Nagao, 1983).

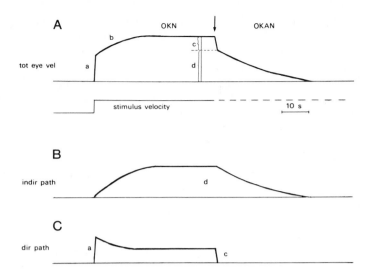

Fig. 2 A-C. A Velocity of the slow phase of the *OKN (tot eye vel)* in response to a step in stimulus velocity *(second line)*. Downward *arrow* lights off; **B** Hypothetical activity within the "indirect" visual-oculomotor pathways with the "velocity storage" or the *OKN*-system *(indir path)*; **C** Hypothetical activity within the "direct" pathways or the smooth pursuit system *(dir path)*

Optokinetic nystagmus (OKN) is composed of two dynamically different processes in primates (Fig. 2A): In response to a step in stimulus velocity the rapid initial change in slow phase velocity (a in Fig. 2A) is followed by a slower rise (b) to a steady state level (c+d; Cohen et al. 1977). Pathways responsible for the fast rise are referred to as "direct" visual-oculomotor pathways (dir path in Fig. 2C; Cohen et al. 1977) or as the smooth pursuit system (Robinson, 1981). Pathways responsible for the slower changes in eye velocity during OKN and for the occurrence of optokinetic after-nystagmus (OKAN) are referred to as "indirect" visual-oculomotor pathways (indir path in Fig. 2B; Cohen et al. 1977; Raphan et al. 1979; Waespe et al. 1983) or as the OKN-system (Robinson, 1981). In Figs. 2B and C the activities are depicted as a function of time and thought to be characteristic for these two pathways. A key element in the "indirect" pathways is a "velocity storage" mechanism shared with the vestibular system (Raphan and Cohen, 1981). In the monkey the initial fast rise reaches velocities of 40-80% to that of the stimulus and maximal constant slow phase velocity of OKN exceeds 100 deg/s, but responses can vary substantially between individual animals (Cohen et al. 1977; Waespe et al. 1980; Lisberger et al. 1981). In the rabbit the initial fast rise is small (1-2 deg/s) and OKN builds up very slowly up to peak velocities of about 20 deg/s (Collewijn, 1981). For further data, especially presumed pathways, see Precht et al. (this Vol.).

Optokinetic after-nystagmus (OKAN) is the continuing nystagmus in darkness after optokinetic stimulation (Fig. 2A). Eye velocity decreases sharply in the first second after lights off (c in Fig. 2A) to a velocity from which it declines slower over a much longer time course. The amount of the initial fast decay in eye velocity is dependent on the preceding stimulus velocity and increases with higher OKN velocities (Cohen et al. 1977). Up to a velocity of 60 deg/s it is very small. The maximal value to which the eye velocity decays in the first second after lights off is called the saturation velocity of the OKAN (d in Fig. 2A; Cohen et al. 1977). Usually it ranges between 50 and 80 deg/s (see also Lisberger et al. 1981) but values up to 120 deg/s have been reported (Cohen et al. 1977). Primary OKAN beats into the same direction as the preceding OKN. Its slow phase velocity declines with a similar time course as VN and T_c ranges between 10 and 40 s. OKAN is very prominent in the rabbit (Collewijn, 1981).

Smooth pursuit eye movements are defined as slow movements in foveate animals generated by a single target object moving in front of the animal. The reaction time of the smooth pursuit system is over 100 ms (man: 125 ms, Robinson, 1965; monkey: 175 ms, Fuchs 1967). Peak velocities can exceed 100 deg/s (Lisberger and Fuchs, 1978a). Smooth pursuit can be elicited by movement of an object over the retina. Determining factors are the object's velocity and eccentricity relative to the fovea (Rashbass, 1961; Robinson, 1965; Kommerell and Klein, 1971). Smooth pursuit eye movements show no substantial after-effects. The rabbit has no fovea but only a visual streak. Under laboratory conditions it does not pursue small moving targets (Collewijn, 1981).

Special stimulus conditions: Conflict stimulation refers to combined visual-vestibular stimulation in which the whole-field visual surround is mechanically coupled to the turntable and both are rotated into the same direction (Waespe and Henn, 1978). The conflict is that the labyrinths signal an acceleration which is not supported by information from the visual system. The vestibular nystagmus is almost completely suppressed up to table accelerations of 10 deg/s^2. When nystagmus cannot be completely suppressed at high accelerations image slip into the same direction as actual motion occurs. The time constant of the residual vestibular nystagmus is below 6 s (Waespe and Henn, 1978; Waespe et al. 1983; Raphan et al. 1979). *VOR-suppression* refers to vestibular stimulation whereby an animal rotated in otherwise complete darkness attempts to foveate a small head-fixed light spot in the center of its visual field thereby suppressing vestibular nystagmus.

2.2 Neuronal Activity in the Vestibular Nerve

The primary vestibular neurons connected to the horizontal semicircular canal are modulated bidirectionally with an activity increase during acceleration towards the ipsilateral side and an activity decrease during acceleration to the contralateral side (Goldberg and Fernández 1981). The activity is not modulated during optokinetic stimulation (cat: Blanks and Precht, 1978; monkey: Keller, 1976; Büttner and Waespe, 1981). Although no visual information is processed in the labyrinth there is one important modification of visually induced eye movements after bilateral labyrinthectomy (mechanical destruction of the labyrinth or cutting of the eighth nerve): OKN is slowed down and less regular, and primary OKAN is abolished (rabbit: Gutman et al. 1964; Collewijn, 1976; monkey: Cohen et al. 1973; man: Zee et al. 1976). In the monkey OKN reaches peak velocities up to 100 deg/s even after labyrinthectomy (Waespe, unpublished), whereas in the rabbit OKN is severely reduced and peak velocities are only 1-2 deg/s (Collewijn, 1981). The interpretation of the effects of labyrinthectomy on OKN and OKAN is that central vestibular neurons which are modulated during OKN and OKAN need the continuous high frequency input of almost 100 imp/s of the primary vestibular neurons in order to function normally.

2.3 Neuronal Activity in the Vestibular Nuclei

Neurons within the vestibular nuclei responsive to angular acceleration in the horizontal plane are classified as type I (activity polarity same as in the nerve) and type II neurons (activity polarity reversed; Duensing and Schaefer, 1958). Neurons are considered to receive a monosynaptic input from horizontal canals if their threshold to angular acceleration is 5 deg/s^2 or below (Waespe and Henn, 1979a, b), and are referred to as central vestibular neurons. Such neuronal activity is modulated during horizontal optokinetic stimulation in a direction specific way (Henn et al. 1974; Waespe and Henn, 1977a, b, 1979a, b) and is also modulated during suppression of the OKN in the alert non-paralyzed monkey (Buettner and Büttner, 1979), or in paralyzed animals when stimulus and image slip velocities correspond (goldfish: Allum et al. 1976; cat: Keller and Precht, 1979; rat: Cazin et al. 1980, rabbit: Barmack and Pettorossi, 1981).

Type I neurons increase their activity during vestibular stimulation to the recording side and during optokinetic stimulation to the contralateral side. In both situations nystagmus is elicited to the recording side. During stimulation into opposite directions type I neurons are inhibited. Type II neurons show a mirrorlike behavior to the type I neurons. Qualitatively, central vestibular neurons have similar responses; quantitatively they differ in their threshold, cut-off, and saturation (Waespe and Henn, 1979a, b). The response after a step of vestibular acceleration during rotation at a constant velocity is characterized by a dominant decaying time constant (T_c) which is similar to that of vestibular nystagmus (VN) and is in the range of 10 to 40 s or greater. Constant velocity optokinetic stimulation leads to a maintained increase in discharge rate up to velocities of an average of 60 deg/s (Waespe and Henn, 1977a). At higher velocities activity does not further increase in contrast to the slow phase velocity of the OKN. During acceleration of the optokinetic stimulus, activity changes follow the instantaneous velocity of the visual surround up to accelerations of an average of 5-10 deg/s^2 (Waespe and Henn, 1979a, b). Most central vestibular neurons will therefore not be modulated during sinusoidal optokinetic stimulation with frequencies above 0.2-0.3 Hz (Büttner et al. 1983). The slow changes in eye velocity during OKAN are faithfully reflected in a similar slow change in the discharge rate of all central vestibular neurons, but the initial fast drop is not (Waespe and Henn, 1977b). Activity of central vestibular neurons is thought not to be modulated during sinusoidal smooth pursuit eye movements (Keller and Daniels, 1975).

Conflict stimulation leads to peak activity changes which are less compared to vestibular stimulation alone. The effect is strongest at low accelerations and minimal at accelerations above 20 deg/s^2. In the presence of a subject-stationary visual surround the threshold of many central vestibular neurons to angular acceleration is raised (Waespe and Henn, 1978). The dominant time constant of neuronal activity changes after an acceleration pulse is less than 8 s (Waespe and Henn, 1978). During suppression of the VOR peak modulation is not attenuated, even at low accelerations (Buettner and Büttner, 1979).

The neural population within the vestibular nuclei is heterogenous. We have selected neurons with high sensitivities to angular acceleration in the horizontal plane. There are other neurons which behave like burst-tonic neurons in the PPRF and the perihypoglossal region (Keller and Kamath, 1975). They are modulated in relation to fast eye movements, to different eye positions and to eye velocity during smooth pursuit eye movements (Keller and Kamath, 1975). Almost nothing is known about the modulation of central vestibular neurons in the rabbit.

2.4 Neuronal Activity in the Flocculus

Mossy fiber (MF) activity is assumed to be reflected in recordings from fibers or granule cells (Lisberger and Fuchs, 1978b; Miles et al. 1980; Waespe et al. 1981; Noda et al. 1977). Llinas has suggested that we have most probably not recorded from granule cells but from MF terminals. We agree as it would be difficult to accept the assumption that a granule cell upon which more than 20 different MFs converge should reflect a behavior which is identical to that of a single MF. Due to this convergence some information processing has to be expected to occur at the level of the granule cells. The activity of many MFs (or MF terminals) is modulated similarly to that of central vestibular neurons during all conditions of visual-vestibular interaction (Waespe et al. 1981). Activity changes saturate at 60 deg/s of constant velocity optokinetic nystagmus on average. There is also modulation during OKAN, but usually none or only little during smooth pursuit in relation to eye velocity (sinusoidal velocity profile; Waespe unpublished).

There are other MF inputs modulated by image slip velocity (Noda, 1981; Waespe et al. 1981) or in relation to different parameters of fast eye movements, eye position, or eye velocity (Noda and Suzuki, 1978; Lisberger and Fuchs, 1978b; Miles et al. 1980; Noda and Warabi, 1982). Activity indicative of vestibular nerve input has not been found in the monkey (see Precht et al. this Volume, for data from non-primates).

In the rabbit, mossy fiber activity has not been recorded. Ito assumes two main inputs: one from primary vestibular fibers, and another one from the accessory optic system (Fig. 1). According to his hypothesis there is no eye velocity MF input (Ito, 1982), but recently such an MF input to the rabbit's flocculus has been suggested (Miyashita, 1983).

Purkinje cells (P-cells) have been recorded in the monkey using several different paradigms (Lisberger and Fuchs, 1978a; Miles et al. 1980). In the untrained monkey, P-cells were selected according to the modulation of their simple spike (SS) activity during optokinetic and conflict stimulation. Such modulation can be observed in 10-20% of the P-cells found in the flocculus. In the responsive group, 40% of the P-cells are not modulated during vestibular stimulation in darkness (modulation less than 20% of the resting discharge), and 60% show some modulation which is always less than during conflict stimulation. During conflict stimulation SS activity is strongly modulated at an acceleration of 40 deg/s^2 but little or not at all at 5 or 10 deg/s^2 except for the most sensitive P-cells, although vestibular nystagmus is comparatively stronger suppressed at lower accelerations. During OKN, SS activity is modulated only at constant velocities above 30-60 deg/s or during rapid changes of nystagmus velocities (above 5-10 deg/s^2), (Waespe and Henn, 1981; Waespe et al. 1985). With lights off during OKN SS activity returns within 1 s to the resting discharge level and is not further modulated during OKAN. About 90% of the P-cells increase SS activity during both conflict and optokinetic stimulation to the ipsilateral side. Whereas optokinetic nystagmus beats with the fast phase to the contralateral side, during conflict stimulation however nystagmus beats to the ipsilateral side. In contrast, type I central vestibular neurons are activated during nystagmus exclusively to the ipsilateral side independently of whether activation is due to optokinetic, vestibular, or conflict stimulation.

SS modulation is uncorrelated with only one parameter such as stimulus, eye, image slip or gaze velocity. Floccular P-cells are always modulated when the activity of central vestibular neurons is not adequate to induce an eye velocity which would minimize image slip (Waespe and Henn, 1981). Lisberger and Fuchs (1978a) and Miles et al. (1980) demonstrated that P-cells in the flocculus are modulated during smooth pursuit eye movements and VOR-suppression and that the level of modulation is similar in both situations. In their experiments, 80-90% of the P-cells were also activated with stimulation to the ipsilateral side. They concluded that the P-cells code gaze velocity (head velocity minus eye velocity). More extensive experiments in our laboratory show that these "gaze-velocity" P-cells are also modulated during conflict stimulation and with high constant velocity optokinetic nystagmus (Büttner and Waespe, 1984). Although these P-cells are strongly modulated during sinusoidal smooth pursuit eye movements with peak velocities of 20-40 deg/s, not one was modulated during constant velocity OKN of the same velocity. The same P-cells were modulated during OKN only at velocities above 40-60 deg/s, i.e. above the OKAN saturation velocity. P-cells were not modulated in relation to image slip velocity.

In the rabbit SS activity of P-cells is deeply modulated by vestibular stimulation in a type I or type II manner. Visual signals have little or no effect on simple spike activity in the absence of vestibular stimulation (Ghelarducci et al. 1975; Ito, 1982). Visual stimulation was very effective in modifying the amplitude and phase angle of SS modulation provoked by simultaneous head rotation. In the alert non-paralysed rabbit many P-cells increase SS activity with optokinetic stimulation to the ipsilateral side (Neverov et al. 1980). Only a few of these P-cells are modulated during secondary OKAN (primary OKAN was not tested; Neverov et al. 1980). Ito (1982) concludes that P-cells are therefore not modulated in relation to eye but rather to image slip velocity during optokinetic stimulation. Further below we offer another hypothesis compatible with monkey data.

Climbing fiber activity recorded as complex spikes in P-cells with a spontaneous activity around 1 imp/s show a behavior which in general is opposite to that of SS modulation. Its modulation seems to be related to image slip velocity only (Waespe and Henn, 1981).

2.5 Functional Interpretation of Activity in the Flocculus and Effects of Surgical Flocculectomy

The changes in SS activity of P-cells in the primate flocculus suggest that the modulation may be directly responsible for inducing (a) high velocity OKN, i.e. above the OKAN saturation velocity of about 60 deg/s, (b) fast changes of OKN velocity, i.e., those exceeding 5-10 deg/s^2, (c) suppression of VN during high acceleration conflict stimulation. These are the functions which are attributed in the Raphan-Cohen model (1981) to the "direct" visual-oculomotor pathways, and in the Robinson model (1981) to the "smooth pursuit" pathways. Robinson's model predicts two further modes of action of floccular P-cells: (d) the generation of smooth pursuit eye movements, (e) the suppression or cancellation of the VOR while animals foveate a single fixation light (VOR-suppression).

Attenuation of these specific functions in lesion experiments supports the hypothesis for an essential floccular role (Takemori and Cohen, 1974; Zee et al. 1981;

Waespe et al. 1983). After bilateral surgical flocculectomy the initial rapid increase in OKN velocity at the onset of stimulation is reduced by 60-90% and the slow increase in OKN velocity has a longer time course than normal. OKN steady state velocities increase approximately up to the pre-operative OKAN saturation velocity of 50-70 deg/s, but cannot reach higher values (Takemori and Cohen, 1974; Waespe et al. 1983). Monkeys are unable to follow adequately an acceleration of the visual surround of 5 deg/s^2 or more. Eye velocity, however, can be decelerated faster than it can be accelerated (Waespe et al. 1983). The transition of OKN to OKAN is smooth after flocculectomy at all stimulus velocities without any or with only a small initial fast velocity drop. OKAN velocities and durations are essentially unchanged. Flocculectomy also has little effect on gain and duration of the vestibular nystagmus (Zee et al. 1981). During conflict stimulation time constants are still below 6 s but peak velocities cannot be attenuated during short pulses of high accelerations. On the other hand, at accelerations below 10 deg/s^2 nystagmus is almost completely suppressed as in the normal animal. Unilateral flocculectomy has similar, but asymmetrical effects. OKN with slow phases to the operated side is more affected as is nystagmus during conflict stimulation with slow phases to the non-operated side. The gain of smooth pursuit eye movements is reduced and the VOR-suppression is impaired (Zee et al. 1981). However, bilateral flocculectomy does not abolish all activity within the "direct" visual-oculomotor pathways and one has to postulate that other brainstem or cerebellar structures contribute to these pathways.

In the rabbit, flocculectomy has similar effects on OKN as in the monkey (Ito et al. 1982; Nagao, 1983). Unfortunately the two different components in the OKN response have not been separated by using constant velocity steps. Probably the "direct" visual pathways account for only 1-2 deg/s during constant velocity OKN. As OKN build-up is severely reduced after flocculectomy, it never reaches adequate velocities using sinusoidal stimulation (for summary see Ito, 1982; Barmack, 1979). However, one would predict an almost normal OKN response during constant velocity stimulation given the weak modulation of P-cells during visual stimulation and assuming that also in the rabbit the "direct" pathways pass through the flocculus. The effect of flocculectomy on OKAN is unknown in the rabbit. It is not yet clear, if the gain of the VOR is always severely reduced after flocculectomy (Ito, 1982) or not (Barmack, 1979; Nagao, 1983). Also it is not yet clear whether unilateral flocculectomy affects only one or both eyes.

The activity of central vestibular neurons is qualitatively unchanged during vestibular, conflict and optokinetic stimulation after flocculectomy (Waespe and Cohen, 1983). During vestibular stimulation the decay time constant (T_c) is unchanged. With optokinetic stimulation neuronal activity increases up to a velocity of approximately 60 deg/s at which it saturates. During OKAN neuronal activity accurately reflects the time course of nystagmus slow phase velocity. In the conflict situation the time constant (T_c) is short. Nothing is known about the modulation of central vestibular neurons after flocculectomy in the rabbit.

2.6 Effects of Bilateral Vestibular Neurectomy on Floccular P-cell Activity

After bilateral neurectomy maximal OKN velocities are reduced, OKAN is abolished and eye velocity no longer increases slowly after the initial fast rise during OKN (Cohen et al. 1982). But even after neurectomy monkeys can produce OKN with constant velocities up to 80-120 deg/s (Waespe unpublished). The deficits can be attributed to a lack of activity within the "indirect" visual-oculomotor pathways or the OKN-system (Fig. 2). Activity to generate nystagmus velocity mainly originates in the "direct" pathways, a part of which seems to go through the flocculus as suggested above. SS activity of P-cells in the flocculus after bilateral neurectomy is already modulated at low OKN velocities of 15 or 30 deg/s. The same P-cells are also modulated during smooth pursuit eye movement in the same way as in the normal monkey. Modulation increases monotonically with eye velocity during OKN and smooth pursuit for all stimulus velocities (Waespe et al. 1985). The behavior of floccular P-cells after labyrinthectomy is unknown in the rabbit. However, after vestibular nuclei lesions with a severe reduction of OKN SS modulation was unchanged (Miyashita and Nagao 1981, cited in Ito 1982).

3 Interpretation and Speculations

3.1 What do P-cells Code?

Ever since Holmes (1917) published his now classical study of clinical deficits after cerebellar lesions, the cerebellum has been perceived as essentially a coordinating and regulatory system of motor functions. Cerebellar deficits cannot be detected in patients who are motionless; therefore cerebellar functions are best investigated experimentally in alert animals performing a specific motor task. One such motor task is the generation and suppression of slow eye movements during vestibular, visual, and various combined stimulations. Evidence now indicates that cellular activity in the cerebellum and the brainstem comprises complex signals during visual-vestibular interactions. They can only be analysed if they are investigated using stimulus conditions which selectively test as many functions as possible. For instance, the examination of OKAN is a powerful tool in the analysis of visual-vestibular interaction both on the level of behavioral phenomena and on the level of single cells. It would be dangerous to draw general conclusions from the results obtained by using a very limited set of stimulus parameters on the overall function of a cell population performing different tasks of visual-vestibular interaction. Results from our experiments show that one cannot relate P-cell activity to only a single input or output parameter: floccular P-cells do not exclusively code eye, gaze, head or image slip velocity. Only the combined output of floccular P-cells and central vestibular neurons can be related to eye velocity. In addition, the participation of other cell populations, for instance, in the vermis or in the nodulus in the generation or suppression of eye velocity is likely.

SS activity of floccular P-cells is not modulated during (a) vestibular stimulation alone, (b) optokinetic stimulation with accelerations below 5-10 deg/s^2 or velocities below 40-60 deg/s, (c) conflict stimulation at accelerations below 5-10 deg/s^2, (d) optokinetic afternystagmus. Under these circumstances eye velocity is reflected in the activity of central vestibular neurons. Eye velocity during these parameters is not affected by bilateral flocculectomy. The activity of central vestibular neurons is assumed not to be modulated during smooth pursuit eye movements (Keller and Kamath, 1975; Keller and Daniels, 1975). The modulation is not attenuated during VOR suppression.

Floccular P-cells are modulated during smooth pursuit and VOR suppression and a close correlation can be established between gaze velocity and SS activity (Lisberger and Fuchs, 1978a; Miles et al. 1980). These authors were therefore led to the interpretation that P-cells code gaze velocity (head minus eye velocity). However, these same P-cells are also modulated during OKN but only at high velocities above 40-60 deg/s and they do therefore not reflect gaze or eye velocity (Büttner and Waespe, 1984). Floccular P-cells are modulated during specific conditions. These include a) optokinetic nystagmus with high accelerations above 5-10 deg/s^2 or high velocities above 40-60 deg/s, i.e. above the OKAN saturation velocity as the activity of central vestibular neurons is then saturated; b) conflict stimulation with accelerations above 5-10 deg/s^2 as the activity of central vestibular neurons is then not attenuated. After bilateral flocculectomy these functions are compromised specifically in the velocity and acceleration ranges as indicated above and suggest that floccular P-cells mediate the signals important for the generation of these parameters.

These experimental results allow us to discuss under what specialized conditions P-cell activity might be related to one of the input or output parameters. Eye velocity is reflected in P-cell SS activity in the normal monkey only during smooth pursuit eye movements, but not during any other condition. In the neurectomized animal it is also reflected during OKN when central vestibular neurons are non-operative. Gaze velocity can be related to P-cell activity during smooth pursuit, during VOR and during VOR suppression (Lisberger and Fuchs, 1978a; Miles et al. 1980). But gaze velocity − in the normal monkey − is not reflected in the SS activity during OKN and OKAN and at low acceleration conflict stimulation. Image slip velocity is not the determining parameter in the modulation of the SS activity of floccular P-cells (Lisberger and Fuchs, 1978a; Miles et al. 1980; Büttner and Waespe, 1984).

The activity changes of central vestibular neurons has been interpreted to reflect the activity within the "indirect" visual-oculomotor pathways and the "velocity storage" mechanism (Raphan and Cohen, 1981). The velocity storage mechanism is independent of the floccular P-cell activity. Floccular P-cells on the other hand exhibit activity changes which are similar to those assumed to be typical for the "direct" visual-oculomotor pathways. Furthermore, the "direct" pathways and the smooth pursuit system converge on the same P-cells, in agreement with the original hypothesis of Robinson (1981; Waespe et al. 1985).

The hypothesis of the existence of two dynamically different mechanisms involved in the generation of OKN and in the visual suppression of vestibular nystagmus has proven to be very useful in analyzing the overall behavior and the activity of different cell populations. However, on the level of single cells, a strict separation cannot always be made. On average, activity of central vestibular neurons is involved in functions of the "indirect" visual-oculomotor pathways, although a few neurons saturate during OKN at velocities well above the OKAN saturation velocity, and although there are eye position-sensitive neurons which are also modulated during smooth pursuit eye movements. On average, SS activity of floccular P-cells is modulated with OKN velocities above the OKAN saturation velocity; yet there also are exceptions. In addition, there are P-cells which are modulated during the VOR. The observed deficits after experimental lesions, however, clearly support the hypothesis of the existence of two such pathways which differ in their dynamic behavior. Bilateral flocculectomy mainly reduces high velocity OKN and affects smooth pursuit eye movements, whereas bilateral labyrinthectomy or neurectomy mainly abolishes OKAN, but seems not to affect smooth pursuit eye movements.

3.2 Unsolved Anatomical Questions

A decisive problem for any conceptual interpretation is the lack of complete anatomical data in the monkey. The flocculus receives an MF input from several brainstem areas, the most important ones from the vestibular nuclei on both sides and the pons (Langer et al. 1985). Theories which are based on a powerful peripheral vestibular input to the flocculus meet the obstacle that as yet most physiologically identified vestibular input seems to originate in the vestibular nuclei (Lisberger and Fuchs, 1978b; Waespe et al. 1981, Fig. 3). Recently Korte and Mugnaini in the cat (1979) and Langer et al. in the monkey (1985) have shown anatomically that probably only a few primary fibers project to the flocculus.

Another classical concept states that P-cells project to the vestibular nuclei to modulate secondary neurons which in turn project to the oculomotor nuclei (Fig. 1). However, activity changes of floccular P-cells during OKN, conflict stimulation and during smooth pursuit are not reflected by corresponding frequency changes in central vestibular neurons. Floccular P-cells for instance are able to change their SS activity to optokinetic stimulation more rapidly than central vestibular neurons. Especially the firing pattern during conflict stimulation can only be interpreted if one assumes complementary rather than serial processing of information in floccular P-cells and central vestibular neurons. A related problem is that although eye velocity is strongly attenuated during VOR-suppression the head velocity signal in central vestibular neurons or MLF fibers is not attenuated (King et al. 1976). A powerful head velocity signal therefore reaches oculomotor neurons which has to be cancelled (Fig. 3).

It is suggested that P-cells do not exert their influence on the class of vestibular neurons described above (in Fig. 3 denoted as "interaction"). Further support for our assumption that the floccular P-cells must have a projection to the oculomotor system bypassing central vestibular neurons comes from labyrinthectomy studies. After labyrinthectomy central vestibular neurons are functionally severely disrupted as indicated by the loss of OKAN. Floccular output mediating OKN and smooth pursuit, however, still reaches the oculomotor system which makes it unlikely to be transmitted via central vestibular neurons. This is puzzling because the only anatomically determined outputs in the monkey are to the lateral cerebellar nuclei region, the Y-group and to the vestibular nuclei (Langer et al. 1985; Haines, 1977). In the cat and the rabbit a pathway to the nucleus prepositus hypoglossi reportedly exists (Yingcharoen and Rinvik, 1983; Alley, 1977; Sato et al. 1983). It is likely that there are several subgroups of secondary vestibular nuclei neurons which have different anatomical connections (Mitsacos et al., 1983) and different functional significance. Our results demonstrate that the reciprocal connection between vestibular nuclei and flocculus requires two different classes of vestibular neurons, those which project to the flocculus and which have been described by us in detail as *central vestibular neurons,* and those which receive floccular output. Furthermore, it is questionable whether the same central vestibular neurons project both to the flocculus and to the abducens nucleus as shown in Fig. 3.

3.3 Comparison of Rabbit and Monkey Data

A decisive difficulty for any comparison is the lack of information for the rabbit about the activity of central vestibular neurons during the different modes of visual-vestibular interaction. The rabbit is a lateral-eyed animal, has no fovea and does not pursue single target objects under laboratory conditions. The gain of the vestibular nystagmus is lower than in the monkey. Despite these differences the principal effects of flocculectomy and labyrinthectomy for both species are remarkably similar as they are for other species too (Precht et al. this Vol.). This suggests that also in the rabbit the OKN has two components with only a small contribution of the "direct" visual pathways and a prominent "velocity storage" mechanism. The lesion studies suggest that in both species the flocculus is mainly involved in the "direct" visual-oculomotor pathways. A further difficulty for a comparison are different experimental setups. All recordings in the monkey have been done in the fully alert animal with eye movements always monitored. Often, animals were trained to fixate a target light. In experiments with non-primates, animals are usually alert but paralyzed (see Precht et al. this Vol.). In the paralyzed state opto-kinetic stimulation operates under open-loop gain which in the rabbit can reach values of 30 (Dubois and Collewijn, 1979). Therefore, the system is already activated maximally at stimulus velocities of a few degrees. In the monkey peak activation is reached under open-loop condition at stimulus velocities of 3-5 deg/s with a gain of 10 (Koerner and Schiller, 1972). The open-loop condition used in many experiments would explain the low saturation velocity of neurons in the vestibular nuclei and the flocculus (Keller and Precht, 1979; Blanks and Precht, 1983). It would also explain the fact that the working ranges of floccular P-cells and of central vestibular neurons are not different (but see Precht et al. this Vol.). It is often assumed that the neuronal modulation in non-primates to optokinetic stimulation reflects only image slip velocity (for discussion, see Precht et al., this Volume), but other explanations cannot be ruled out. Neuronal modulation could reflect a slow eye velocity signal which is still generated even under open-loop condition as the central structures are not affected by the paralyzing drug. An illustrative example is the behavior of central vestibular neurons which are activated differently during optokinetic stimulation in the alert non-paralyzed and paralyzed cat (Keller and Precht, 1979). At low stimulus velocities neuronal modulation is about double in the paralyzed cat and modulation increases monotonically up to stimulus velocities of 10 deg/s only instead of 40-60 deg/s as in the non-paralyzed cat. In con-clusion, the data available in subprimates are not complete enough to prove Ito's hy-pothesis.

3.4 Implication for Adaptation Studies

The flocculus constitutes a crucial link in inducing plastic changes of the VOR by altered visual input (Ito, 1972; Robinson, 1976). There is no agreement yet concerning the possible mechanism for this phenomenon. Are the plastic modifiable elements localized within the flocculus itself (review: Ito, 1982) or do floccular P-cells only carry an "error signal" necessary for the induction of the adaptation process which takes place some-where else (Miles and Lisberger, 1981)? Ito's hypothesis is that the plastic changes in the rabbit take place in the floccular cortex through the activity of climbing fibers

Fig. 3. Main functional connections important during the immediate and adaptive visual adjustment of the VOR and in the generation of OKN and OKAN slow phase velocity in the primate. There is no direct MF input from the eighth nerve to the flocculus. CF inputs are not shown. *Interaction* denotes the not yet localized target cells of P-cell output. These cells are different from vestibular MF input, but could also be localized within the vestibular nuclei. The *visual* MF input carries information about image slip velocity and/or eye velocity itself

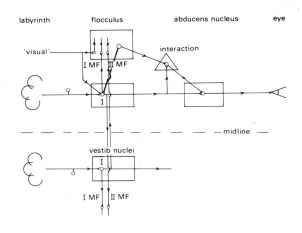

which modify the strengths of parallel fiber synapses on P-cell dendrites. According to Miles and coworkers the primate flocculus has an inductive role by providing visually derived signals indicating the existence and magnitude of errors in the VOR. Unclear are the pathways which transmit the "error signal", and what the functional role of the proposed direct connection of floccular P-cells to central vestibular neurons is. There seems to be no functional role for this direct connection in the immediate adjustment of the VOR by visual inputs, and in transmitting the signals for rapid changes or high velocity OKN. The floccular projection to central vestibular neurons (heavy line in Fig. 3) however, could be crucial during long-term adjustments of the VOR. Signals of the same P-cells which are modulated during OKN, smooth pursuit and suppression of the VOR may at the same time constitute "error signals" which are effective only when occurring either repetitively or continuously over long periods. Central vestibular neurons receiving such an "error signal" may project back to the flocculus and may reduce this signal via a feedback loop. Lisberger et al. (1981) showed that in the monkey VOR gain adaptation is reflected by gain changes in the "indirect" pathways. With a VOR gain of 1.6 the OKAN saturation velocity is enhanced to 90 deg/s and for a VOR gain of 0.3 it is reduced to 30 deg/s. It was specifically pointed out that changes in the "direct" visual-oculomotor pathways were not seen. This suggests that the signals driving them on a short-term basis do not access the final oculomotor pathways through central vestibular neurons. This reasoning further supports the general outline of our scheme in Fig. 3. Adaptation of the OKAN should always be reflected in the activity of central vestibular neurons and also in the SS activity of floccular P-cells. An increase in the saturation velocity of the OKAN to 90 deg/s for instance would also increase the saturation velocity of central vestibular neurons and the threshold at which floccular P-cells would start to be modulated during OKN to about the same value of 90 deg/s. This hypothesis has to be tested yet.

4 Conclusion

The microanatomy of the cerebellar cortex repeats itself in the flocculus. The one feature which makes it different from other parts of the cerebellum is the input-output connections, and thereby the information it processes. However, the anatomical connections of the flocculus are not yet fully explored. Ito put forward a very fruitful hypothesis of how visual and labyrinthine inputs combine to modify central-vestibular output (1972). At the same time lesion experiments specified deficits of visual-vestibular interaction after flocculectomy (Takemori and Cohen, 1974).

After a decade of single unit recordings in alert monkeys we now face a much more complex, yet still experimentally accessible picture of information processing. The stimulus parameters can be precisely controlled, and oculomotor output can be monitored. Probably all vestibular input to the flocculus is of central origin. These neurons, mostly one synapse away from the labyrinths, already transform activity in the nerve into a complex signal (reviews Waespe and Henn, 1979b; Henn et al. 1980). Therefore, it is not surprising that signals in the flocculus cannot directly be related to input or output parameters of the behaving animal. Instead, they represent internal parameters which can be understood only in terms of the activity of the corresponding brainstem circuits with which they interface.

This actually fits the clinical picture: cerebellar lesions do not lead to palsies or sensory deficits, but the smooth performance of movements becomes impossible because of tremor, dysmetria, dysdiadochokinesia, and decomposition of movement (Holmes, 1917). In descriptive clinical terms, oculomotor deficits after cerebellar lesions show a similar list of dysfunctions of slow eye movements such as saccadic pursuit, gaze evoked nystagmus, reduction of optokinetic nystagmus velocity, and failure to visually suppress vestibularly evoked nystagmus. These dysfunctions appear after floccular lesions alone and some can be reduced to deficits within the "direct" visual-oculomotor pathways.

References

Alley K (1977) Anatomical basis for the interaction between cerebellar flocculus and brainstem. In: Baker R, Berthoz A (eds) Control of gaze by brainstem neurons. Dev Neurosci 1: 109-117

Allum JHJ, Graf W, Dichgans J, Schmidt CL (1976) Visual-vestibular interaction in the vestibular nuclei of the goldfish. Exp Brain Res 26: 463-485

Angaut P, Brodal A (1967) The projection of the "vestibulo-cerebellum" onto the vestibular nuclei in the cat. Arch Ital Biol 105: 441-479

Barmack NH (1979) Immediate and sustained influences of visual olivocerebellar activity on eye movement. In: Talbott RE, Humphrey DR (eds) Posture and movement. Raven Press, New York, pp 123-168

Barmack NH, Pettorossi VE (1981) Influence of visual olivocerebellar inactivation on the optokinetic properties of neurons in the vestibular nuclei of rabbits. In: Fuchs AF, Becker A (eds) Progress in oculomotor research. Dev Neurosci 12: 455-464

Batini C, Ito M, Kado RT, Jastreboff PJ, Misashita Y (1979) Interaction between the horizontal vestibulo-ocular reflex and optokinetic response in rabbits. Exp Brain Res 37: 1-15

Blanks RHI, Precht W (1978) Response properties of vestibular afferents in alert cats during optokinetic and vestibular stimulation. Neurosci Lett 10: 225-229

Blanks RHI, Precht W (1983) Responses of units in the rat cerebellar flocculus during optokinetic and vestibular stimulation. Exp Brain Res 53: 1-15

Brodal A, Høivik B (1964) Site and mode of termination of primary vestibulocerebellar fibers in the cat. Arch Ital Biol 101: 1-21

Buettner UW, Büttner U (1979) Vestibular nuclei activity in the alert monkey during suppression of vestibular and optokinetic nystagmus. Exp Brain Res 37: 581-593

Büttner U, Waespe W (1981) Vestibular nerve activity in the alert monkey during vestibular and optokinetic nystagmus. Exp Brain Res 41: 310-315

Büttner U, Waespe W (1984) Purkinje cell activity in the primate flocculus during optokinetic stimulation, smooth pursuit eye movements and VOR-suppression. Exp Brain Res 55: 97-104

Büttner U, Boyle R, Schreiter U (1983) Vestibular nuclei activity in the alert monkey during constant velocity and sinusoidal optokinetic stimulation. Soc Neurosci Abstr 9: 315

Carpenter MB, Stein BM, Peter P (1972) Primary vestibulo-cerebellar fibers in the monkey: distribution of fibers arising from distinctive cell groups of the vestibular ganglia. Am J Anat 135: 221-250

Cazin L, Precht W, Lannou J (1980) Pathways mediating optokinetic responses of vestibular nucleus neurons in the rat. Pflüger's Arch 384: 19-29

Cohen B, Uemura T, Takemori S (1973) Effects of labyrinthectomy on optokinetic nystagmus (OKN) and optokinetic after-nystagmus (OKAN). Equil Res 3: 88-93

Cohen B, Matsuo V, Raphan T (1977) Quantitative analysis of the velocity characteristics of optokinetic nystagmus and optokinetic after-nystagmus. J Physiol 270: 321-344

Cohen B, Suzuki J, Raphan T, Matsuo V, deJong V (1982) Selective labyrinthine lesions and nystagmus induced by rotation about off-vertical axis. In: Lennerstrand G, Keller E, Zee DS (eds) Functional basis of ocular motility disorders. Pergamon Press, Oxford New York, pp 337-346

Collewijn H (1976) Impairment of optokinetic (after-)nystagmus by labyrinthectomy in the rabbit. Exp Neurol 52: 146-156

Collewijn H (1981) The optokinetic system: In: Zuber BL (ed) Models of oculomotor behavior and control. CRC Press, West Plam Beach, Fla, pp 111-137

Dow RS (1938) Efferent connections of the flocculo-nodular lobe in macacca mulatta. J Comp Neurol 68: 297-305

Dubois MFW, Collewijn H (1979) The optokinetic reactions of the rabbit: relation to the visual streak. Vision Res 19: 9-17

Duensing F, Schaefer KP (1958) Die Aktivität einzelner Neurone im Bereich der Vestibulariskerne bei Horizontalbeschleunigung unter besonderer Berücksichtigung des vestibulären Nystagmus. Arch Psychiat Nervenkr 198: 225-252

Fuchs AF (1967) Saccadic and smooth pursuit eye movements in the monkey. J Physiol 191: 609-631

Fukuda J, Highstein SM, Ito M (1972) Cerebellar inhibitory control of the vestibulo-ocular reflex investigated in rabbit 3rd nucleus. Exp Brain Res 14: 511-526

Ghelarducci B, Ito M, Yagi N (1975) Impulse discharges from flocculus Purkinje cells of alert rabbits during visual stimulation combined with horizontal head rotation. Brain Res 87: 66-72

Goldberg JM, Fernandez C (1981) Physiological mechanisms of the nystagmus produced by rotations about an earth-horizontal axis. Ann NY Acad Sci 374: 40-43

Gonshor A, Melvill Jones G (1976) Extreme vestibulo-ocular adaptation induced by prolonged optical reversal of vision. J Physiol 256: 381-414

Gutman J, Zelig S, Bergmann F (1964) Optokinetic nystagmus in the labyrinthectomized rabbit. Confin Neurol 24: 158-162

Haines DE (1977) Cerebellar corticonuclear and corticovestibular fibers of the flocculonodular lobe in a prosimian primate (Galago senegalensis). J Comp Neurol 174: 607-630

Henn V, Young L, Finley C (1974) Vestibular nucleus units in alert monkeys are also influenced by moving visual fields. Brain Res 71: 144-149

Henn V, Cohen B, Young LR (1980) Visual-vestibular interaction in motion perception and the generation of nystagmus. Neurosci Res Progr Bull 18: 459-651

Holmes G (1917) The symptoms of acute cerebellar injuries due to gunshot injuries. Brain 40: 461-535

Ito M (1972) Neural design of the cerebellar motor control system. Brain Res 40: 81-84

Ito M (1976) Cerebellar learning control of vestibulo-ocular mechanisms. In: Desirayu T (ed) Mechanisms in transmission of signals for conscious behavior. Elsevier, Amsterdam New York, pp 1-22

Ito M (1982) Cerebellar control of the vestibulo-ocular reflex, around the flocculus hypothesis. Annu Rev Neurosci 5: 275-296

Ito M, Jastreboff PJ, Miyashita Y (1982) Specific effects of unilateral lesions in the flocculus upon eye movements in albino rabbits. Exp Brain Res 45: 233-242

Keller EL (1976) Behavior of horizontal semicircular canal afferents in alert monkey during vestibular and optokinetic stimulation. Exp Brain Res 24: 459-471

Keller EL, Daniels PD (1975) Oculomotor related interaction of vestibular and visual stimulation in vestibular nuclei cells in alert monkeys. Exp Neurol 46: 187-198

Keller EL, Kamath BY (1975) Characteristics of head rotation and eye movement-related neurons in alert monkey vestibular nucleus. Brain Res 100: 182-187

Keller EL, Precht W (1979) Visual-vestibular responses in vestibular nuclear neurons in intact and cerebellectomized, alert cat. Neuroscience 4: 1599-1613

King WM, Lisberger SG, Fuchs AF (1976) Responses of fibers in medial longitudinal fasciculus (MLF) of alert monkeys during horizontal and vertical conjugate eye movements evoked by vestibular or visual stimuli. J Neurophysiol 39: 1135-1149

Koerner F, Schiller PH (1972) The optokinetic response under open and closed loop conditions in the monkey. Exp Brain Res 14: 318-330

Kommerell G, Klein U (1971) Über die visuelle Regelung der Okulomotorik: die optomotorische Wirkung exzentrischer Nachbilder. Vision Res 11: 905-920

Korte GE, Mugnaini E (1979) The cerebellar projection of the vestibular nerve in the cat. J Comp Neurol 184: 265-278

Langer T, Fuchs AF, Chubb MC, Scudder CA (1985) Floccular efferents in the rhesus macaque as revealed by autoradiographic and horseradish peroxidase. (submitted)

Lisberger SG, Fuchs AF (1978a) Role of primate flocculus during rapid behavioral modification of vestibulo-ocular reflex. I. Purkinje cell activity during visually guided horizontal smooth-pursuit eye movements and passive head rotation. J Neurophysiol 41: 733-763

Lisberger SG, Fuchs AF (1978b) Role of primate flocculus during rapid behavioral modification of vestibulo-ocular reflex. II. Mossy fiber firing patterns during horizontal head rotation and eye movement. J Neurophysiol 41: 764-777

Lisberger SG, Miles FA, Optican LM, Eighmy B (1981) Optokinetic response in monkey: underlying mechanisms and their sensitivity to long-term adaptive changes in vestibuloocular reflex. J Neurophysiol 45: 869-890

Lorente de Nó R (1933) Vestibulo-ocular reflex arc. Arch Neurol Psychiat 30: 245-291

Maekawa K, Takeda T (1976) Electrophysiological identification of the climbing and mossy fiber pathways from the rabbit's retina to the contralateral cerebellar flocculus. Brain Res 109: 169-174

Miles FA, Lisberger SG (1981) Plasticity in the vestibulo-ocular reflex: a new hypothesis. Annu Rev Neurosci 4: 273-299

Miles FA, Fuller JH, Braitman DJ, Dow BM (1980) Long term adaptive changes in primate vestibulo-ocular reflexes. III. Electrophysiological observations in flocculus of adapted monkeys. J Neurophysiol 43: 1437-1476

Mitsacos A, Reisine H, Highstein SM (1983) The superior vestibular nucleus: An intracellular HRP study in the cat. II. Non-vestibular-oculor neurons. J comp Neurol: 215, 92-107

Miyashita Y (1983) Eye velocity inputs to the cerebellar flocculus of rabbits. Neursci Lett Suppl 13: Abstr S25

Miyashita Y, Nagao S (1981) Signal contents of Purkinje cell responses in rabbit flocculus to optokinetic stimuli. J Jpn Physiol Soc 43: 317

Mowrer OH (1937) The influence of vision during bodily rotation upon the duration of post-rotational vestibular nystagmus. Acta Otolaryngol 25: 351-364

Nagao S (1983) Effects of vestibulocerebellar lesions upon dynamic characteristics and adaptation of vestibulo-ocular and optokinetic responses in pigmented rabbits. Exp Brain Res 53: 36-46

Neverov VP, Šterc J, Bureš J (1980) Electrophysiological correlates of the reversed postoptokinetic nystagmus in the rabbit: Activity of vestibular and floccular neurons. Brain Res 189: 355-367

Noda H (1981) Visual mossy fiber inputs to the flocculus of the monkey. In: Cohen B (ed) Vestibular and oculomotor physiology. Ann NY Acad Sci 374: 465-475

Noda H, Suzuki DA (1978) The role of the flocculus of the monkey in saccadic eye movements. J Physiol 294: 317-334

Noda H, Warabi T (1982) Eye position signals in the flocculus of the monkey during smooth-pursuit eye movements. J Physiol 324: 187-202

Noda H, Asoh R, Shibagaki M (1977) Floccular unit activity associated with eye movements and fixation. In: Baker R, Berthoz A (eds) Control of gaze by brain stem neurons. Elsevier, Amsterdam, pp 371-380

Raphan T, Cohen B (1981) The role of integration in oculomotor control. In: Zuber B (ed) Models of oculomotor behavior and control, CRC Press, West Palm Beach, Fla, pp 91-109

Raphan T, Matsuo V, Cohen B (1979) Velocity storage in the vestibulo-ocular reflex arc (VOR). Exp Brain Res 35: 229-248

Rashbass C (1961) The relationship between saccadic and smooth tracking eye movements. J Physiol 159: 326

Robinson DA (1965) The mechanics of human smooth pursuit eye movement. J Physiol 180: 569-591

Robinson DA (1976) Adaptive gain control of vestibuloocular reflex by the cerebellum. J Neurophysiol 39: 954-969

Robinson DA (1981) Control of eye movements. In: Brooks VB (ed) Handbook of physiology, sect 1: the nervous system, vol II. Am Physiol Soc (Bethesda), pp 1275-1320

Sato Y, Kawasaki T, Ikarashi K (1983) Zonal organization of the floccular Purkinje cells projecting to the vestibular nucleus in cats. Brain Res 232: 1-15

Takemori S, Cohen B (1974) Loss of suppression of vestibular nystagmus after flocculus lesion. Brain Res 72: 213-224

Waespe W, Cohen B (1983) Effects of flocculectomy on unit activity in the vestibular nuclei during visual-vestibular interactions. Exp Brain Res 51: 23-35

Waespe W, Henn V (1977a) Neuronal activity in the vestibular nuclei of the alert monkey during vestibular and optokinetic stimulation. Exp Brain Res 27: 523-538

Waespe W, Henn V (1977b) Vestibular nuclei activity during optokinetic after-nystagmus (OKAN) in the alert monkey. Exp Brain Res 30: 323-330

Waespe W, Henn V (1978) Conflicting visual-vestibular stimulation and vestibular nucleus activity in alert monkeys. Exp Brain Res 33: 203-211

Waespe W, Henn V (1979a) The velocity response of vestibular nucleus neurons during vestibular, visual, and combined angular acceleration. Exp Brain Res 37: 337-347

Waespe W, Henn V (1979b) Motion information in the vestibular nuclei of alert monkeys: Visual and vestibular input vs. optomotor output. In: Granit R, Pompeiano O (eds) Reflex control of posture and movement. Prog Brain Res 50: 683-693

Waespe W, Henn V (1981) Visual-vestibular interaction in the flocculus of the alert monkey. II. Purkinje cell activity. Exp Brain Res 43: 439-360

Waespe W, Henn V, Isoviita V (1980) Nystagmus slow-phase velocity during vestibular, optokinetic, and combined stimulation in the monkey. Arch Psychiat Nervenkr 228: 275-286

Waespe W, Buettner U, Henn V (1981) Visual-vestibular interaction in the flocculus of the alert monkey. I. Input activity. Exp Brain Res 43: 337-348

Waespe W, Cohen B, Raphan T (1983) Role of the flocculus and paraflocculus in optokinetic nystagmus and visual-vestibular interactions: effects of lesions. Exp Brain Res 50: 9-33

Waespe W, Rudinger D, Wolfensberger M (1985) Floccular Purkinje cell activity after bilateral neurectomy during optokinetic nystagmus (OKN) and smooth pursuit eye movements in primates (in preparation)

Westheimer G, McKee SP (1975) Visual acuity in the presence of retinal image motion. J Opt Soc Am 65: 847-850

Yingcharoen K, Rinvik E (1983) Ultrastructural degeneration of a projection from the flocculus to the nucleus prepositus hypoglossi in the cat. Exp Brain Res 51: 192-198

Zee DS, Yee RD, Robinson DA (1976) Optokinetic responses in labyrinthine-defective human beings. Brain Res 113: 423-428

Zee DS, Yamazaki A, Butler PH, Gucer G (1981) Effects of ablation of flocculus and paraflocculus on eye movements in primate. J Neurophysiol 46: 878-899

Clinical Evidence for Functional Compartmentalization of the Cerebellum

J. DICHGANS and H.C. DIENER [1]

1 Introduction

The unique structure of the cerebellum suggests a specific function of this part of the brain. Its nature, however, is poorly understood. Given the anatomical uniformity of the cerebellar cortex one may wonder whether it will be possible to localize functions of a principally different type within the cerebellar mantle. Even, if this were not the case, it is important to realize that there may exist functional localization as the result of the very specific afferent and efferent connections of a particular cerebellar area. Aside from these questions of a more basic significance, it is of clinical importance to know whether there are symptoms that allow for localization. This paper reports on the literature treating the subject and a number of our own studies on patients with postural ataxia and cerebellar disorders of eye movements. A major part of this review has already been published elsewhere (Dichgans 1984). So far the literature mainly contains studies with lesions in animals and rather few studies on patients with lesions that are well limited and precisely localized, e.g. by CT-scanning in recent years.

Many explanations previously offered for the function of the cerebellum and correlations of dysfunction with clinical signs of disease of this structure have been based on the present knowledge about the areas of termination of particular types of afferents and their reciprocal target regions of efference in conjunction with phylogenetic considerations (Dow and Moruzzi 1958; Brodal 1981; Gilman et al. 1981). These two aspects are summarized in Fig. 1, which at the same time, may be used to clarify the nomenclature employed in this article. Figure 1 also indicates some of the frequent inaccuracies in terminology. Thus, for example, the equation of the anterior lobe with the spinocerebellum is incorrect since spino-cerebellar afferents terminate not only in the more medial parts of the anterior lobes, but also in the posterior lobes, while pontocerebellar afferents project to the more lateral parts of both lobes. Reciprocal (spino-cerebello-spinal) loops are suggested by anatomy and probably are involved in updating ongoing motor programs via the intermediate and vermal cerebellum (follow-up assistance). In addition, non-reciprocal circuits, originating in prefrontal (Brodmann's area 9+10) and premotor (6) areas of the cerebral cortex exist that involve the lateral cerebellum in the initiation of movement and in motor programming (see also Sasaki, this Volume). One such circuit was originally proposed by Evarts and Thach (1969) and by Allen and Tsukahara (1974). The function of this circuit has further been interpreted by Eccles (1977). The interpretations given by Eccles with respect to clinical evidence

[1]   Department of Neurology, University of Tübingen 7400 Tübingen, FRG

Cerebellar Functions
ed. by Bloedel et al.
© Springer-Verlag Berlin Heidelberg 1984

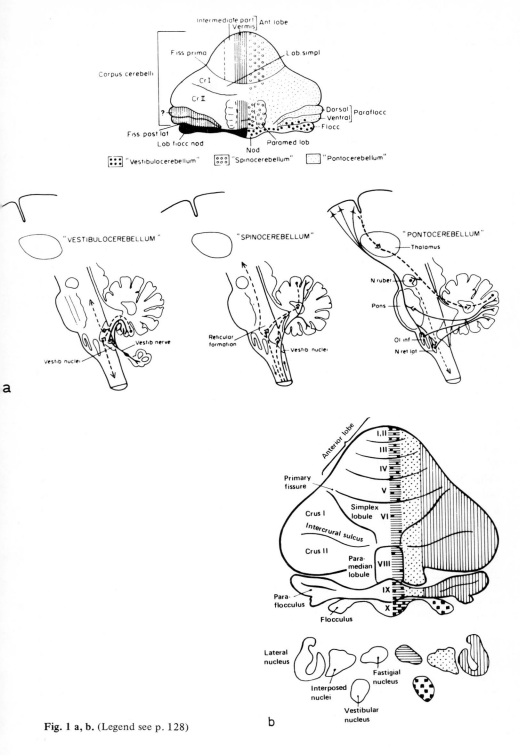

Fig. 1 a, b. (Legend see p. 128)

are based largely on the splendid work of Holmes (e.g. 1917, 1939) of whom Walshe correctly wrote in his obituary notice (1966, quoted after Eccles 1977): "His clinical studies still remain the most careful and detailed record of dysfunction in the human cerebellum". Holmes mainly studied patients with lesions of the cerebellar hemisphere, due to gunshot injury, and therefore studied and described mainly the consequences of damage to the lateral, neocerebellar hemisphere. The clinical symptoms of neocerebellar damage are invariably more pronounced in the arm than in the leg and in brief comprise the following features.

2 Symptoms of Damage to the Lateral Cerebellar Hemispheres

2.1 Hypotonia, Hyporeflexia, and Asthenia

Hypotonia, hyporeflexia, and asthenia are most prominent after an acute lesion. Muscular power may be reduced to as low as half the control (Holmes 1917). Affected limbs tire more quickly than their fellows. Power can be felt to be jerky. Asthenia was found to be more prominent in proximal muscles than in distal ones (Holmes 1917). The possible reasons for hypotonia and hyporeflexia and the relevant literature have extensively been discussed by Gilman (1969) and Gilman et al. (1981). In brief, the depressed excitability of stretch reflexes in the affected limbs and the hypotonia have been both ascribed to a reduction of the proprioceptive inflow due to a decrease in the resting discharge of both static and dynamic fusimotor fibers. The extensor rigidity following complete cerebellar ablation or ablation of the anterior lobe only (in the cat) stems from an increase in the excitatory action of descending pathways directly on alpha motoneurons rather than gamma motoneurons. Extensor rigidity can also be produced in deafferented preparations by ablation of the cerebellar anterior lobe (Pollock and Davis, 1930). The marked extensor rigidity in subprimates results from interrupting the tonic inhibitory action of a large direct projection from the cerebellar anterior lobe to the vestibular nuclei. A comparably developed projection from the cerebellar cortex to the vestibular nuclei has not been found in primates. In primates the output projections of the cerebellar hemispheres are more fully developed and provide a much greater proportion of the total cerebellar output (Gilman et al. 1981). The output of the neocerebellum can increase the excitability of alpha motoneurons by way of the cerebello-cortical pathway to gamma-motoneurons from motor cortex to the anterior horn.

Fig. 1 a, b. A simplified diagram of the mammalian cerebellum. (After Brodal 1981). In the *left half* of the *upper diagram* the three main subdivisions, which can be recognized on a comparative anatomical basis. *Black* Archicerebellum (flocculo-nodular lobe); *hatched* paleocerebellum (vermis of the anterior lobe, pyramis, uvula, and paraflocculus); *white* neocerebellum. In the *right half* the main terminal areas of spinocerebellar pathways *(open circles)*, pontine afferents *(small dots)* and vestibular afferents *(filled circles)*. *Below* three simplified diagrams illustrating that each of the main functional subdivisions, by way of its efferent projections, will influence first and foremost the part of the nervous system from which it receives its main input; b The three sagittal zones of the cerebellum, each of which specifically connects with the deep cerebellar or vestibular nuclei, as shown in the lower part (projections of Purkinje cells in cat, after Brodal 1981). The cortical sites of origin of fibers to the various intracerebellar nuclei and the vestibular nuclei are indicated by symbols corresponding to those in the nuclei. *Stippled* area largely corresponds to what in the text is termed intermediate zone

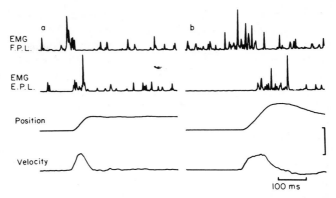

Fig. 2 a, b. Effect of ingestion of alcohol sufficient to cause cerebellar ataxia on fast ballistic thumb flexion (from Marsden et al. 1977). The records in **a** were taken in the morning prior to alcohol, those in **b** were obtained 90 min after oral intake of 200 ml of 50% ethanol. The signal to move occurred 50 ms in **a** and 100 ms in **b** prior to the start of the sweep. Note the delay in onset of movement, the slower movement, the overshoot of the target, and inability to hold the final position and the prolongation of the bursts of rectified *EMG* activity in the agonist (flexor poll. long). and antagonist (extensor poll. long.). The calibration is $20°$ resp. $250°/s$)

2.2 Abnormalities in Timing and Build-up of Force

Intentional movements, such as grasping or pointing, but also withdrawals in reaction to pain are slower in the affected arm, but not in the leg (Holmes 1917). Build-up and relaxation of intended force and consequent displacement upon command occur with a delay and more slowly in the affected limb. The frequent overshoot dysmetria may be interpreted conceptually as the consequence of delayed termination of ongoing force in a ballistic or ramp movement. Among other factors involved, it is this difficulty in timing and build-up of force that contributes to the slowness of alternating movements: dysdiadochokinesis. That the lateral cerebellum indeed participates in initiation of movement has been shown by Meyer-Lohmann et al. (1977), who, by cooling of the dentate nucleus, caused a delay in both the initiation of movement and the discharge of pyramidal tract neurons linked to motor activity. Delayed termination of muscle action may also be induced by cooling of the dentate nucleus (Conrad and Brooks 1975). Human cerebellar ataxia with overshoot, due to delayed termination, is characterized by a pronounced delay in or absence of the agonist pause and antagonist burst (Fig. 2) resulting in inappropriate deceleratory forces (Terzuolo and Viviani 1974; Hallett et al. 1975; Marsden et al. 1977). The use of proprioceptive loops for braking actions in triceps brachii via the cerebellum may also explain the rapid stop of elbow flexion when an opposed flexion is suddenly released in normals and its delay in the cerebellar patient. It is the lack of the normal rebound phenomenon that is characteristic for a cerebellar lesion.

2.3 Decomposition of Movement

Errors in direction, deviations from proper course, discontinuity, dysmetria (mostly overshoot), and tremor (increasing with proximity to the target) illustrate the decomposistion of voluntary movements. This, with hemispherical lesions, is again more striking in the upper limbs than in the lower extremity and more pronounced in complex than in simple movements. Control of movements by vision has no influence on their accuracy. Decomposition of movement according to Holmes (1917) is partly due to "the absence or disturbance of the proper synergic association in the contraction of agonists, antagonists, and fixating muscles, which assures that the different components of an act follow in proper sequence at the proper moment and are of the proper degree. There is often a tendency to an irregular spread of the innervation to other muscles than those which under normal conditions execute the act". Here again, it is the temporal composition of the orderly time sequence of a complex program involving multiple functional subunits of agonist-antagonist interaction composing a coordinate action that is deranged. The individual command concerning the various protagonist muscles might come from the motor cortex, the function of the cerebellum being to superimpose the functional synergies necessary for the achievement of the motor act (Rondot et al. 1979). Considerations like these have stimulated the conceptual interpretation of cerebellar anatomy by Braitenberg (1967). This author viewed the parallel fibers of the cerebellar cortex as a delay line with the ability to transform spatial into temporal patterns.

2.4 Tremor and Myoclonus

Both intention — tremor, and intention — myoclonus are markers of dysfunction of the loops involving the intermediate and lateral corticonuclear zones. Myoclonus characterizes some dentate lesions (e.g. in the Ramsey-Hunt Syndrome). Lesions of the lateral cerebellar nuclei and brachium conjunctivum induce tremor most markedly during limb movements (intention or kinetic tremor, Gilman et al. 1981). Carrea and Mettler (1955) showed that interrupting the ventral portion of the crossed ascending limb of the brachium conjunctivum produces tremor while lesions interrupting the descending limb result in ataxia. L-dopa has been reported to relieve postural tremor following cerebellar ablations in animals, but not the kinetic tremor (Goldberger and Growdon 1971). This finding was interpreted to indicate that different mechanisms may underly the two kinds of tremor. Kinetic tremor can be provoked by having the patient perform the finger-nose and heel-shin tests. The amplitude of the oscillation usually increases as the finger approaches the target. Postural tremor can be demonstrated by asking the patient to extend the arms parallel to the floor. Usually this position can be sustained steadily for some seconds, but then oscillation develops. Llinas and Volkind (1973) relating the limb tremor induced by harmaline intoxication in animals to the physiological action of olivocerebellar projections concluded that the inferior olive generates the phasic movements associated with tremor through its action on neurons in the cerebellar nuclei. The evidence speaking for and against one of the two leading hypotheses explaining tremor (the central neural network behaving as an oscillator or decreased damping of oscillation by instability of long loop reflexes (Neilson and Lance 1978, Vilis and Hore 1977, 1980) has been discussed by Gilman et al. (1981). Some clinical and neuropathological evidence indicating the role of the inferior olive may be added: Palatal myorrhythmia which is characterized by the delayed appearance of rhythmical movements at a frequency of 2-3/s is caused by olivary hypertrophy which is thought to be the consequence of transsynaptic degeneration following removal of the input to the inferior olive presumably due to lesions of the dentate nuclei or tegmental tracts. The surviving neurons are enlarged and frequently vacuolated and present elaborate dendritic expansions (Koeppen et al. 1980). Patients complain if muscles of pharynx, larynx, floor of the mouth, and lower part of the face are also involved. — A similar tremor of the head and hand may develop within two to threee months after an acute cerebellar lesion.

3 Ataxia of Gait and Stance

Ataxia of the arm or hand originates from lesions of the lateral neocerebellar hemispheres or their output via the dentate nucleus, the brachium conjunctivum, and the ventro-lateral nucleus of the thalamus. Ataxia of gait and stance, however, results from lesions of the more medial structures within the cerebellum, the anterior lobe, and vestibulo-cerebellar vermis. Cerebellar ataxia of gait includes difficulties in walking on a straight line and difficulties in precise placement of the feet, mostly with placement too widely apart. Dysmetria is common, but the elevation of the leg is not as exaggerated as it is observed with impaired position sense. Vision greatly eases walking of the ataxic patient; stance usually is on a broad base.

Earlier investigations indicated that lesions of the different parts of the cerebellum lead to specific patterns of postural instability (Dichgans et al. 1976; Mauritz et al. 1979; Diener et al. 1984b). In order to further substantiate the topodiagnostical significance of these sway patterns 122 patients with cerebellar disorders were investigated using a posturographic platform for measurement. Patients with severe paresis due to additional lesions of the pyramidal tract and patients with multiple sclerosis were excluded. Six different groups of patients were formed according to the site of their lesion. Their results were compared with those of normals (N = 30). From the recording of the movement of the center of foot pressure on the platform sway path (SP, Fig. 3), sway area, the amount of anterior-posterior and lateral sway per unit time, both with open and closed eyes, were calculated. The amount of visual stabilization was calculated from the quotient of sway path and sway area with the eyes closed and open (Romberg quotient). In order to construct the sway direction histogram (SDH) of the CFP we divided the full circle of possible sway directions into eight intervals of 45° each. The single vectors of the displacement of the CFP within each sampling interval were assorted according to their directions and summed up (Fig. 3). Fourier analysis of the displacements of the CFP was also performed. Head and hip movements were recorded by means of goniometers attached to the head and the hip by rigid belts.

3.1 Lesions of the Spinocerebellar Part of the Anterior Lobe

Lesions of the spinocerebellar (upper vermal and intermediate) part of the anterior lobe were observed in 42 patients. This disease, the late cortical cerebellar atrophy, originates from a combination of chronic alcoholism and malnutrition (Victor et al. 1959). It causes abnormalities in gait and stance with mild or absent ataxia of the upper limbs tested with the finger-to-nose-test, but prominent ataxia if tested with the heel-to-knee-manoeuvre. Polyneuropathy is only mild when present. The syndrome of postural instability in these patients is quite specific and may easily be differentiated from that

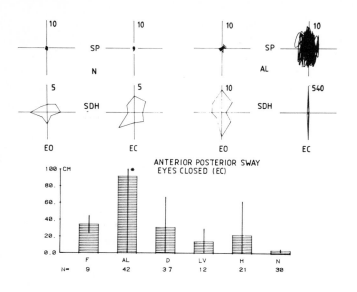

Fig. 3. Sway path *(SP)* and sway direction histograms *(SDH)*, the latter summing up the direction of vectors of sway within each of 8 bins of the 360 deg full circle. Data from a normal *(upper left)* and a patient with anterior lobe atrophy *(upper right)*. Note the different scales of SDH and the strong preference of anterior-posterior sway in the patient with anterior lobe atrophy. In the lower part of the figure means and standard deviations of the anterior-posterior sway component with eyes closed are shown. *F* Friedreich's ataxia; *AL* anterior lobe atrophy; *D* diffuse cerebellar lesion; *LV* lower vermis lesion; *H* cerebellar hemispherical lesion; *N* normal controls

due to other cerebellar lesions. Patients with anterior lobe atrophy as a group exhibit the largest amount of sway path. Body sway is predominantly in the anterior posterior direction (Fig. 3). It contains a very conspicuous high frequency sway component around 3 Hz (Silfverskiöld 1969; Dichgans et al. 1976). This "tremor" is provoked by eye closure (Fig. 4). Recordings from head and hip show an increased amplitude of inter-segmental stabilization of head versus trunk versus legs (see also Mauritz et al. 1979) which, although opposite in phase, occurs at the same frequency of 3 Hz at all three levels recorded (Fig. 4). This is in contrast to other cerebellar lesions, where head and trunk tremor sometimes have different frequencies. In incipient cases tremor may be provoked by suddenly unbalancing the body by a rapid push to the trunk or the rapid tilt of a platform preferably toe-up (Diener et al. 1984c). The body tremor frequency was reported to decrease with progression of the disease (Mauritz et al. 1981). Our own follow-up study in 11 patients indicates no systematic correlation of sway frequency neither with the duration of the illness nor the amount of ataxia in terms of the length of the sway path or the area covered by sway of the body's center of force.

A second follow-up study in 17 patients with late atrophy of the anterior lobe (average time interval 18.5 months) showed a significant, sometimes dramatic, decrease of body sway in patients who were abstinent (N = 11) and an increase of body sway in the six patients who continued drinking (Diener et al. 1984d).

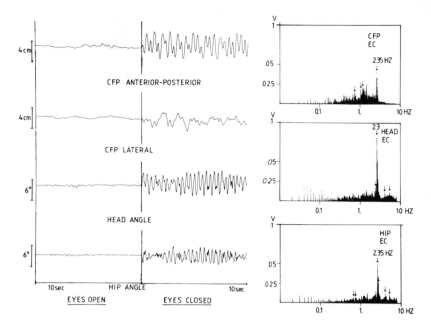

Fig. 4. Original recording of anterior and lateral displacement of the center of foot pressure, head, and hip angle with eyes open and eyes closed in a patient with anterior lobe atrophy on the *left*. Note the predominantly anterior posterior body sway (frequency 2.3 Hz) when the eyes are closed. This dominant frequency can also be observed in the Fourier power spectra of the CFP, the head and the hip, on the *right*

3.2 Lesions of the Vestibulocerebellum

Lesions of the vestibulocerebellum mainly due to medulloblastoma or bleeding from an angioblastoma in our sample (N = 12) cause postural ataxia of head and trunk while sitting, standing, and walking. Dysmetria of the upper and lower limbs is not prominent, if tested separately. Posturography shows omnidirectional body sway (Fig. 5), sometimes of excessive amplitude predominantly containing frequencies below 1 Hz. Mauritz et al. (1979) described a diminished intersegmental stabilization of upright stance in these patients. Visual stabilization as evaluated by the Romberg quotient is less than in the other groups of cerebellar patients. One may be tempted to conclude that visual afferents to the vestibulocerebellum not only serve the well documented stabilization of retinal images on the eye (see below), but also the visual stabilization of posture. Based on the observation that patients with a vestibulocerebellar lesion tend to fall even when sitting with their eyes open we assume that the vestibular graviceptive set value for spatial orientation versus gravity as elaborated by the vestibulocerebellum is unaccessible for postural stabilization in these patients causing drifts and poor control activity. In contrast, patients with anterior lobe atrophy although heavily oscillating almost never fall. In them the correct position seems to be known to the system, but the control loops oscillate because of increased gain and poor control of the duration of postural reflexes (see below).

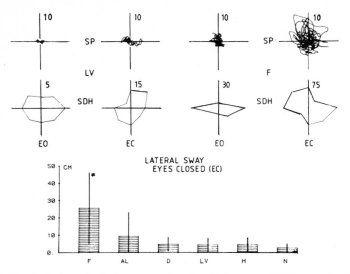

Fig. 5. Sway path *(SP)* and sway direction histograms *(SDH)* in a patient with a lesion of the lower vermis *(upper left)* and a patient with Friedreich's ataxia *(upper right)*. Note the different scaling and the strong preference of lateral sway in the patient with Friedreich's disease. Means and standard deviations of the lateral sway component in the different groups of cerebellar lesions are shown in the lower part of the figure

3.3 Lesions of the Neocerebellum

In patients in whom a tumor or ischemic lesion was limited to the *lateral cerebellar hemisphere* (N = 21) postural stability although occasionally somewhat less was not affected to a statistically significant amount with respect to all the parameters tested so far. Mauritz (1979) showed abnormal ataxic deviations in these patients if they attempted to follow with their bodycenter of force displayed on an oscilloscope a sinusoidally moving target displayed on the same scope. This observation nicely fits the assumption that the lateral cerebellar hemisphere subserves the fine spatio-temporal organization of pursuit by limb and trunk movements. Holmes (1917) studying patients with acute hemispherical lesions described an inclination of head and trunk to the injured side with the patients spine concave to it. In addition head and trunk occasionally showed a tendency to be rotated towards the opposite side. Placing of the affected foot was irregular, dysmetric, and gait stumbling with a tendency to deviate and fall towards the side of the lesion. Patients "threw their weight" as little as possible on the unsafe leg. Holmes (1917) noted that patients being in danger of falling do not move either trunk or arms naturally or adequately in attempting to regain equilibrium, an observation that is reminiscent of what we have seen in patients with a vestibulocerebellar lesion.

3.4 Friedreich's Disease

Friedreich's disease (N = 9) was considered to be paradigmatic for a spinal ataxia. In its early stages the disease mainly affects spinocerebellar afferents and the posterior columns. We observed in most of these patients a low frequency large amplitude sway with most of its power below 1.1 Hz (Fig. 5). The lateral component of sway was significantly larger than in normals and other patients when the eyes were closed (Fig. 5). Visual stabilization was preserved. These patients never exhibit a high frequency peak within the Fourier power spectrum of body sway, but may show high frequency tremor of the head (Dichgans et al. 1983).

Patients with diffuse cerebellar lesions (N= 37) including heriditary late cerebellar atrophy, olivo-ponto-cerebellar atrophy, and atrophy due to toxic agents like bromides and hydantoin do not exhibit a specific pattern of postural instability. Statistically they may be clearly separated from normals, but not from the other cerebellar patients.

4 Operation of Long Latency EMG Responses in Cerebellar Patients

Three successive EMG responses can be recorded after the sudden application of a perturbation to a limb. They were named M1, M2, and M3 by Lee and Tatton (1975). M1 is equivalent to the segmental stretch reflex. The occurance of M2 and M3 has been thought to depend on the functional integrity of supraspinal structures. They are probably wired through sensorimotor cortex (see review by Wiesendanger and Miles 1983) with a possible contribution of the cerebellum (Lee and Tatton 1975; MacKay and Murphy 1979). The circuits involved and their physiology are, however, still far from being understood. The clinical literature concerning long-loop responses in cerebellar patients is very small. Marsden et al. (1978) described a loss or diminuation of the initial component of the long latency stretch reflex in the long flexor of the thumb with relative preservation or delay of the later component in four patients with a unilateral cerebellar lesion. In an experiment with acute alcohol intoxication they also observed a loss of the early part of the long-loop reflex. Experiments of Diener et al. (1983b) hint that it is the possible influence of alcohol on spinal afferents that causes the delay of the late component of long latency responses. MacKay and Murphy (1979) observed a striking reduction or delay of the medium latency response in wrist muscles in a patient with a pontine angle tumor.

With the experimental paradigm most frequently used M2 and M3 both occur in the same stretched muscle. It is often difficult to separate them clearly. We therefore also evoked long latency reflexes in standing subjects by a sudden tilt toe-up of the support. With this manoeuvre, the short (SL) and medium (ML) latency response are evoked in the stretched triceps surae muscle (TS). They destabilize posture and are followed by the posture stabilizing long latency response (LL) in the antagonist, the anterior tibial muscle (TA), (Fig. 6). In order to clarify whether EMG recordings from finger muscles are comparable to those from leg muscles we recorded short-, medium-, and long latency responses after stretch of the first dorsal interosseus muscle (FDI) and of the triceps surae in 40 patients with cerebellar lesions (see Friedemann et al. 1984). In the remaining 82 patients we applied only platform tilts. The latency of M1 in the first dorsal interosseus muscle (FDI) and of the SL response in the triceps surae muscle was normal in most of the patients, except those with an additional polyneuropathy (mostly alcoholics, Figs. 6, 7). Due to the severe demyelination of the most proximal segment of the afferent fibers the stretch reflex was missing or considerably delayed in patients

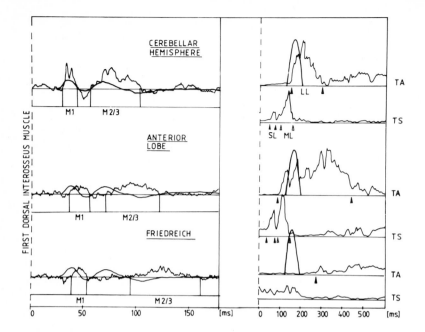

Fig. 6. EMG-responses to stretch of the first dorsal interosseus muscle, on the left, and to platform tilt toe-up in the anterior tibial *(TA)* and triceps surae *(TS)* muscles, on the right. *Heavy line* on the *left* shows the grand average of 20 normal subjects. Note the increased M 2/3-complex in the patient with anterior lobe disease, and the marked delay of the M 2/3 response in the patient with Friedreich's disease. *Arrows* on the *right* indicate beginning and end of the three EMG-responses with short, medium, and long latency. Note the increase of the long latency response in the patient with anterior lobe disease and the marked delay of the long latency response in the patient with Friedreich's disease

with Friedreich's ataxia. The integral of the SL response was normal in more than 85% of the patients. M2 and M3 could not clearly be separated in most of the normals and patients in FDI and therefore were treated as an M2/3 complex. The latency of this complex was sometimes slightly delayed in patients with anterior lobe atrophy, but considerably delayed in patients with Friedreich's ataxia (Fig. 7). The occurence of ML in the triceps surae was also markedly delayed when present in Friedreich's disease, but normal in the other groups (Fig. 6).

The integral of the M2/M3 complex in FDI was increased in patients with vermal and hemispherical cerebellar lesions. The integral of the ML response in TS was always normal, but the integral of the LL response in TA was markedly increased in patients with anterior lobe atrophy, hemispherical, and diffuse cerebellar lesions. The latency of LL was within normal limits as long as the lesion was restricted to the cerebellum itself. It was massively delayed from 119.7+/-14.2 to 255.5+/-50 ms in patients with Friedreich's disease. The lack of a training effect on latency in repeated trials, small intraindividual variance, and the correlation of the delay with the severity of the disease were considered in favor of the assumption of a delayed LL response in Friedreich's disease and against a voluntary contraction (Diener et al. 1984a, c).

Healthy subjects submitted to an acute alcohol intoxication in addition to signs of spinocerebellar dysfunction show a significant delay in the stabilizing LL response to

Fig. 7. Means and standard deviations of the latency of short, medium, and long latency responses in the triceps surae *(SL, ML)* and the anterior tibial muscle *(LL)*. *F* Friedreich's disease; *AL* anterior lobe atrophy; *D* diffuse cerebellar lesions; *LV* lower vermal lesion; *H* hemispherical cerebellar lesion; *N* normal population. Note the increase in latency of the ML and LL response in patients with Friedreich's disease

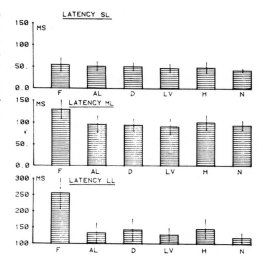

platform tilt toe-up of the anterior tibial muscle thereby indicating that alcohol also affects afferent pathways involved in the generation of long-loop postural responses (Diener et al. 1983b; Woollacott 1983).

We are aware of the difficulties which arise from the comparison of long-loop reflexes from finger and leg muscles. Since nearly all of the patients exhibiting a lesion confined to the cerebellum showed normal latencies of M2/3 and ML/LL one may be tempted to conclude that the cerebellum does not generate these long-loop responses. The clear delay of long-loop responses in patients with Friedreich's ataxia, as to our understanding, must be due to the predominant involvement of afferent (and efferent) spinal pathways in these patients. This assumption is supported by the observation of increased latencies of the LL response in patients with multiple sclerosis presenting with delayed sensory evoked potentials (Diener et al. 1984e) and patients with spinal tumors or cervical myelopathy (unpublished observation). The most striking effect of a cerebellar lesion is the increase in amplitude and, more so, in duration of long-loop responses. Obviously the cerebellum participates in the control of gain and duration of long-loop responses, whereas the basal ganglia modulate M2 as evidenced by its increase in patients with Parkinson's disease (Lee and Tatton 1975; Scholz et al. 1984) and its absence or decrease in patients with chorea (Noth et al. 1983). Since ML is normal in the triceps surae, but LL is increased we assume that it is the M3 component of the M2/M3 complex in FDI responses that is increased in cerebellar diseases.

The stabilizing long-loop response of the anterior tibial muscle after a rapid tilt of the supporting platform toe-up, although mostly normal in latency, is significantly increased in amplitude and prolonged in duration from an average of about 80ms to 185 ms when vision is occluded in patients with anterior lobe atrophy (Diener et al. 1984c). The increase in duration and amplitude of the antagonist response and the obvious increase in amplitude of intersegmental movements may constitute the 3 Hz body tremor. Despite the tremor and a considerable increase in sway path and sway area the patients with anterior lobe atrophy generally are able to keep upright, even with rapid tilts of a supporting platform. The 3 Hz body tremor per se stabilizes posture and filters imposed disturbances (Fig. 4).

Our results are in contrast to the ones obtained by Marsden et al. (1977) in arm muscles where cerebellar dysfunction resulted in a loss or diminution of the initial component of M2 and a delay of M3. A delay in onset of the antagonist activity terminating the reflexive response to stretch of the biceps brachii muscle was also found by Vilis and Hore (1980) after cooling the dentate and interpositus nuclei in monkeys. Whereas this could not be confirmed in the anterior tibial muscle of humans with cerebellar lesions their observation of an increased duration was repeated.

We have never observed adaptation of the ML response to stretch of the triceps surae with platform tilt in normals and the patients recorded by now (Diener et al. 1983a). This is in disagreement to the finding of Nashner and Grimm (1978) who observed adaptation of this functionally destabilizing response in normals and a loss of adaptation of this reflex in 11 of 15 of their cerebellar patients when they changed platform movement from a horizontal backward motion to platform rotation toe-up. Both manoeuvres stretch the triceps surae. But with linear motion, ML stabilizes whereas it destabilizes with platform tilt. The reasons of this disagreement are not clear to us. One possibility is the much higher speed of angular displacement used in our experiments ($50°/s$ versus $8°/s$). Nashner and Grimm (1978) also reported abnormalities in static and dynamic vestibular control of posture. These were present also in patients with a slight to moderate ataxia of gait.

A further subject of interest is to investigate to what extent the cerebellum participates in the generation of anticipatory postural adjustments (Belenkii et al. 1967; Bouisset and Zattara, 1981; Cordo and Nashner 1982) preceeding voluntary movement of the arm. Patients with Parkinson's disease invariably show missing or greatly reduced anticipation. A few patients with cerebellar truncal ataxia of varying origin showed diminution only in severe cases (Traub et al. 1980). Paltsev and Elner (1967) have measured an appreciable phase lag in the supportive reactions of the ipsilateral leg muscles in response to forward arm extension in patients with unilateral cerebellar damage.

5 Dysarthria — Dysprosodia

Cerebellar dysarthria has been given the following descriptors: staccato, hesitant, explosive, scanning, slurring, slow, or garbled. The sum of the difficulties with the regulation of speech in cerebellar diseases is called dysprosody (Holmes 1917; Cole 1971). Deranged speed and transition from one syllable or one word to the next, inappropriate accentuation and intonation, pauses where unnecessary and slurred transitions instead of pauses as well as tremulous voice are characteristic features consequent to ataxia of the respiratory and oral-buccal-lingual musculature. They reflect the inability to appropriately program and control force, velocity, and timing of muscle activity involved in enunciation. Localization of speech function in the cerebellum has been attempted by only a few authors. Weisenburg (1927) inferred that the superior vermis portion of the cerebellum is important in the regulation of speed. But Holmes (1917) also collected cases in whom the lesion was confined to the cerebellar hemisphere (see also Brown 1959). Amici et al. (1976) found cerebellar dysarthria most often in patients with damage to the paravermal and lateral elements of the hemispheres. Lechtenberg and

Gilman (1978) finally observed a statistically significant association between lesions of the left cerebellar hemisphere and dysarthria. The area of encroachment that repeatedly appeared in patients with speech disorders was the superior paravermal segment of the left hemisphere, about Larsell's lobules H VI and H VII (see Fig. 1b). Gilman et al. (1981), however, concede that, although the present evidence implicates a focal lesion in the paravermal segment of the left cerebellar hemisphere in cerebellar speech disorders, it is unlikely that only one cerebellar locus is responsible for all the facets of speech disorder occurring with cerebellar diseases. — The differences in disordered speech between patients suffering from Friedreich's disease and those suffering from olivo-ponto-cerebellar atrophy have been analyzed by Gilman and Klein (this Volume).

6 Oculomotor Symptoms

The oculomotor symptoms of cerebellar diseases have been widely studied both by basic scientists performing single unit recordings and ablation studies, and by clinicians. The results demonstrate a nice example of a very advanced analysis of motor behavior and its partial organization by the cerebellum. A recent review by Dichgans and Jung (1975) and the excellent summary of the current knowledge and concepts by Zee (1982) provide sufficient information about the relevant literature. Because of the enormous wealth of information now available the following paragraphs can only deal with some highlights of recent clinical and physiological research on the cerebellar contribution to oculomotor function (see also Waespe and Henn and Precht et al., this Vol.).

Apparently, oculomotor functions can now at least tentatively be relegated to two particular portions of the cerebellum: the vestibulocerebellum and the posterior vermis. The dorsal cerebellar vermis and underlying fastigial nuclei function in the control of

Table 1. Hypothetical scheme of cerebellar localization of ocular motor functions and eye movement abnormalities. (After Zee 1982)

Structure:	Vestibulocerebellum	Dorsal vermis/ fastigial nuclei
Function:	Retinal-image stabilization (smooth tracking, suppression of inappropriate vestibular nystagmus, holding positions of gaze, long-term adjustments in VOR gain and the saccadic pulse-step match)	Immediate and longterm control of saccadic pulse amplitude
Disorder:	Impaired smooth pursuit, VOR cancellation and fixation suppression of caloric nystagmus; gaze-evoked, rebound and downbeat nystagmus; postsaccadic drift; inappropriate VOR	Enduring saccadic dysmetria

VOR = vestibulo-ocular reflex

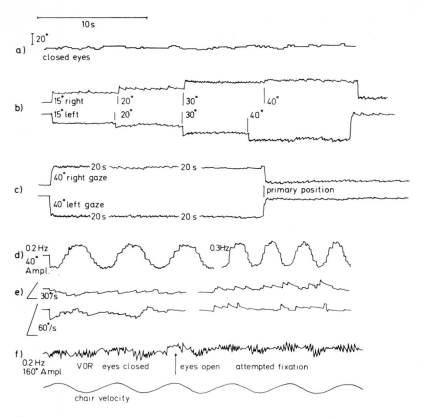

Fig. 8 a-f. Disorders of oculomotor function in a patient with a bilateral lesion of the cerebellar flocculus; **a** Increased number and amplitude of square wave jerks; **b** Gaze paretic nystagmus increasingly active with increasing deviation from the straight ahead position; **c** Rebound nystagmus: progressively decreasing activity of gaze paretic nystagmus with prolonged eccentric fixation and reversed direction of nystagmus upon return to the midline; **d** Cogwheeled smooth pursuit (low gain of pursuit, catch-up saccades); **e** Marked diminuition of slow phase velocity of OKN; **f** Well-preserved VOR *(left)* absence of the ability to suppress vestibular nystagmus by fixation of a target that is stationary with respect to the subject *(right)*. It is the dissociation of OKN and smooth pursuit deficits and preserved *VOR* that is characteristic for a floccular lesion, whereas all three functions are impaired with a lesion of the paramedian pontine reticular formation (Dichgans 1984)

a number of retinal image stabilizing reflexes including smooth pursuit, visual modulation of the vestibulo-ocular reflex, holding positions of gaze and suppression of post-saccadic drift (see Table 1 and Fig. 8).

Lasting deficits in smooth pursuit and optokinetic nystagmus are created by total cerebellectomy in adult monkeys (Westheimer and Blair 1973; Burde et al. 1975). Hemicerebellectomy causes a pursuit and gaze holding deficit towards the ipsilateral side. Pursuit gain is reduced to 65% after bilateral flocculectomy and paraflocculectomy in the monkey (Zee et al. 1981). The reduction in gain is more pronounced (gain less than 20%) with total cerebellectomy (Optican and Robinson 1980), a fact that indicates that, besides the flocculus, another, yet unknown, site within the cerebellum exists, that participates in pursuit. Whether this second representation of pursuit resides in areas VI and VII of the dorsal vermis, as indicated by single unit recordings of, Suzuki et al. (1981) remains open until pursuit gain and phase are systematically studied after lesioning this region. Optican and Robinson (1980), upon gross inspection, saw no pursuit deficit after selectively ablating this region. Tracking deficits in gain (Fig. 8d) usually roughly correspond to the deficit in cancelation of the vestibulo-ocular reflex (Robinson 1982) while fixating a target moving with the observer (Fig. 8f). This has been observed in patients (Dichgans et al. 1978; Halmagyi and Gresty 1979) and in flocculectomized monkeys (Zee et al. 1981). It has been suggested that the mechanisms of pursuit and cancelation have similar dynamics and share a common pathway at least to the level of the cerebellar flocculus. Thereafter, there is presumably an anatomical dissociation of the signals mediating the two functions (Chambers and Gresty 1983). The gain of optokinetic nystagmus (OKN) at high stimulus velocities is also reduced after flocculectomy in primates (Takemori and Cohen 1974). Vestibulo-cerebellar lesions in patients with Arnold-Chiari malformations or with isolated atrophy of the lower vermis (Baloh et al. 1981) not only cause a decrease in OKN gain (Fig. 8e), but also a prolonged rise of the slow phase velocity to a steady state after sudden exposure to the stimulus. The similarity in the time course of OKN, when adjusted for initial retinal slip, and in gain, saturation level, and time course of optokinetic afternystagmus before and after bilateral flocculectomy in the monkey indicates that the lesion did not significantly alter the coupling of the visual system to the velocity storage integrator in the brainstem of monkeys, but rather affected the pursuit system responsible for the initial rapid rise in velocity (Waespe et al. 1983, also this Volume).

The smooth pursuit deficit towards the ipsilateral side and a corresponding reduction in gain of OKN slow-phase velocity in patients with *cerebello-pontine angle tumors* (von Reutern and Dichgans 1977) may be explained by compression of the cerebellar flocculus situated immediately adjacent to the eighth nerve. The almost complete absence of pursuit and OKN in humans with a global cerebellar cortical atrophy (Dichgans and Jung 1975; Dichgans et al. 1978; Baloh et al. 1975; 1979; Zee et al. 1976; Avanzini et al. 1979) indicates that the vast majority of visual-oculomotor pathways involved in these functions travel via the cerebellum (mainly the flocculus and possibly paraflocculus) and that the indirect pathway via the brainstem storage mechanism plays a minor role in humans.

Interesting, but still poorly understood information arises from the recent observation of Westheimer and Blair (1974) who found an almost complete compensation of various transient deficits within a few weeks, if ablation of the cerebellum was performed in a juvenile monkey. This observation was confirmed and extended by Eckmiller and Westheimer (1983) who found a permanent deficit only if the cerebellar nuclei were bilaterally included in the ablation. Regarding this, one may be tempted to speculate that at least some of the seemingly normally behaving cases of congenital cerebellar malformation secure motor function by way of their preserved cerebellar nuclei that in early stages of ontogeny may show a considerable ability of rearrangement.

A decreased capability of *short-term adaptation of vestibuloocular reflex* (VOR) gain has been documented in cerebellar patients (Yagi et al. 1981) and in the cerebellectomized cat (Robinson 1976). As expected from its wiring, the vestibulocerebellum executes this control. Ablation of the cerebellar flocculus and paraflocculus in monkeys variably affects the gain, modulating it up or down (Zee et al. 1981). The VOR gain is frequently increased in human patients with vestibulocerebellar lesions (Baloh et al.

1981; Zee et al. 1974). Anomalies of the VOR gain in cerebellar patients may result in perceived motion of the world every time the head is actively moving or passively such as while walking. These findings indicate the role of the cerebellum in calibration and *adaptive gain control* of the vestibulo-ocular reflex. A much more impressive illustration of this is given by experiments using reversing prisms or magnifying (minifying) spectacles, so as to modify the gain of the VOR (Gonshor and Melvill-Jones 1971 and followers, recent review by Miles 1982). A number of recent behavioral studies by Miles and his group and neurophysiological recordings from Purkinje cells in the flocculus (e. g. Lisberger and Fuchs 1978; Miles et al. 1980) suggest that the gaze velocity Purkinje cells have been assigned two quite separate functions, i.e. to form a part of the pursuit system and part of the system regulating VOR gain.

Saccadic dysmetria has been demonstrated by Ritchie (1976) after ablation of the cerebellar vermis (Larsell's lobules VI-VII). Ritchie observed a saccadic hypermetria of centripetal saccades and hypometria with centrifugal saccades. His interpretation assumes that this part of the cerebellum receiving a projection from stretch receptors within the eye muscles (Fuchs and Kornhuber 1969) subserves the parametric adjustment of saccadic force in relation to the starting position. Similar observations of dysmetria depending on the initial position of the saccading eye have been made in patients with advanced cerebellar atrophy (Zee et al. 1976). Their saccades showed normal velocity and latencies.

An inability to hold an excentric position of gaze with a tendency of the eyes to drift back exponentially towards the midline or the neutral position ("gaze paretic nystagmus") (Fig. 8b) has been observed in patients with a suspected floccular lesion due to cerebellar atrophy (Zee et al. 1981) or cerebello-pontine angle tumor with floccular compression (von Reutern and Dichgans 1977) and also in monkeys with bilateral flocculectomy (Zee et al. 1981). According to Optican and Robinson (1980) it is the *"pulse-step mismatch"* of force that by way of too low an amplitude of the step determining final eye position causes the postsaccadic drift back to the midline. Their concept implies that the pulse determining saccadic velocity and amplitude is generated at a place not identical with the one ultimately determining the size of step in discharge frequency of the oculomotor nuclei determining permanent eye position. This was supported by an experiment in which the isolated ablation of the posterior vermis led to a lack of the ability to adapt the size of the saccadic pulse. The lesion resulted in permanent saccadic dysmetria, but not a deficit in suppression of postsaccadic drift in response to a surgically induced ocular muscle weakness.

Differences in the saccadic dysmetria between the two eyes were produced by reversible cooling of the medial cerebellar nuclei on one side (Vilis et al. 1983). If cooling was performed on the left side, the right eye made larger amplitude and higher velocity saccades to the right and smaller amplitude and lower velocity saccades to the left than the left eye. Differences were largest when the saccade was directed away from the center. The results suggest that the cerebellum can compensate for differences in muscles strength by selectively adjusting the strength of the pulse-step innervation to each muscle of a yoked muscle pair.

Holmes (1917) reported that with acute unilateral cerebellar lesions the eyes are no longer spontaneously positioned in the midline, but rather are conjugately displaced contralateral to the side of the lesion in a position he termed: *the new rest point.* One can conceive that this finding results from unilateral loss of cerebellar inhibition on the vestibular nuclei. This is a transient phenomenon. During recovery, gaze paretic nystagmus toward the lesioned side may appear.

Taken together, the results of Optican and Robinson (1980) and of Zee et al. (1981) suggest that the dorsal cerebellar vermis and/or underlying fastigial nuclei are important for plastic adjustments of saccadic pulse amplitude, but not for appropriately matching the size of the saccadic step to the pulse necessary to prevent postsaccadic drift. This latter function appears to be relegated to the flocculus that obtains the appropriate afferent information about retinal slip. No disorder of saccadic latency has been described with vermal or fastigial lesions. Cooling of the fastigial nucleus in the monkey causes no increase in saccadic latency, but causes dysmetria, which by Vilis and Hore (1981) is attributed to a defect in termination of the saccadic pulse.

A special case of holding deficit is the *inability to hold stable fixation,* even in the resting position of the eyes (Fig. 8a). Many of the cerebellar patients, particularly patients with cerebellar atrophy, show an increased number and amplitude of fixation saccades termed "Gegenrucke" in the German literature and "square wave jerks" in the English speaking literature. Whereas the intersaccadic interval is invariably present with square wave jerks, it is constantly missing with *opsoclonus* a chaotic sequence of conjugate saccades seen in patients with myoclonic encephalopathy, a disease that probably involves the dentate (and other?) cerebellar nuclei (see review by Dichgans and Jung 1975).

Some additional symptoms indicating the difficulty with holding a stable position of gaze may finally be mentioned: A rather poorly understood, but probably specific oculomotor sign of cerebellar involvement is *rebound nystagmus* (Fig. 8c). After a prolonged attempt at holding excentric gaze, upon returning to the primary position, a nystagmus occurs counter in direction to the prior gaze nystagmus that disappeared with the prolonged attempt to fixate excentrically (Hood et al. 1973). A more recent paper of Hood (1981) reports repeated reversals of rebound nystagmus upon return to the midline, if the prior excentric fixation was attempted long enough. This observation is interpreted to be analogous to vestibular hyperexcitability with repeated reversals of postrotatory nystagmus. Gaze paretic nystagmus, rebound nystagmus, and *downbeat nystagmus* accentuated on lateral gaze — all three cardinal features of the human oculomotor cerebellar syndrome — have been found in flocculectomized monkeys (Zee et al. 1981). Downbeat nystagmus may relate to a loss of inhibition of the anterior semicircular canal VOR (which mediates upward slow phases) or a pursuit imbalance or an imbalance of the vertical integrators stabilizing eye position (Zee 1982).

In writing this paper it was frequently difficult to resist the temptation to give a more complete description of clinical symptoms and of the wealth of observations made after ablations in animals. The principle of organization largely followed was to point out specific functional disturbances that help to localize a lesion within the cerebellum and to simultaneously interpret them within the framework of current concepts of functional cerebellar organization. Symptoms of localizing significance clearly exist within this structure. It is certainly true that their specificity is mostly determined by the most miraculous arrangement of afferent and efferent connections. The question of whether or not cerebellar cortex locally performs in a principally different way could not be answered.

References

Allen GJ, Tsukahara N (1974) Cerebellar communication systems. Physiol Rev 54: 957-1006

Amici R, Avancini G, Pacini L (1976) Cerebellar tumors. Monographs in neural sciences, vol IV. Karger, Basel

Avanzini G, Girotti F, Crenna P, Negri S (1979) Alterations of ocular motility in cerebellar pathology. Arch Neurol 36: 274-280

Baloh RW, Konrad HR, Honrubia V (1975) Vestibulo-ocular function in patients with cerebellar atrophy. Neurology 25: 160-168

Baloh RW, Jenkins HA, Honrubia V, Yee RD, Lau CGY (1979) Visual-vestibular interaction and cerebellar atrophy. Neurology 29: 116-119

Baloh RW, Yee RD, Kimm J, Honrubia V (1981) Vestibulo-ocular reflex in patients with lesions involving the vestibulocerebellum. Exp Neurol 72: 141-152

Belenkii VYE, Gurfinkel VS, Paltsev YEI (1967) Elements of control of voluntary movements. Biophyzika 12: 135-141

Bouisset S, Zattara M (1981) A sequence of postural movements precedes voluntary movement. Neurosci Lett 22: 263-270

Braitenberg V (1967) Is the cerebellar cortex a biological clock in the millisecond range? Prog Brain Res 25: 334-346

Brodal A (1981) Neurological anatomy. Oxford Univ Press, New York Oxford

Brown JR (1959) Degenerative cerebellar ataxias. Neurology (Minneapolis) 9: 799-805

Burde RM, Stroud MH, Roper-Hall G (1975) Ocular motor dysfunction in total and hemicerebellectomized monkeys. Br J Ophthalmol 59: 560-565

Carrea RME, Mettler FA (1955) Function of the primate brachium conjunctivum and related structures. J Comp Neurol 102: 151

Chambers BR, Gresty MA (1983) The relationship between disordered pursuit and vestibulo-ocular reflex suppression. J Neurol Neurosurg Physiat 46: 61-66

Cole M (1971) Dysprosody due to posterior fossa lesions. Trans Am Neurol Assoc 96: 151-154

Conrad B, Brooks V (1975) Cerebelläre Bewegungsstörungen im Tierversuch. Vergleich rascher Alternativbewegungen und langsamer Zielbewegungen während reversibler Dentatusausschaltung. J Neurol 209: 165-179

Cordo PJ, Nashner LM (1982) Properties of postural adjustments associated with rapid arm movements. J Neurophysiol 47: 287-302

Dichgans J (1984) Clinical symptoms of cerebellar dysfunction and their topodiagnostical significance. Human Neurobiol 2: 269-279

Dichgans J, Jung R (1975) Oculomotor abnormalities due to cerebellar lesions. In: Lennerstrand G, Bach-y-Rita P (eds) Basic mechanisms of ocular motility and their clinical implications. Pergamon Press, Oxford New York, pp 281-298

Dichgans J, Mauritz KH, Allum JHJ, Brandt TH (1976) Postural sway in normals and ataxic patients. Agressologie 17C: 15-24

Dichgans J, Reutern von GM, Römmelt U (1978) Impaired suppression of vestibular nystagmus by fixation in cerebellar and noncerebellar patients. Arch Psychiat Nervenkr 226: 183-193

Dichgans J, Diener HC, Mauritz KH (1983) What distinguishes the different kinds of postural ataxia in patients with cerebellar diseases. Adv Otorhinolaryngol 30: 285-287

Diener HC, Bootz F, Dichgans J, Bruzek W (1983a) Variability of postural "reflexes" in humans. Exp Brain Res 52: 423-428

Diener HC, Dichgans J, Bacher M, Hülser J, Liebich H (1983b) Mechanisms of postural ataxia after intake of alcohol. Z Rechtsmed, 90: 159-165

Diener HC, Dichgans J, Bootz F, Bacher M (1984a) Early stabilization of human posture after a sudden disturbance: Influence of rate and amplitude of displacement. Exp Brain Res 56: 126-134

Diener HC, Dichgans J, Bacher B, Gompf B (1984b) Quantification of postural sway in normals and patients with cerebellar diseases. Electroencephalogr Clin Neurophysiol 57: 134-142

Diener HC, Dichgans J, Bacher B, Guschlbauer P (1984c) Characteristic alterations of long loop "reflexes" in patients with Friedreich's disease and late atrophy of the cerebellar anterior lobe. J Neurol Neurosurg Psychiat 47:679-685

Diener HC, Dichgans J, Bacher M, Guschlbauer B (1984d) Improvement of ataxia in late cortical cerebellar atrophy through alcohol abstinence. J Neurol (in press)

Diener HC, Dichgans J, Hülser PJ, Buettner UW, Bacher M, Guschlbauer B (1984e) The significance of long loop "reflexes" for the diagnosis of multiple sclerosis. Electroenceph Clin Neurophysiol 57: 336-342

Dow RS, Moruzzi G (1958) The physiology and pathology of the cerebellum. Univ of Minnesota Press, Minneapolis

Eccles JC (1977) Cerebellar function in the control of movement. In: Rose F (ed) Physiological aspects of clinical neurology. Blackwell, Oxford, pp 157-178

Eckmiller R, Westheimer G (1983) Compensation of oculomotor deficits in monkeys with neonatal cerebellar ablations. Exp Brain Res 49: 315-326

Evarts EV, Thach WTS (1969) Motor mechanisms of the CNS: cerebro-cerebellar interrelations. Ann Rev Physiol 31: 451-498

Friedemann HH, Noth J, Diener HC, Bacher M (1984) Long latency EMG responses in hand and leg muscles. I. Cerebellar disorders. J Neurol Neurosurg Psychiat (submitted)

Fuchs AF, Kornhuber HH (1969) Extraocular muscle afferents to the cerebellum of the cat. J Physiol 200: 713-722

Gilman S (1969) The mechanism of cerebellar hypotonia: an experimental study in the monkey. Brain 92: 621-638

Gilman S, Bloedel JR, Lechtenberg R (1981) Disorders of the cerebellum. Davis, Philadelphia

Goldberger ME, Growdon JH (1971) Tremor at rest following cerebellar lesions in monkeys: effect of L-dopa administration. Brain Res 27: 183-187

Gonshor A, Melvill-Jones G (1971) Plasticity in the adult human vestibulo-ocular reflex arc. Proc Can Fed Biol Soc 14: 11

Hallett M, Shahani BT, Young RR (1975) EMG analysis of patients with cerebellar deficits. J Neurol Neurosurg Psychiat 38: 1163-1169

Halmagyi GM, Gresty MA (1979) Clinical signs of visual-vestibular interaction. J Neurol Neurosurg Psychiat 42: 931-939

Holmes G (1917) The symptoms of acute cerebellar injuries due to gunshot injuries. Brain 40: 461-535

Holmes G (1939) The cerebellum of man. (The Hughlings Jackson memorial lecture). Brain 62: 1-30

Hood JD (1981) Further observations on the phenomenon of rebound nystagmus. In: Cohen B (ed) Vestibular and oculomotor physiology. Ann NY Acad Sci 374: 532-539

Hood JD, Kayan A, Leech J (1973) Rebound nystagmus. Brain 96: 507-526

Koeppen AH, Baron KD, Deutinger MP (1980) Olivary hypertrophy in man. In: Courville J et al. (eds) The inferior olivary nucleus: anatomy and physiology. Raven Press, New York, pp 309-314

Lechtenberg R, Gilman S (1978) Speech disorders in cerebellar disease. Ann Neurol 3: 285-290

Lee RG, Tatton WG (1975) Motor responses to sudden limb displacements in primates with specific CNS lesions and in human patients with motor system disorders. Can J Neurol Sci 2: 285-293

Lisberger SG, Fuchs AF (1978) Role of primate flocculus during rapid behavioural modification of vestibulo-ocular reflex. I. Purkinje cell activity during visually guided horizontal smooth pursuit eye movements and passive head rotation. J Neurophysiol 41: 733-763

Llinas R, Volkind RA (1973) The olivo-cerebellar system: Functional properties as revealed by harmaline-induced tremor. Exp Brain Res 18: 69-87

MacKay WA, Murphy JT (1979) Cerebellar influence on proprioceptive control loops. In: Massion J, Sasaki K (eds) Cerebro-cerebellar interactions. Elsevier, Amsterdam, pp 141-162

Marsden CD, Merton PA, Morton HB, Hallett M, Adam J, Rushton DM (1977) Disorders of movement in cerebellar disease in man. In: Rose F (ed) Physiological aspects of clinical neurology. Blackwell, Oxford, pp 179-199

Marsden CD, Merton PA, Morton HB, Adam J (1978) The effect of lesions of the central nervous system on long-latency stretch reflexes in the human thumb. In: Desmedt JE (ed) Cerebral motor control in man: Long loop mechanisms. Karger, Basel, pp 334-341

Mauritz KH (1979) Standataxie bei Kleinhirnläsionen. Untersuchungen zur Differentialdiagnostik und Pathophysiologie gestörter Haltungsregulation. Habilitationsschr, Med Fak, Univ Freiburg

Mauritz KH, Dichgans J, Hufschmidt A (1979) Quantitative analysis of stance in late cortical cerebellar atrophy of the anterior lobe and other forms of cerebellar ataxia. Brain 102: 461-482

Mauritz KH, Schmitt C, Dichgans J (1981) Delayed and enhanced long latency reflexes as the possible cause of postural tremor in late cerebellar atrophy. Brain 104: 97-116

Melvill-Jones G, Watt DGD (1971) Observations on the control of stepping and hopping movement in man. J Physiol 219: 709-727

Meyer-Lohmann J, Hore J, Brooks VB (1977) Cerebellar participation in generation of prompt arm movements. J Neurophysiol 40: 1038-1050

Miles FA (1982) Adaptive gain control in the vestibulo-ocular reflex. In: Lennerstrand G, Zee DS, Keller EL (eds) Functional basis of ocular motility disorders, vol 37. Wenner Gren Symp Pergamon Press, Oxford, pp 325-337

Miles FA, Fuller JH, Braitman DJ, Dow BM (1980) Long-term adaptive changes in primate vestibulo-ocular reflex. III. Electrophysiological observations in flocculus of normal monkeys. J Neurophysiol 43: 1437-1476

Nashner LM, Grimm KJ (1978) Analysis of multiloop dyscontrols in standing cerebellar patients. In: Desmed JE (ed) Cerebral motor control in man: Long loop mechanims. Karger, Basel Progr Clin Neurophysiol, vol IV, pp 300-319

Neilson PD, Lance JW (1978) Reflex transmission characteristics during voluntary activity in normal man and patients with movement disorders. In: Desmedt JE (ed) Cerebral motor control in man: Long loop mechanisms, Karger, Basel (Progr Clin Neurophysiol, vol IV, pp 263-299)

Noth J, Friedemann HH, Podol HK, Lange HW (1983) Absence of long latency reflexes to imposed finger displacements in patients with Huntington's disease. Neurosci Letters 35: 97-100

Optican LM, Robinson DA (1980) Cerebellar dependent adaptive control of the primate saccadic system. J Neurophysiol 44: 1058-1076

Paltsev YJ, Elner AM (1967) Preparatory and compensatory period during voluntary movement in patients with involvement of the brain of different localization. Biophys J 12: 142-147

Pollock LJ, Davis L (1930) Studies in decerebration VI. The effect of deafferentation upon decerebrate rigidity. Am J Physiol 98: 47

Reutern von GM, Dichgans J (1977) Augenbewegungsstörungen als cerebelläre Symptome bei Kleinhirnbrückenwinkeltumoren. Arch Psychiat Nervenkr 223: 117-130

Ritchie L (1976) Effects of cerebellar lesions on saccadic eye movements. J Neurophysiol 39: 1246-1252

Robinson DA (1976) Adaptive gain control of vestibuloocular reflex by the cerebellum. J Neurophysiol 39: 954-969

Robinson DA (1982) A model of cancellation of the vestibulo-ocular reflex. In: Lennerstrand G, Zee DS, Keller EL (eds) Functional basis of ocular motility disorders, vol. 37. Wenner Gren Symp, Pergamon Press, Oxford New York, pp 5-13

Rondot P, Bathien N, Toma S (1979) Physiopathology of cerebellar movement. In: Massion J, Sasaki K (eds) Cerebro-cerebellar interactions. Elsevier, Amsterdam New York, pp 203-230

Scholz E, Diener HC, Dichgans J, Noth J, Friedemann H (1984) Long latency EMG responses in hand and leg muscles II Parkinson's disease. J Neurol Neurosurg Psychiat (in press)

Silfverskiöld BP (1969) Romberg's test in the cerebellar syndrome occurring in chronic alcoholism. Acta Neurol Scand 45: 292-302

Suzuki DA, Noda H, Kase M (1981) Visual and pursuit eye movement-related activity in posterior vermis of monkey cerebellum. J Neurophysiol 46: 1120-1139

Takemori S, Cohen B (1974) Loss of visual suppression of vestibular nystagmus after flocculus lesions. Brain 72: 213-224

Terzuolo CA, Viviani P (1974) Patterns of motion and EMG activities during some simple motor tasks in normal subjects and cerebellar patients. In: Cooper IS, Riklan M, Snider RS (eds) The cerebellum, epilepsy and behavior. Plenum Press, New York, pp 173-215

Traub MM, Rothwell JC, Marsden CD (1980) Anticipatory postural reflexes in Parkinson's disease and other akinetic-rigid syndromes and cerebellar ataxia. Brain 103: 393-412

Victor M, Adams RD, Mancall EL (1959) A restricted form of cerebellar cortical degeneration occurring in alcoholic patients. Arch Neurol 1: 579-688

Vilis T, Hore J (1977) Effects of changes in mechanical state of limb on cerebellar intention tremor. J Neurophysiol 40: 1214-1224

Vilis T, Hore J (1980) Central neural mechanisms contributing to cerebellar tremor produced by limb perturbations. J Neurophysiol 43: 279-291

Vilis T, Hore J (1981) Characteristics of saccadic dysmetria in monkeys during reversible lesions of medial cerebellar nuclei. J Neurophysiol 46: 828-838

Vilis T, Snow R, Hore J (1983) Cerebellar saccadic dysmetria is not equal in the two eyes. Exp Brain Res 51: 343-350

Waespe W, Cohen B, Raphan T (1983) Role of the flocculus and paraflocculus in optokinetic nystagmus and visual-vestibular interactions: effects of lesions. Exp Brain Res 50: 9-33

Weisenburg TH (1927) Cerebellar localization and its symptomatology. Brain 50: 357

Westheimer G, Blair SM (1973) Oculomotor defects in cerebellectomized monkeys. Invest Opthalmol Vis Sci 12: 618-621

Westheimer G, Blair SM (1974) Functional organization of primate oculomotor system revealed by cerebellectomy. Exp Brain Res 21: 463-472

Wiesendanger M, Miles TS (1982) Ascending pathway of low-threshold muscle afferents to the cerebral cortex and its possible role in motor control. Physiol Rev 62: 1234-1270

Woollacott MH (1983) Effects of ethanol on postural adjustments in humans. Exp Neurology 80: 55-68

Yagi T, Shimizu M, Sekine S, Kamio T, Suzuki J-I (1981) A new neurotological test for detecting cerebellar dysfunction. In: Cohen B (ed) Vestibular and oculomotor physiology. Ann NY Acad Sci 374: 526-531

Zee DS (1982) Ocular motor control: the cerebellum. In: Lessel S, Dalen van JTW (eds) Neuro-opthalmology, vol II. Excerpta Medica, Amsterdam Oxford, Princeton, pp 136

Zee DS, Friendlich AR, Robinson DA (1974) Mechanisms of downbeat nystagmus. Arch Neurol 30: 227-237

Zee DS, Yee RD, Cogan DG, Robinson DA, Engel WK (1976) Oculomotor abnormalities in hereditary cerebellar ataxia. Brain 99: 207-234

Zee DS, Yamazaki A, Butler P, Gücer G (1981) Effect of ablation of flocculus and paraflocculus on eye movement in primate. J Neurophysiol 46: 878-899

Perceptual Analysis of Speech Disorders in Friedreich Disease and Olivopontocerebellar Atrophy

S. Gilman[1] and K. Kluin[2]

1 Introduction

Motor speech production is highly sensitive to alterations in function of the nervous system (Darley et al. 1975; La Pointe 1975). Dysarthria, a frequent symptom of neurological disorders, is a collective term for a group of related speech disorders resulting from involvement of the muscular control of the speech mechanisms owing to impairment of any of the basic motor speech processes involved in the execution of speech (Darley et al. 1969a, b, 1975). Dysarthria can result not only from abnormalities of articulation but also from disorders of respiration, phonation, resonance, and prosody.

Darley et al. (1969a, b, 1975) designed a classification system of the basic abnormalities of speech ("deviant dimensions") underlying dysarthria and related these to disorders involving various regions of the nervous system. In a study of 30 patients with cerebellar lesions, these investigators identified 10 deviant speech dimensions which were rated high (above 1.50) on their scale of severity: (1) imprecise consonants; (2) excess and equalized stress; (3) irregular articulatory breakdowns; (4) distorted vowels; (5) harsh voice; (6) prolonged phonemes; (7) prolonged intervals; (8) monoton of pitch; (9) monotony of loudness; and (10) slow rate. They found other deviant speech characteristics which ranked lower on their scale of severity but occurred in as many as 14 of their 30 patients: (1) low pitch; (2) excess loudness variations; (3) hypernasality; (4) strained-strangled sound; (5) pitch breaks; and (6) voice tremor. In their studies of speech disorders with cerebellar disease, the investigators did not specify the types of cerebellar disease processes affecting their patients and did not comment upon the presence of other neurologic disorders in them.

Darley et al. (1969a, b, 1975) also described the deviant speech dimensions in 30 patients with spastic dysarthria owing to pseudobulbar palsy. The characteristics which ranked high (above 1.50) on their scale of severity were: (1) imprecise consonants; (2) monotony of pitch; (3) reduced stress; (4) harsh voice quality; (5) monotony of loudness; (6) low pitch; (7) slow rate; (8) hypernasality; (9) strained-strangled quality; (10) short phrases; (11) distorted vowels; (12) pitch breaks; (13) breathy voice (continuous); and (14) excess and equal stress.

In the course of clinical examinations of speech in patients with neurologic disorders, we have found that patients with cerebellar disease without other neurological disturbances do not manifest some of the deviant speech characteristics (continuously

[1]   Departments of Neurology and [2]Physical Medicine and Rehabilitation, The University of Michigan, Ann Arbor, Michigan, USA

Cerebellar Functions
ed. by Bloedel et al.
© Springer-Verlag Berlin Heidelberg 1984

low pitch, monotony of pitch, monotony of loudness, and strained-strangled sound) found in the patients with cerebellar lesions in the series of Darley et al. (1969a, b, 1975). In contrast, we have noted that these four deviant speech characteristics appear in conjunction with the other characteristics of cerebellar speech disorders in patients with a combination of cerebellar disease and pseudobulbar palsy. We have begun an investigation to determine whether continuously low pitch, monotony of pitch, monotony of loudness, and strained-strangled sound result from cerebellar disease alone by examining with perceptual speech analysis patients with "pure" cerebellar disorders, i. e., those without signs of upper motor neuron disease of the cranial nerve musculature such as pseudobulbar palsy (hyperactive gag reflex, enhanced jaw muscle stretch reflex, limited range of facial movement, or inappropriate laughter or weeping). In the present communication we report the results of perceptual speech analysis in a group of patients with Friedreich disease who had signs of cerebellar disorder without signs of pseudobulbar palsy. We have compared the findings with those in patients with a combination of cerebellar disorder and pseudobulbar palsy resulting from a progressive degenerative disease, olivopontocerebellar atrophy.

2 Methods

Six patients were studied, three with Friedreich disease and three with olivopontocerebellar atrophy. The patients with Friedreich disease were white and English speaking, consisting of two females and one male, ages 24, 26, and 18 (Table 1). The duration of the illness ranged from 5 to 20 years. One patient (CK) had mild deficits of muscular coordination and the remaining 2 had moderate to severe deficits. The diagnosis of Friedreich disease was based upon the onset in childhood to adolescence of a progressive ataxia of gait and limb movements with kyphoscoliosis, areflexia, extensor plantar reflexes, and loss of vibration and position sense. One patient (LT) had an affected sibling but the others had no family history of a similar illness. The patients were thoroughly studied to exclude other causes of cerebellar dysfunction in this age group (Gilman et al. 1981).

The three patients with olivopontocerebellar atrophy were white and English speaking, though one patient (SS) was Hawaiian and of Japanese descent. They ranged in age between 57 and 70 years, consisting of two females and one male (Table 2). The duration of symptoms ranged from 3 to 5 years. One patient (JR) was mildly impaired and two were moderately to severely impaired with a combination of ataxia, spasticity, and pseudobulbar palsy. Apart from the finding of cogwheel rigidity in an upper limb of one patient, none of the patients showed clinical features of Parkinson disease or the Shy-Drager syndrome. None were tested for the presence of glutamate dehydrogenase deficiency. None of the patients had a family history of a similar illness. The diagnosis of olivopontocerebellar atrophy was based upon the development in middle age of a progressive disturbance of cerebellar function along with disturbances of corticobulbar and corticospinal function, with or without evidence of cerebellar atrophy on CT scan. Other causes of cerebellar disorder in this age group were excluded through comprehensive evaluations in the hospital. No evidence was adduced of inflammatory, demyelinative, metabolic, endocrinologic, or neoplastic disease.

Table 1. Summary of clinical findings in three patients with Friedreich disease

Patient	Sex	Age of Onset of Symptoms	Symptoms	Age Studied	Mental Status	Cranial Nerves	Motor System	Reflexes	Sensation
LP	F	6	Clumsiness walking and running Poor handwriting Slurred speech Unable to walk after age 16	26	Intact	Opsoclonus Voluntary facial movements slow, irregular Tongue movements slow, decreased strength, elevation, poor RAM Gag reflex active	Ataxia of trunk and limbs Dysmetria with FNF, HKS Slow RAM of limbs Unable to walk alone Hypotonia of limbs, trunk and neck Scoliosis	Absent DTR Plantars upgoing	Absent PS, VS in all limbs distally Positive Romberg
CK	F	19	Clumsiness walking and running Frequent falls Slurred speech	24	Intact	Slow EOM with poor pursuit Tongue movements slow, poor RAM Lag of palate with phonation Palatal asymmetry Mildly hypernasal speech with nasal air emission	Ataxia of trunk and limbs Dysmetria with FNF, HKS Slow RAM of limbs Hypotonia of limbs, trunk and neck Scoliosis	Absent DTR Plantars downgoing	Absent PS, VS distally in the legs Positive Romberg

Table 1. (continued)

Patient	Sex	Age of Onset of Symptoms	Symptoms	Age Studied	Mental Status	Cranial Nerves	Motor System	Reflexes	Sensation
LT	M	13	Clumsiness walking and running Frequent falls Slurred speech	18	Intact	Slow EOM with saccadic pursuits and end-gaze nystagmus Static tremor of the head Decreased RAM, elevation and strength of tongue Lag of palate with phonation Palatal asymmetry Mildly hypernasal speech with nasal air emission	Ataxia of trunk and limbs Dysmetria with FNF, HKS Slow RAM of limbs Gait spastic and ataxic Mild spasticity of legs Scoliosis Pes cavus	Absent DTR Plantars upgoing	Absent PS, VS distally in all limbs Positive Romberg

Abbreviations: RAM – rapid alternating movements; EOM – extraocular movements; DTR – deep tendon reflexes; FNF – movement of an index finger alternately between patient's nose and examiner's finger; HKS – movement of the heel of 1 leg from the knee down along the shin of the other leg; PS – position sense; VS – vibration sense (perception of vibration of a 128 cps tuning fork)

Table 2. Summary of clinical findings in 3 patients with olivopontocerebellar atrophy. Abbreviations as in Table 1

Patient	Sex	Age of Onset of Symptoms	Symptoms	Age Studied	Mental Status	Cranial Nerves	Motor System	Reflexes	Sensation
JR	F	65	Poor balance Poor coordination	70	Intact	Overshoot dysmetria with EOM Facial movements irregular with reduced range Tongue movements slow, decreased range of movement and extension, RAM Palatal droop and asymmetry Hyperactive gag reflex Altered nasality of speech	Ataxia of trunk and limbs Dysmetria with FNF, HKS Slow RAM Ataxic Gait Hypotonia of limbs	2+ upper limbs 2-3+ lower limbs Clonus both knees Plantars downgoing	Distal loss of PS and VS
MT	F	54	Staggering with walking Slurred speech	59	Intact	Facial and mandibular movements slow with decreased range Tongue movements slow, decreased strength, range of movement, RAM Palatal droop and asymmetry Hyperactive gag reflex Altered nasality of speech Positive jaw jerk	Ataxia of trunk and limbs Dysmetria with FNF, HKS Ataxic gait Cogwheel rigidity left arm	3+ upper limbs 1+ lower limbs Plantars downgoing	Intact

Table 2. (continued)

Patient	Sex	Age Onset of Symptoms	Symptoms	Age Studied	Mental Status	Cranial Nerves	Motor System	Reflexes	Sensation
SS	M	54	Poor coordination with walking Deterioration of handwriting Slurred speech	57	Intact	Saccadic pursuit movements Gaze paretic nystagmus Facial and mandibular movements slow with decreased range Tongue movements slow, decreased range, strength, RAM Palatal droop and asymmetry Hyperactive gag reflex Altered nasality of speech	Ataxia of trunk and limbs Dysmetria with FNF, HKS Slow RAM Ataxic wide based gait Mild spasticity in the limbs	2+ all limbs Unsustained ankle clonus Plantars downgoing	Intact

Conventional neurological examinations were performed and recorded. Evaluation of the dysarthria included oral motor assessment and perceptual speech analysis. The two authors analyzed and rated the severity of the dysarthria from videotaped samples of spontaneous speech, oral reading of the "grandfather passage", tests of alternate motion rates and sequential motion rates/diadochokinetic rates, attempts to sustain the vowels "ah" and "e", and examples of counting from 1 to 50. Data for comparison were obtained from videotaped samples of speech production by a normal 26-year old woman. We used the deviant speech dimensions defined by Darley et al. (1975). Speech samples were assessed in multiple listening sessions, with each session focused upon a single deviant dimension. All patients had a high resolution CT scan, study of EMG activity and peripheral nerve conduction velocities and studies of cerebral glucose utilization and cerebral blood flow in the Positron Emission Tomography (PET)/Cyclotron Facility. PET studies were performed using intravenous injections of ^{18}F-2-deoxyglucose to evaluate cerebral glucose metabolic activity and H_2 [15]O to examine cerebral blood flow. A full description of the rationale, methodology, and results of the PET studies will be presented elsewhere.

3 Results

The patients with Friedreich disease on clinical examination showed mild to severe degrees of the type of muscular incoordination typically seen with cerebellar disease without signs of disturbance in function of corticobulbar pathways (Table 1). One patient (LT) had mild spasticity in the legs. CT scans in the patients with Friedreich di-

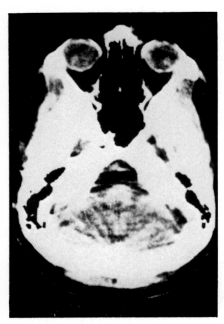

Fig. 1. Computerized axial tomography (CT) scan through the posterior fossa of a 26-year-old woman with Friedreich disease (LP) showing mild atrophy

Fig. 2. CT scan through the posterior fossa of a 70-year-old woman (JR) with olivopontocerebellar atrophy showing no abnormality

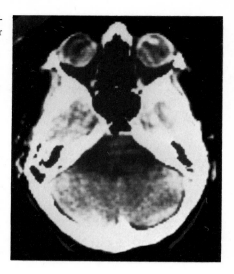

sease either were normal or showed mild atrophy (Fig. 1, Table 5). Study of peripheral nerve conduction revealed marked abnormalities of sensory nerve function in all three patients (Table 5). Examination of speech production in these patients revealed findings compatible with an ataxic dysarthria without continuously low pitch, monotony of pitch, monotony of loudness, or strained-strangled sound (Table 6). Diadochokinetic studies revealed slow alternate motion rates, impaired sequential motion rates in two of the three cases, and limited breath support in all three (Table 3). Two patients (LP, LT) had a mild and the third (CK) had a subtle to mild degree of dysarthria.

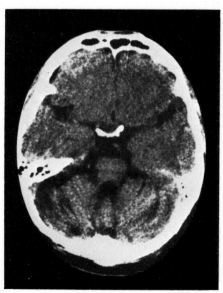

Fig. 3. CT scan through the posterior fossa of a 57-year-old man (SS) with olivopontocerebellar atrophy showing moderate atrophy of the brain-stem and cerebellum

Table 3. Summary of diadochokinetic rates and breath support scores in three patients with Friedreich disease

Patient	Alternate motion rates per 5 s	Sequential motion rates per 5 s	Duration of "ah" (s)
(Normal values)	pa = 28 ta = 28 ka = 25	pataka = 8-10	16-20
LP	pa = 15 ta = 15 ka = 14	pataka = 7.5	6
CK	pa = 25.5 ta = 22.5 ka = 11	pataka = 8.5	8.5
LT	pa = 18.5 ta = 19.5 ka = 16.5	pataka = 7.5	7.5

The patients with olivopontocerebellar atrophy on clinical examination showed mild to moderate degrees of muscular incoordination with signs of disturbance in function of corticobulbar pathways (limited range of facial movements, active jaw jerk, hy-

Table 4. Summary of diadochokinetic rates and breath support scores in three patients with olivopontocerebellar atrophy. Normal values are given in Table 3

Patient	Alternate motion rates per 5 s	Sequential motion rates per 5 s	Duration of "ah" (s)
JR	pa = 26 ta = 23 ka = 21	pataka = 9	8
MT	pa = 16 ta = 16 ka = 10.5	pataka = 5.5	8.5
SS	pa = 16 ta = 14 ka = 12	pataka = 7	17

Table 5. Selected laboratory investigations

A. Friedreich disease

Patient		Investigations
LP	CT scan:	mild, generalized atrophy; EMG: normal; NCS: absent SEP
CK	CT scan:	normal; EMG: normal; NCS: reduced amplitude SEP
LT	CT scan:	mild atrophy of cerebellum and brainstem; EMG: normal; NCS: reduced amplitude SEP

B. Olivopontocerebellar atrophy

Patient		Investigations
JR	CT scan:	normal
MT	CT scan:	mild cerebellar cortical and brainstem atrophy
SS	CT scan:	mild cerebral cortical atrophy; moderate cerebellar and brainstem atrophy

Abbreviations: CT — computerized axial tomography; EMG — electromyographic examination; NCS — nerve conduction studies; SEP — sensory evoked potentials

Table 6. Summary of deviant speech dimensions in three patients with Friedreich disease and three patients with olivopontocerebellar atrophy

			Friedreich disease	Olivopontocerebellar atrophy
I.	Respiration:		Audible inspirations Abnormal synchrony	Occasional audible inspirations Occasional abnormal synchrony
II.	Phonation:	Pitch:	Fluctuating levels	Low pitch, monopitch
		Quality:	"Explosive"⌐ Harsh voice ⎤-transient Breathiness ⌐	Strained-strangled sound Harsh voice
		Volume:	Alternating loudness	Alternating loudness Low volume
III.	Resonance:		Normal to mildly hypernasal	Hypernasal
IV.	Articulation:		Occasional imprecise consonants Irregular breakdown	Imprecise consonants Irregular breakdown Distorted vowels
V.	Prosody:	Rate:	Slow, dysrhythmia	Slow, dysrhythmia
		Stress:	Excess and equalized patterns Prolonged phonemes Prolonged intervals	Equalized, occasionally broken by excess patterns Prolonged phonemes Prolonged intervals

peractive gag reflex), though none had pseudobulbar laughter or weeping (Table 2). These patients had either normal CT scans (Fig. 2, Table 5) or mild to moderate degrees of atrophy (Fig. 3, Table 5). Examination of speech production revealed findings compatible with a mixed ataxic-spastic dysarthria including continuously low pitch, monotony of pitch, monotony of loudness, and strained-strangled sound (Table 6). Diadochokinetic studies revealed slow alternate motion rates, impaired sequential motion rates in two of the three cases, and limited breath support in two of the three cases (Table 4). Two patients (MT, SS) had a moderate and the third had a mild degree of dysarthria.

Only preliminary results of PET scanning are available at this time. Thus far the results indicate that glucose metabolic activity in the cerebellum is essentially normal in patients with Friedreich disease but markedly reduced in patients with olivopontocerebellar atrophy, both in the presence (Figs. 3 and 6) and absence (Figs. 2 and 5) of cerebellar atrophy.

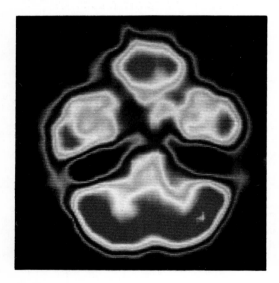

Fig. 4. Positron emission tomography (PET) scan with ^{18}F-2-deoxyglucose of a 42-year-old male volunteer with no neurologic abnormality. *Darkest areas* in the scan indicate the highest rates of glucose utilization. *Bottom half* of the scan shows the cerebellum and *top half* shows the ventral portion of the frontal lobes (the midline structure) and the ventral portions of both temporal lobes. *Left side* of the scan is on the reader's left

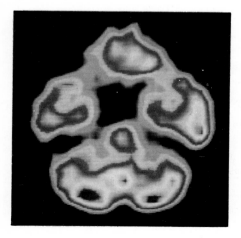

Fig. 5. PET scan with ^{18}F-2-deoxyglucose of a 70-year old woman (JR) with olivopontocerebellar atrophy. *Darkest areas* in the scan indicate the highest rates of glucose utilization. *Bottom half* of the scan shows the cerebellum and *top half* shows the ventral portions of the frontal lobes (the midline structure) and the ventral portions of both temporal lobes. *Left side* of the scan is on the reader's left. Glucose utilization rates in the cerebellum of this patient are approximately 50% of those of the control subject in Fig. 4. The CT scan of the patient is shown in Fig. 2

Fig. 6. PET scan with ^{18}F-2-deoxyglucose of a 57-year-old man (SS) with olivopontocere-bellar atrophy. *Darkest areas* in the scan indicate the highest rates of glucose utilization. *Bottom 1/3* of the scan shows the cerebellum and *top 2/3* shows the temporal and frontal lobes. *Left side* of the scan is on the reader's left. This scan was made at a different plane than the scans shown in Figs. 4 and 5, which were made parallel to the orbitomeatal line. The scanning plane in this patient was needed because of the degree of atrophy of the cere-bellum. Glucose utilization rates in the cere-bellum of this patient are approximately 50% of those in the control subject in Fig. 4. The CT scan of the patient is shown in Fig. 3

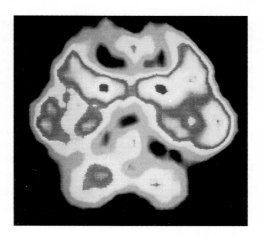

4 Discussion

In this sample of patients with Friedreich disease we found deviant speech dimensions compatible with ataxic dysarthria without continuously low pitch, monotony of pitch, monotony of loudness, or strained-strangled sound. In contrast, patients with olivo-pontocerebellar atrophy showed a mixed ataxic-spastic dysarthria which included con-tinuously low pitch, monotony of pitch, monotony of loudness and strained-strangled sound. We selected patients with Friedreich disease who had no clear physical signs on clinical neurological examination of corticobulbar disease or lower motor neuron disease affecting the cranial musculature and concluded consequently that these cases had speech disorders resulting chiefly from disturbed cerebellar function. These findings are compatible with the notion that continuously low pitch, monotony of pitch, mono-tony of loudness, and strained-strangled sound are deviant speech characteristics en-countered not with cerebellar disease, but with disease of other components of the nervous system.

Disease restricted to the cerebellum results in a constellation of signs including dis-ordered stance and gait, truncal titubation, rotated postures of the head, disturbances of extraocular movements, hypotonia, dysarthria, dysmetria, dysdiadochokinesis, dys-rhythmokinesis, ataxia, tremor, check, rebound, and limb weakness (Holmes 1922; Gilman et al. 1981). These abnormalities stem from several fundamental pathophysio-logical processes in motor control, including hypotonia, mild degrees of weakness and fatigability of muscles, and abnormalities of the rate and regularity of projected move-ments (Holmes 1922; Gilman 1970). "Pure" cerebellar disease in the human does not lead to the clinical characteristics of spasticity (abnormally enhanced resistance to pas-sive movement of the limbs, hyperactive deep tendon reflexes, clonus, and extensor plantar reflexes). On the contrary, cerebellar disease in the human leads to diminished resistance to passive manipulation of the limbs (hypotonia) rather than increased resist-ance to passive manipulation of the limbs (Brooks and Thach 1981; Gilman et al. 1981). The deviant speech dimensions observed in the patients with Friedreich disease in this study can be explained by the fundamental abnormalities of motor function from cerebellar disease as applied to the oral, pharyngeal, laryngeal, and respiratory musculature. Thus, hypotonia, muscular fatigability, and weakness, and abnormalities of the rate and range of movement of the musculature involved in speech can account for the abnormalities detected (imprecise consonants, excess and equalized stress, irregular articulatory breakdowns, distorted vowels, harsh voice, prolonged phonemes, prolonged intervals and slow rate) (Brown et al. 1968; Darley et al. 1969a, b, 1975; Kent and Netsell 1975). The additional characteristics observed in patients with olivopontocerebellar atrophy, low pitch, monotony of pitch, monotony of loudness, and strained-strangled sound, were not seen with Friedreich disease and cannot be explained easily by the motor disturbances occurring with cerebellar disease. Rather, these abnormalities most likely stem from limitations of muscular control due to spasticity and are known to be prominent features of the speech disturbances in pseudobulbar palsy (Darley et al. 1975).

The neuropathological findings in Friedreich disease correspond closely to the clinical findings of an ataxic disorder of speech without elements of pseudobulbar palsy. The principal pathological changes consist of degeneration of the dorsal root ganglia, dorsal roots, dorsal columns, dorsal spinocerebellar tracts, and corticospinal tracts in the spinal cord (Greenfield 1954). Although degenerative changes in the motor cortex have been described, the medullary pyramids are usually preserved and only the spinal projections of the corticospinal tracts show degeneration. Thus, the corticobulbar projections are not regularly involved. The principal changes in the brainstem consist of degeneration in the central tegmental tract, medial longitudinal fasciculus, fascicularis solitarius, root of the vagus, descending trigeminal root, and nuclei of the vestibular, vagus, glossopharyngeal, and hypoglossal nerves. The cerebellum is usually normal although some investigators have found loss of Purkinje cells and degenerative changes in the dentate nucleus and the middle and superior cerebellar peduncles (Greenfield 1954).

The widespread neuropathological abnormalities in olivopontocerebellar atrophy are consistent with the clinical findings of a mixed ataxic-spastic disorder of speech. The most prominent findings on gross examination of the nervous system consist of marked shrinkage of the ventral half of the pons, disappearance of the olivary prominences on the ventral surface of the medulla, and reduction in size of the cerebellum. Histological changes regularly found include loss of nerve cells in the pontine nuclei, inferior olives, cerebellar cortex, and dentate nucleus (Greenfield 1954). Other pathological abnormalities frequently found include degenerative changes in the dorsal and lateral columns of the spinal cord, cerebral cortex, cerebellar peduncles, lower cranial nerve nuclei, retinae, and basal ganglia (Konigsmark and Weiner 1970; Gilman et al. 1981). The neuropathological changes vary considerably between patients in sporadic cases of the disease but tend to follow similar patterns within individual families in familial cases.

A limited number of observations have been made on the speech disorders in Friedreich disease. DeJong (1979) described sudden pitch changes and ataxic, staccato and explosive elements as the remarkable speech abnormalities. Joanette and Dudley (1980) described the speech disturbances in 22 patients with Friedreich disease between the ages of 19 and 49 years. They found two groups of speech characteristics: (1) a "general dysarthric factor" and (2) a pattern of phonatory stenosis. They related the two characteristics to two distinct speech mechanisms, the first to articulation and the second to laryngeal function. They concluded that their study clearly defined two distinct subgroups of subjects who represent two different manifestations of the same underlying pathology. The "phonatory-stenosis" involved harshness and pitch breaks, but not monotony of pitch, monotony of loudness or strained-strangled sound. We also found transient harshness in our patients with Friedreich disease, but link this to the fluctuating pitch level, since a harsh voice generally has a low pitch (Boone 1979). Moreover, fluctuations in pitch may be due not to phonatory stenosis, but to ataxia of respiration. Respiratory function influences phonatory characteristics in part through changes in subglottic air pressure (Hixon 1973). Vocal loudness and pitch depend upon constant subglottic pressure. A sudden change of subglottic pressure from ataxia of the respiratory muscles (Nielsen 1951) may produce irregular, inappropriate changes in pitch and loudness by altering vocal cord tension and length (Aronson 1980).

A number of investigators recently have developed objective recordings of the acoustic and physiologic abnormalities in ataxic dysarthria (Kent and Netsell 1975; Hirose et al. 1978; Kent et al. 1979). Using cineradiographic and spectrographic analyses in patients with a variety of neurologic disorders causing ataxic dysarthria, Kent and Netsell (1975) and Kent et al. (1979) found disturbances of timing patterns which resulted in a tendency to equalize syllable durations and extend a variety of segments and abnormal contours of the fundamental frequency. In words with a consonant-vowel-consonant sequence, the measures of vowel format frequency were normal except for transitional segments. Although vowel distortions occurred in connected speech, with sufficient time, the patients could reach the appropriate vowel target. The physiologic findings in these studies indicated articulation errors of direction, range and speed. The occurrence of the dysrhythmia of alternate repetitive movements paralleled the occurrence of irregular articulatory breakdown. The authors identified instances of marked and inappropriate changes, including upward and downward sweeps in the fundamental frequency. They raised the possibility that patients with ataxic dysarthria are more variable in the control of intonation than in the control of articulation. In contrast, Darley et al. (1969a, b, 1975) rated articulation as the most deviant dimension in patients with cerebellar lesions. Murray (1983) described the speech in Friedreich disease as more explosive than in ataxic dysarthria with bizarre phonatory characteristics including a rough or harsh quality along with a strained-strangled sound and a tendency to increase pitch.

In our study, the patients with mixed ataxic-spastic dysarthria from olivopontocerebellar atrophy had disturbances of articulation, including vowel distortions, as the most prominent abnormality. In contrast, we found the phonatory and prosodic dimensions to be the most aberrant in the patients with ataxic dysarthria from Friedreich disease. In the patients with Friedreich disease, we did not perceive strained-strangled sounds with elevations of pitch, nor did we find evidence for increased resistance of the vocal cords, effortful squeezing of the voice through the glottis, or obstruction of the exhaled airstream, all of which may result in a strained-strangled sound. Our patients with Friedreich disease did not have vowel distortions, probably because the ataxic dysarthria was mild in two patients and the third had received speech pathology services with emphasis upon maintaining a slow rate. Our findings support DeJong's observations and, in part, Murray's observations of the speech disorders in Friedreich disease. Our findings are compatible also with the acoustic and physiologic observations of ataxic dysarthria.

A significant problem in defining the speech disturbances in cerebellar disease is in finding patients with cerebellar disease and no other disturbance in neurological function. This problem has interfered with the results in many previous studies. Patients with multiple sclerosis, although often showing marked abnormalities of speech (Darley et al. 1972; Haggard 1969), are not good subjects for evaluation of the effects of pure cerebellar lesions upon speech since multiple sclerosis characteristically affects many regions of the nervous system. Patients with cerebellar degeneration of undetermined cause may present similar problems since corticobulbar disturbances often occur in combination with disorders of cerebellar function. Careful selection, investigation and description of the patient population is essential in such studies.

Acknowledgement. We are indebted to Drs. Richard Ehrenkaufer, Richard Hichwa, and Larry Junck for assistance in PET studies of these patients. We are also grateful to Pamela Hendee for her secretarial assistance. This research was supported in part by NIH Grant NS15655.

References

Aronson AE (1980) Clinical voice disorders. Thieme-Stratton, New York

Boone (1979) The voice and voice therapy. Prentice-Hall, Englewood Cliffs

Brooks VB, Thach WT (1981) Cerebellar control of posture and movement. In: Brookhart JM, Mountcastle VB, Brooks VB (eds) Handbook of physiology Sect I: The nervous system, vol II, part 2. Am Physiol Soc (Bethesda)

Brown JR, Darley FL, Aronson AE (1968) Deviant dimensions of motor speech in cerebellar ataxia. Trans Am Neurol Assoc 93: 193-196

Darley FL, Aronson AE, Brown JR (1969a) Differential diagnostic patterns of dysarthria. J Speech Hear Res 12: 246-269

Darley FL, Aronson AE, Brown JR (1969b) Clusters of deviant speech dimensions in the dysarthrias. J Speech Hear Res 12: 462-496

Darley FL, Brown JR, Goldstein NP (1972) Dysarthria in multiple sclerosis. J Speech Hear Res 15: 229-245

Darley FL, Aronson AE, Brown JR (1975) Motor speech disorders. Saunders, Philadelphia

DeJong RN (1979) The neurologic examination, 4th edn. Harper & Row, Hagerstown

Gilman S (1970) The nature of cerebellar dyssynergia. In: Williams D (ed) Modern trends in neurology, vol V. Butterworths, London, pp 60-79

Gilman S, Bloedel JR, Lechtenberg R (1981) Disorders of the cerebellum, Davis, Philadelphia

Greenfield JG (1954) The spino-cerebellar degenerations. Blackwell, Oxford

Haggard MP (1969) Speech waveform measurements in multiple sclerosis. Folia Phoniatr 21: 307-312

Hirose H, Kiritani S, Ushijima T, Sawashima M (1978) Analysis of abnormal articulatory dynamics in two dysarthric patients. J Speech Hear Disord 63: 96-105

Hixon (1973) Respiratory function in speech. In: Minifie FD, Hixon TJ, Williams F (eds) Normal aspects of speech, hearing, and language. Prentice-Hall, Englewood Cliffs

Holmes G (1922) The Croonian lectures on the clinical symptoms of cerebellar disease and their interpretation. Lancet 1: 1177-1231 and 2: 59-111

Joanette Y, Dudley JG (1980) Dysarthric symptomatology of Friedreich's ataxia. Brain Lang 10: 39-50

Kent RD, Netsell R (1975) A case study of an ataxic dysarthric: cineradiographic and spectrographic observations. J Speech Hear Disord 40: 115-134

Kent RD, Netsell R, Abbs JH (1979) Acoustic characteristics of dysarthria associated with cerebellar disease. J Speech Hear Res 22: 627-648

Konigsmark BW, Weiner LP (1970) The olivopontocerbellar atrophies: a review. Medicine 49: 227-241

LaPointe LL (1975) Neurologic abnormalities affecting speech. In: Tower DB (ed) Human communication and its disorders, vol III. Raven Press, New York

Murray T (1983) Friedreich's ataxia. In: Perkins W (ed) Current therapy of communication disorders – dysarthria and apraxia. Thieme-Stratton, New York

Nielsen JM (1951) A textbook of clinical neurology, 3rd edn. Hoeber, New York

Cerebellar Hemispherectomy at Young Ages in Rats

A. Gramsbergen and J. IJkema-Paassen[1]

Early animal experiments suggested that brain lesions at an early stage of brain maturation have less severe effects on later behavior than similar lesions in adult animals. From this so-called Kennard principle the notion has been derived that the capacity for functional compensation after brain trauma is greater for the immature than for the mature brain. However, more recent investigations — often involving a meticulous analysis of short and long term behavioral sequelae — rather provides evidence against the existence of any simple relation between early lesions and increased compensational capacity.

Against this background we decided to study the effects of cerebellar hemispherectomy on locomotor behavior in rats. Operations were performed on the 5th, 10th, 20th, or 30th day after birth. The rats, behavior was studied systematically, and after the last test at 360 days the extent of the lesion was verified histologically. Before the age of 14 days no signs of major neurological handicaps were apparent despite cerebellar hemispherectomy at the 5th or 10th day. This result seems to argue against the cerebellum playing any important role in neurological functioning up to that age. After this age neurological abnormalities started to appear in the rats lesioned at the 5th or 10th day (while handicaps were immediately present after the operation in rats operated at the 20th or 30th day). Total recovery occurred in none of the experimental groups even 1 yr after lesioning. The most unexpected result, however, was that effects on locomotor behavior were more severe in the groups of rats lesioned at the 5th or 10th day than in those operated on the 20th or 30th day, the earlier lesioned rats scoring lower in a standardized locomotion test and showing more evidence of specific handicaps such as ataxia, increased gait width and hypermetria of paws. (For a detailed description of the experiments on which these conclusions are based see: Gramsbergen 1982, Gramsbergen and IJkema-Paassen 1984).

Why should the earlier operated animals be more handicapped in their locomotor behavior than those operated later? Several investigators, including ourselves have studied neuronal rearrangement after early cerebellar hemispherectomy. Castro (1978) and Leong (1978a) found aberrant projections emanating from the remaining lateral and interposed cerebellar nuclei onto the ipsilateral red nucleus after lesions up to the 10th day (see number 1 in Fig. 1; in normal rats only contralaterally projecting cerebello-rubral fibers occur). We studied the relative numbers of these ipsi- and contralaterally projecting cerebello-rubral fibers in relation to the age at lesioning

[1] Department of Developmental Neurology, University Hospital, Oostersingel 59, Groningen, The Netherlands

Cerebellar Functions
ed. by Bloedel et al.
© Springer-Verlag Berlin Heidelberg 1984

by means of the double labeling technique. Cerebellar hemispherectomy was performed in rats on the 2nd, 5th, 10th, 20th, or 30th day. At adult age retrogradely transported fluorescent tracers (True Blue and Nuclear Yellow) were injected in the left and right red nucleus respectively. We found that the presence of aberrantly projecting fibers was clearly age-dependent, their relative numbers decreasing from 20-30% after lesioning at the 2nd day, to 12-18% after lesioning at the 5th or 10th day to less than 2% in rats operated at the 20th or 30th day. This latter value corresponds to what we have found in normal adults (Gramsbergen and IJkema-Paassen, 1982). Other aberrant cerebello-fugal projections include *ipsilateral* (instead of contralateral) projections onto several thalamic nuclei (ventralis medialis, ventralis anterior, ventralis lateralis, and medio ventralis), the zona incerta and the lateral geniculate (Leong, 1978a; see numbers 2, 3, and 4 respectively in Fig. 1).

Neuronal rearrangement after early hemicerebellectomy is not limited to efferent projections from the remaining cerebellar hemisphere. Leong (1977; 1978b; 1980) reported aberrant projections from the sensori-motor cortex contralateral to the cerebellar lesion onto pontine nuclei in rats operated neonatally (see number 5 in Fig. 1). Leong (1978b) also studied the projection from the sensori-motor cortex onto the red nuclei but did not find any aberrantly projecting fibers. Recently we reinvestigated this projection and used the double labeling technique. Preliminary findings confirmed that in normal adult rats pyramidal cells in the sensori-motor cortex project onto the ipsilateral red nucleus, as earlier reported by Brown (1974). In rats lesioned at the 2nd or 5th day we found aberrantly projecting cells in the sensori-motor cortex contralateral to the cerebellar lesion (see number 6 in Fig. 1).

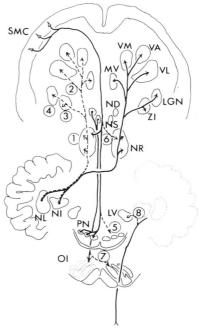

Fig. 1. Schematic drawing of aberrant fiber connections found after cerebellar hemispherectomy up to the 10th day of life in rats based on findings in literature and on our own results. *Dotted lines* removed cerebellar hemisphere (the inferior olivary complex contralateral to the cerebellar lesion degenerates secondarily).
Continuous lines normally occurring projections; *discontinuous lines* aberrant projections, *numbers* passages in the text. Abbreviations: *LGN* n. geniculate lateralis; *LV* n. vestibularis lateralis; *MV* n. medialis ventralis thalami; *ND* n. of Darkschewitsch; *NI* n. interpositus cerebelli; *NL* n. lateralis cerebelli; *NR* n. ruber; *NS* n. subparafascicularis; *OI* inferior olivary complex; *PN* pontine nuclei; *VA* n. ventralis anterior thalami; *VL* n. ventralis lateralis thalami; *VM* n. ventralis medialis thalami; *ZI* zona incerta

However, although consistently occurring, the incidence of these projections is low (less than 5%). In rats operated after the 10th day no such wrongly projecting fibers have been found. In the sensori-motor cortex ipsilateral to the cerebellar lesion no neuronal rearrangement was found at all at any experimental age.

Neuronal remodelling has been shown by others to occur in diencephalic afferents onto the inferior olivary complex ipsilateral to the lesion (Swenson and Castro. 1982; see number 7 in Fig. 1). Castro and Smith (1979) reported an abnormally dense spinal projection onto the lateral vestibular nucleus, ipsilateral to the cerebellar lesion (number 8 in Fig. 1). They claim these fibers to be rerouted from their normal trajectory onto the removed cerebellar hemisphere.

The common denominator in all experiments cited above is that lesions inflicted after the 10th day hardly produce any aberant fiber projections. Before this cerebellar hemispherectomy leads to neuronal remodelling in several structures involved in motor control. Moreover, strong indications exist that aberrant fiber connections are functional and that remodelling leads to abnormal electrical activity in the red nuclei (Yamamoto et al., 1981; Gramsbergen et al., 1984). Taken in conjunction with the more impaired locomotor behavior in rats lesioned before the 10th day this leads us to conclude that neuronal rewiring is a causal factor in locomotor impairment. Our data show furthermore that the dogma attributing a greater compensational capacity to the immature brain is not generally valid.

Acknowledgment. This research is supported by a programme grant, 13-51-91 from the Foundation for Medical Research FUNGO, which is subsidized by the organization for the Advancement of Pure Research (ZWO).

References

Brown LT (1974) Corticorubral projections in the rat. J Comp Neurol 154: 149-168

Castro, A.J. (1978) Projections of the superior cerebellar peduncle in rats and the development of new connections in response to neonatal hemicerebellectomy. J Comp Neurol 178: 611-628

Castro, A.J., Smith, D.E. (1979) Plasticity of spinovestibular projections in response to hemicerebellectomy in newborn rats. Neurosci Lett 12: 69-74

Gramsbergen, A. (1982) The effects of cerebellar hemispherectomy in the young rat, I. Behavioural sequelae. Behav Brain Res 6: 85-92

Gramsbergen, A., IJkema-Paassen, J (1982) CNS plasticity after hemicerebellectomy in the young rat. Quantitative relations between aberrant and normal cerebellorubral projections. Neurosci Lett 33: 129-134

Gramsbergen, A., IJkema-Paassen, J (1984) The effects of early cerebellar hemispherectomy in the rat. Behavioral, neuroanatomical and electrophysiological sequelae. In: Almli C R, Finger S (eds) Early brain damage, vol 2. Academic Press, London New York 155-177

Gramsbergen, A., Schuling, F.H., Vos, J.E. (1984) Electrical activity in the red nuclei of rats and the effects of hemicerebellectomy at young ages. Behav Brain Res 12: 91-90

Leong, S.K. (1977) Sprouting of the corticopontine fibres after neonatal cerebellar lesion in the albino rat. Brain Res 123: 164-169

Leong, S.K. (1978a) Plasticity of cerebellar efferents after neonatal lesions in albino rats. Neurosci Lett 7: 281-289

Leong, S.K. (1978b) Effects of deafferenting cerebellar or cerebral inputs to the pontine and red nuclei in the albino rat. Brain Res 155: 357-361

Leong, S.K. (1980) A qualitative electron microscopic study of the corticopontine projections after neonatal cerebellar hemispherectomy. Brain Res 194: 299-310

Swenson, R.S., Castro, A.J. (1982) Plasticity of meso-diencephalic projections to the inferior olive following neonatal hemicerebellectomy in rats. Brain Res 244: 169-172

Yamamoto, T., Kawaguchi, S., Samejima, A. (1981) Electrophysiological studies on plasticity of cerebellothalamic neurons in rats following neonatal hemicerebellectomy. Jpn J Physiol 31: 217-224

Cerebellar Control of Movement in Fish as Revealed by Small Lesions

K. BEHREND[1]

An attempt was made to quantify the effects of a cerebellar lesion on a specific simple motor task called "probing" of the electric fish Eigenmannia. Probing serves to improve the "electric image" of objects (Heiligenberg 1975, Bacher 1983). It is a smooth bending of the body towards the object. Using a coordinate system as in Fig. 1 the bending could be described by $y(t) = f(x) \cdot \sin(9.8t - \gamma(x))$, the lesion resulted in a change of the probing such that the above expression differed only in the sign of the phase becoming $y(t) = f(x) \cdot \sin(9.8t + \gamma(x))$. The difference in the sign of the phase means, that the movement in a normal fish starts at the tip of the tail whereas in a lesioned one at the head. Lesions resulting in this effect had to

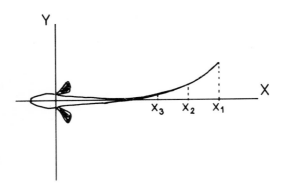

Fig. 1. The coordinate system as defined by the tip of the snout and pectoral fin insertion. $Y(t)$ is measured at the x_i locations

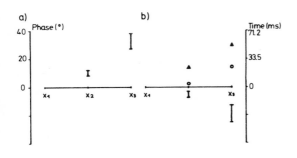

Fig. 2 a,b. Phase versus body position X_i **a** normal animals **b** lesioned animals. Bars cover values calculated from several (at least 8) probing sequences of ten fish in **a** and eight in **b**. *Open circles* and *triangles* in **b** show values of two animals where the lesion covered a part of the cerebellum (lobus caudalis) sparing the electrosensitive area

[1] Inst. f. Zoologie, Univ. Mainz, 65 Mainz

Cerebellar Functions
ed. by Bloedel et al.
© Springer-Verlag Berlin Heidelberg 1984

cover at least part of the region where electrosensitive units have been recorded (Bastian 1974, Behrend 1977). Sparing this region did not alter the normal behavior (see Fig. 2 open triangles and circles). The effect showed no dependency on wether the lesion was unilateral or bilateral nor was there evidence of differential effects for differently located lesions. This is certainly due to the collection of Y-values from a frozen TV picture limiting the accuracy since, as described below, minute changes in segmental timing probably caused by any lesion should manifest quite different overall movements. This order of onset of segmental activity accounting for the movement was calculated using a fish model. It turned out that the movement of a normal animal required a contraction of all segments simultaneously on one side, whereas in the lesioned animal a delay of 0.5 ms between the segments was needed. Considering the cerebellum as a predictive motor space-time metric as formulated by Pellionisz and Llinás (1982) the phase shift is exactly what one would predict in a type of movement where the single components – the segmental muscles – work in a sinusoidal fashion. It results from the missing "lookahead" normally provided by the cerebellar metric.

References

Bacher M (1983) A new method for the simulation of electric fields, generated by electric fish, and their distorsions by objects. Biol Cybernet 47: 51 - 58

Bastian J (1974) Electrosensory input to the corpus cerebelli of the high frequency electric fish *Eigenmannia virescens*. J Comp Physiol 90: 1 - 24

Behrend K (1977) Processing information carried in a high frequency wave: Properties of cerebellar units in a high frequency electric fish. J Comp Physiol 118: 357 - 371

Heiligenberg W (1975) Theoretical and experimental approaches to spatial aspects of electrolocation. J Comp Physiol 103: 247 - 272

Pellionisz A, Llinás R (1982) Space-time representation in the brain. The cerebellum as a predictive space-time metric tensor. Neuroscience 7: 2949-2970

Functional Significance of the Basic Cerebellar Circuit in Motor Coordination

R. Llinás[1]

1 Introduction

Probably the most striking example of uniformity in the neuronal fabric of the brain is that present in the cerebellar cortex. Its connectivity and neuronal circuitry have an almost crystal-like structural organization. An example of the former is the precise distribution of the synaptic inputs onto the soma and dendrites of the cerebellar cortical neurons at the most superficial stratum, the molecular layer (cf. Palay and Chan-Palay 1974). At the neuronal circuit level the parallel fibers course in parallel to the cerebellar surface, the basket cell axons run orthogonally with respect to the direction of the parallel fibers, and all dendrites in the molecular layer run radially towards the surface of the cortex. This organization gives the cerebellar cortex a tridimensional matrix structure. As observed from the surface, the x axis is the direction of the parallel fibers, the y axis the direction of the basket cell axons, and the z axis the direction of the Purkinje cell dendrites (Ramón y Cajal 1911). In addition, since the descriptions by Ramón y Cajal (1888) it has been well known that the Purkinje cell dendrites are close to isoplanar and that the dendritic plane is oriented orthogonally with respect to the parallel fibers (Fig. 1).

Amongst the neurons in this cortex, the Purkinje cell (its only output element) has one of the most extensive dendritic trees in the central nervous system. This dendritic arbor receives an extremely large number of synaptic boutons (Eccles et al. 1967). The excitatory synaptic inputs arise from two different types of afferent systems which, in addition, are clearly segregated spatially such that they cover two different portions of the Purkinje cell surface (Ramón y Cajal, 1911). These are the climbing (CF) and parallel fiber (PF) systems. The parallel fiber input is restricted to the most peripheral dendritic branches (the so-called spiny branchlets) while the climbing fiber system terminates on spines located on the main dendritic trunk. Because the mossy fiber-parallel fiber-Purkinje cell system and the climbing fiber-Purkinje cell system are present in all cerebella so far studied, the concept of the basic cerebellar circuit was proposed some 15 years ago (Llinás 1969 a,b); the other elements present in this cortex (i.e. stellate, basket, Golgi and Lugaro cells) were viewed accordingly as elaborations of the rather ancient theme of this basic cerebellar circuit. At that time it was the prevailing view that, due to the rather complete characterization of both the morphological organization of these inputs and the well understood nature of

[1] Dept. of Physiology and Biophysics New York University Medical Center 550 First Avenue, New York 10016 USA

Cerebellar Functions
ed. by Bloedel et al.
© Springer-Verlag Berlin Heidelberg 1984

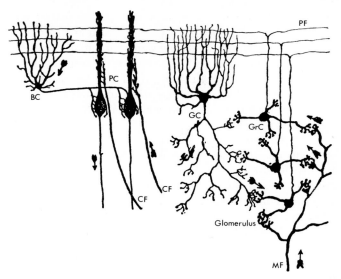

Fig. 1. Diagram of the basic cerebellar circuit. Mossy and climbing fibers comprise inputs to Purkinje cells. Activity of mossy fiber *(MF)* is relayed through granule cells *(GrC)* via parallel fibers *(PF)* to Purkinje cells *(PC)*. Axons of these cells are the only output system from cerebellar cortex. Second afferent is a climbing fiber *(CF)*, which establishes a monosynaptic input to Purkinje cell dendrites. The two basic inhibitory systems are also shown. Basket cell *(BC)* axon contacts the somata and dendrites of Purkinje cells. Stellate cells (not shown) establish direct contact with *PC* dendrites. Both basket and stellate cells receive input via parallel fibers *(PF)* and constitute the inhibitory systems of the molecular layer. Golgi cell *(GC)* receives input from parallel fibers *(PF)*, mossy fibers *(MF)* and climbing fibers (not shown), and relays inhibition onto dendrites of granule cells *(GrC)* in granule layer. Note orthogonal organization of parallel fibers, with respect to isoplanar characteristics of dendrites of Purkinje cells and basket cells and that axons of basket and stellate cells run at right angles with respect of parallel fibers and that dendritic tree of Golgi cell is close to cylindrical rather than isoplanar. (after Ramón y Cajal, 1909-1911)

their electrophysiological characteristics, the functional significance of these two different inputs on the Purkinje cell would be comprehended rather quickly. It was also believed that understanding this functional significance would be the central key in understanding the ultimate function of the cerebellar cortex. However, almost two decades later we find ourselves still quite puzzled with regard to the meaning of these two afferent systems in the overall role of the cerebellum and even at odds as to their immediate significance with regard to the function of Purkinje cells. Indeed, while the electrophysiological consequences of these inputs was already quite well described in the 1960's (Eccles et al. 1967, Llinás 1969 a,b), precious little has been uncovered since to reveal their ultimate significance in cerebellar function.

2 The Role of the Climbing Fiber System

The excitatory nature of this afferent input was described in the mid-sixties (Eccles et al. 1966 a,b). At that time it was considered that this cerebellar afferent was capable of generating short bursts of action potentials transmitted down the Purkinje cell axon. Subsequently bursts of spikes were recorded at the axonal terminals of the Purkinje cells (Ito and Simpson 1971) and were found to be correlated with IPSPs in their target nuclei (Bruggencate et al. 1972). Since these initial observations, much effort has been invested in discovering whether this afferent has long-term effects on the excitability of Purkinje cells. Attempts were made to determine the existence of possible plastic changes on the Purkinje cell following climbing fiber activation, as envisaged for example by Marr (1969) and by Albus (1958). Indeed, this view deflected the attention of neurophysiologists from studying this afferent as a throughput pathway towards studying the climbing fiber role in "cerebellar learning". In fact, in order to give validity to the hypothesis that climbing fibers may exercise a long-term effect on Purkinje cells, it was even assumed that the climbing fiber systems were incapable of activating Purkinje cell axons. This meant that the olivo-cerebellar system was denied a role as a true afferent to the cerebellar cortex and instead was given as its sole function the long-term modification of the parallel fiber Purkinje cell synapse (cf. Ito et al. 1982).

While this view continues to have acceptance, several lines of research demonstrate that the olivocerebellar system has a clear role as a cerebellar afferent. The first demonstration was the original description of the climbing fiber activation of Purkinje cells which already indicated that action potentials were generated by this input (Eccles et al. 1966 a,b). In the early seventies it was shown, as stated above, that activation of the climbing fiber system would produce one or more action potentials recorded at the axon of the Purkinje cells at the level of the cerebellar or vestibular nuclei (Ito and Simpson 1971) and that such activation produces a powerful inhibition on their target cells (Bruggencate et al. 1972). Another important experimental finding relates to the fact that direct electrical stimulation of the inferior olive (I.O.) was shown to produce eye movements in the rabbit (Barmack 1979). More importantly, these movements were shown to have a rather clear short-term relation to moving visual stimuli. This activation of the I.O. was clearly related to specific aspects of sensory information processing, requiring that the CF input be considered as capable of serving as an afferent system. Moreover, drugs such as harmaline were shown to produce tremor by directly affecting I.O. neurons (de Montigny and Lamarre 1973); Llinás and Volkind 1973).

While all of the above experiments verified the role of the I.O. as a component of a sensory-motor pathway, earlier experiments employing olivary lesions had already demonstrated the role of the I.O. in motor coordination independently of any "learning function". Indeed, Wilson and Magoun (1945) showed that acute ataxia follows I.O. lesions.

More recently, with the development of techniques capable of producing quite complete chemical lesions of the I.O. (Desclin and Escubi 1974; Llinás et al. 1975), it was demonstrated that such damage produces distinct abnormalities of coordination which could be demonstrated to be related to the specific I.O. lesion. Following damage of this nucleus, abnormal gait occurs (Llinás et al. 1975). This particular syndrome may be acutely obtained following partial chemical lesions of the I.O., if the remaining olive is inactivated by drugs such as harmaline (Walton 1980).

Another reason for considering the olivo-cerebellar system as a true afferent system is the fact that motor activity such as the compensation following a unilateral vestibular lesion (cf. Schaefer and Meyer 1973) requires the presence of the olivo-cerebellar pathway for the acquisition and retention of such motor learning. Unilateral lesion of the vestibular nerve is followed by rotation of the body and abnormal posture; this lasts in the rat for a period of about 1/2 to 1 h at which point the animal begins to compensate, reaching full compensation approximately 48 hr after the lesion (Llinas and Walton 1977). It was also demonstrated that, if the I.O. of these animals is damaged prior to lesion, the animals never compensate from acute vestibular asymmetries produced by severing the vestibular nerve (Llinás and Walton 1977). This finding, when first observed, was thought to add credence to the notion that the I.O. is necessary for acquisition of motor learning. However, following the acquisition of vestibular compensation after a unilateral lesion, damage of the I.O. produced a return of the animal to the precompensated state (Llinâs and Walton 1977). This implied that with destruction of the olive the animal had lost not only the ability to acquire, but also to maintain this previously acquired motor skill. Thus, the indication is that the presence of the I.O. is not necessary to modify the cerebellar cortex, as would be expected from the hypothesis of Marr or Albus, but rather that it is actually required for the maintenance of such acquired motor activity. This finding implied that whatever the function of the I.O., its role is a continuous one rather than one to be activated only during the period of acquisition of a learned behavior. A similar set of findings was in fact reported more recently using a similar paradigm by Demer and Robinson (1982). That is, the I.O. must continue to function and therefore must be considered as an afferent carrying particular information to the cerebellum and brainstem.

In a second set of experiments it was actually demonstrated that vestibular compensation could occur following cerebellar cortical lesions, implying that the climbing fiber input to the cerebellar nuclei was the pathway utilized for this compensation (Llinás and Walton 1979). Furthermore, following compensation in the decerebellocorticate animals, damage of the I.O. once again generated a total reversion to the uncompensated state.

Another proposal concerning the question of the role ot the climbing fibers was that of Ito and co-workers who suggested that the climbing fiber input regulates the amount of inhibition exercised by the Purkinje cells on the cerebellar nuclear cells (Ito et al., 1978, 1979, 1982).

More recently, however, the statement that the climbing fiber system is necessary for the inhibitory effect of Purkinje cells has met with rather serious criticism. It was found that transient, pharmacological removal of the I.O. does not actually affect the response of these neurons to physiological input (Leonard and Simpson 1982). However, de-afferentation (prolonged elimination of the climbing fiber input) does produce long-term change in Purkinje cell spontaneous activity (Montarolo et al. 1982; Leonard and Simpson 1982; Benedetti et al. 1983 a,b). This increase in Purkinje cell spontaneous activity is then the most probable reason that Ito et al. (1979) observed less inhibition following I.O. lesion. The mechanism for this decrease is probably three fold: (a) The target neurons are already under tonic inhibition due to the increased Purkinje cell background activity and thus further inhibition will be difficult to observe. (b) The background activity will produce a change in the driving force for the IPSP since the E_{C1} would be kept slightly more positive than normal due to the rather continuous chloride influx. (c) The amount of transmitter released by a given presynaptic Purkinje cell spike would be reduced due to the transmitter depletion resulting from the elevated discharge rate of Purkinje cells. These three different mechanisms are thoroughly discussed in this volume in the paper by Strata.

At a more fundamental level, however, in tissue culture, where Purkinje cell and nuclear cells can be co-cultured in the absence of climbing fibers, the inhibitory effect of Purkinje cells has been shown to be quite powerful (Marshall and Hendelman 1982). In short, the experimental results do pose serious doubts regarding the olivo-cerebellar system as a mere modulator of Purkinje cell activity rather than as a true cerebellar afferent. It is also true that the above data, while questioning the validity of the hypothesis that the olivo-cerebellar system is not a true afferent, does not provide any direct insight into the role of the climbing fiber system as an afferent pathway.

3 If the Climbing Fiber is Not Present to Modify a Parallel Fiber-Purkinje Cell Synapse, What Then is its Function?

This rather central question may be divided into two parts: (1) What do we know about the properties of the climbing fiber activation of Purkinje cells and of the cells of origin of the climbing fiber system? (2) How does that knowledge relate to the ultimate role of the inferior olive in motor coordination?

3.1 Electrophysiology of Climbing Fiber Activation of Purkinje Cells and of the Inferior Olivary Neurons

Electrophysiological analysis of the climbing fiber input under in vitro conditions has shown that this afferent generates a powerful depolarization of the Purkinje cell dendrites which is accompanied by a rather substantial calcium influx (Llinás and Sugimori 1982). It has also been demonstrated that this calcium influx produces a sizeable increase in potassium conductance. Indeed, as seen in Fig. 2, activation of this afferent produces an "early excitation" followed by a "late inhibition". The early excitation is produced by the plateau calcium current observed in these cells, the late inhibition produced by a calcium-dependent potassium conductance increase. The biophysical consequences of the ionic conductance triggered by the climbing fiber activation actually go quite far in explaining much of what is seen following climbing fiber activation. Indeed, the results obtained by Bloedel and Roberts (1971) in which climbing fiber excitation is followed by an inhibitory period can be explained, at least in part, by the presence of a depolarizing voltage-dependent calcium influx and a late potassium conductance which hyperpolarizes this cell. Purkinje cells can also be inhibited through the activation of interneurons through climbing fiber collaterals (Bloedel and Roberts 1971).

The effect of climbing fibers on the background activity of Purkinje cells may be related to the same mechanism. If the climbing fiber input is removed, some of the calcium influx to the Purkinje cell is reduced. Consequently the membrane resistivity

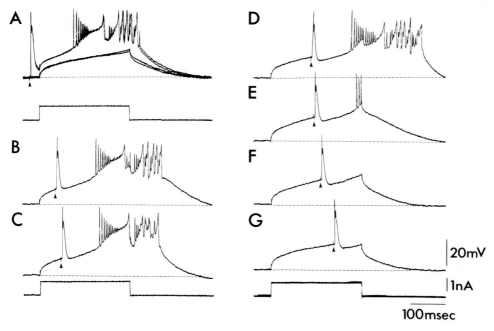

Fig. 2 A-G. Intradendritic recording of changes in excitability produced by climbing fiber *(CF)* activation. In *A* subthreshold depolarization of a dendrite by a square pulse and increased excitability of the dendrite when the square pulse is preceded by CF activation *(arrowhead)*. Note superimposed traces. In **B** to **G** the biphasic excitability change which follows CF activation is illustrated. The CF first decreases excitability and then produces a rebound excitation. This is illustrated by displacing the onset of CF activation *(arrowhead)* over the square current pulse, which is kept stationary. (Llinás and Sugimori, 1982)

of the cell increases, while the resting potential becomes less negative. This explains the increased background activity seen in these cells following climbing fiber de-afferentation (Strata, this volume; Leonard and Simpson 1982). The point remains, nevertheless, that the climbing fiber afferent fires at a slow frequency (less than 15/s) and, for the most part, in a manner that is difficult to correlate with the onset of any particular sensory input or with the generation of any particular motor activity. How then can we understand the activity of this rather powerful but infrequently activated afferent system? A most surprising aspect concerning this input is that almost regardless of the stimulus utilized, the system seems incapable of responding to high frequencies of synaptic or electrical stimuli. In fact, the highest frequency ever attained is that following injection of harmaline in which case the frequency may be as high as 15/s (Llinás and Volkind 1973). One may ask then why and by what mechanism is the activity of this afferent limited to such a low firing frequency? The answer is clearly illustrated in Fig. 3 where an intracellular recording from an inferior olivary neuron is shown. Indeed, the activation of this cell both in vivo (Llinás et al. 1974) and in vitro (Llinás and Yarom 1981) is known to be followed by a powerful after-hyperpolarization which was first assumed to be produced by inhibitory collaterals (Llinás et al.

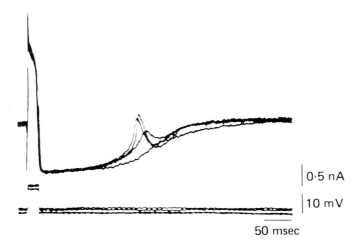

0·5 nA

10 mV

50 msec

Fig. 3. Rebound calcium spike in the presence of tetrodotoxin. Direct stimulation of an inferior olivary neuron produces a dendritic calcium spike, followed by an after-hyperpolarization and a rebound spike. Small changes in d.c. hyperpolarization (note current record) facilitates the rebound spike, which becomes larger and moves to the left. (Llinás and Yarom 1981)

1974) but which was later shown to be due to a calcium-dependent potassium conductance increase (Llinás and Yarom 1980, 1981). Because of the rather powerful activation of this calcium/potassium system, once the inferior olivary cell fires the cell is refractory for a least 100 ms, explaining the usual spontaneous firing frequency of approximately 10/s.

A secondary but rather important finding relating to the olivo-cerebellar system is the fact that I.O. cells tend to show a powerful rebound excitation (arrow, Fig. 3) produced by the activation of a calcium-dependent somatic conductance which is normally inactive at resting membrane potential (Llinás and Yarom 1981). This conductance is de-inactivated by hyperpolarization and tends to produce oscillatory behavior of the I.O. with a rhythm of approximately 10/s. This is particularly significant when considering that in mammals inferior olivary neurons are electrotonically coupled at gap junctions between their dendrites (Sotelo et al. 1974; King et al. 1976).

3.2 Considerations of the Role of the Inferior Olive in Motor Coordination

The electrophysiological properties of the inferior olive and the one-to-one relation between a Purkinje cell and its climbing fiber does suggest that the olivo-cerebellar system cannot be understood by the detailed study of individual cells only (Llinás 1974). Indeed, the rather powerful activation of the Purkinje cell by the climbing fiber renders this neuron incapable of integrative activity during the period of repetitive firing. At this time the Purkinje cell behaves as a simple inhibitory interneuron firing high frequency (500/s) bursts of spikes rather than as a large integrative "super neuron" capable of firing only at slower rates due to a current load. This is of significance if one assumes that the synaptic action of Purkinje cells on the target nuclear neurons may be facilitated when 3 or 4 spikes enter the presynaptic terminal at a frequency of 500/s. This could ultimately result in different transmitter release properties than observed if the same preterminal were activated at the usual frequency of 10-15 spikes/s observed following parallel fiber activation of these neurons.

Secondly, the olivo-cerebellar pathway may function as a distributed system where an ensemble of Purkinje cells rather than a single cell is the functional unit. Both anatomical and physiological considerations point clearly in this direction. First, the activation of any I.O. cell must be followed by the simultaneous activation of at least 10 Purkinje cells since it is known that a single olivary neuron may generate as many as 10 distinct climbing fiber terminals onto 10 different Purkinje cells (Moatomed 1966; Faber and Murphy 1969; Armstrong 1974). Secondly, the fact that I.O. neurons are electrotonically coupled would mean that, at least in principle, there is the possibility that larger numbers of Purkinje cells may be simultaneously activated (Bloedel et al.. 1983).

This has recently been indicated by work in our laboratory in which as many as 15 Purkinje cells were simultaneously studied. Under these conditions, two rather important findings were encountered. (1) Analysis of the spontaneous firing of complex spikes demonstrated that there is a very high probability of Purkinje cells firing within a given time interval. Thus, autocorrelogram analysis reveals a clear set of true correlations between successive spikes in Purkinje cells. This time correlation has a peak at 100 ms, in agreement with similar results obtained by Bell and Kawasaki (1972). (2) If cross-correlation analysis (Ebner and Bloedel 1981) is done of the electrical activity generated by climbing fiber inputs to pairs of Purkinje cells at given sites, a rather powerful correlation is observed among a large proportion of the units of the ensemble (Bower and Llinás 1983; Bloedel et al. 1983). These results indicate that the understanding of the climbing fiber system will necessitate a better understanding of the properties of the Purkinje cell ensembles, rather than the simple circuitry approach which has been utilized so far. The theoretical approach which stimulated the above experiments has led Pellionisz and I to suggest that the ultimate role of the climbing fiber system is to modify characteristics of the Purkinje cells, as a group, for short periods of time. This transient modification of Purkinje cell output leads to what we refer to as "changing the curvature" of the metric tensor hyperspace (Pellionisz and Llinás 1982). While this may seem a rather recondite statement, the activation of climbing fibers does force Purkinje cells to be active in a burst manner at particular moments in time, independent of the activity of other inputs. Thus, the firing patterns of Purkinje cells at the cerebellar nuclei (the coordination vector, merge with the inputs arriving from the direct excitatory afferents to generate the sensory motor transformation underlying motor coordination. The climbing fiber-Purkinje cell system then represents, as viewed some years ago, the more phasic component of this transformation (Llinás 1974).

4 The Organization of the Mossy Fiber/Parallel Fiber Input

In contrast to the simplicity which the climbing fiber system displays in connectivity and distribution, the mossy fiber-granule cell system must be considered, from the view point of numbers alone, as among the more complex systems in the brain. First, the enormous number of granule cells in the cerebellar cortex (10^{10} to 10^{11} in man, Braitenberg and Atwood 1958; 2.2×10^9 for cat, Palkovits et al. 1971) gives this structure a richness unparalleled in almost any other brain region. Indeed, one of the enigmas in the understanding of the structure-function relationship in the cerebellum is the contrast between the order displayed by the parallel fiber/Purkinje cell system and the apparently near chaotic interlacing of connectivity within the granule cell layer. On first impression, one feels that this almost free-for-all organization of the granule cells must be considered as a rather permissive and nondiscriminating relay between the Purkinje cells and rest of the nervous system.

However, as we learn more about the anatomy and physiology of the mossy fiber system, it becomes clear that the mossy fiber input is organized into rather complex sets of patterns (see, for example, Oscarsson 1980) which do not follow the usual somatotopy which earlier anatomists indicated. Rather, a multiplicity of mosaic-like representations (as first envisaged by Dow, 1939) seems to be present, as clearly illustrated in the experiments of Shambes et al. (1978). Indeed, in those areas in which the distribution of afferent inputs is well known, such as the flocculo-nodular lobe, we learn that the granule cells receive input not only from the vestibular system (Brodal and Hoivik 1964; Precht and Llinás 1969; Shinoda and Yoshida 1975; cf. Precht 1978) but from a large variety of other sources including the visual system (Maekawa and Takeda 1975), neck (Wilson et al. 1975) and oculomotor system (Simpson et al. 1974; Hess and Simpson 1978). This implies that the rather simplistic assumption that each area of the cerebellum relates to a specific system or subsystem (e.g. vestibulo-cerebellum) is probably quite incorrect (cf. Llinás and Simpson 1981; Bloedel and Courville 1981). Parallel rather than serial organization appears to be the rule in this system. Mossy fibers probably course medio-laterally over wide regions of the cortex forming rosettes along folia and covering many folia as if attempting to embody every permutation and combination of afferent input onto the granular layer. In the cat there are 98.8×10^3 mossy fiber glomeruli/mm^3 which, for a total granule cell volume of 355/mm^3, gives a total of 3.5×10^7 glomeruli (Palkovits et al. 1971). Each mossy fiber forms contacts with 16-17 glomeruli/folium, so indeed a large number of mossy fibers may contact a given Purkinje cell.

The mossy fiber system is organized in a parallel and distributed manner, and activation of a given set of mossy fibers will generate activity in large groups of Purkinje cells over wide areas of the cerebellar cortex (Bloedel and Courville 1981). Considering the through-put delay which may be calculated from the field potentials (Eccles et al. 1966b), it is interesting to note that activity coming into the cerebellum persists for only a short time (about 5ms). We could say then that, as in the case of the mossy fiber input, the cerebellum is a sheet of neuronal circuitry [in man about 10 cm wide and one meter long (Braitenberg and Atwood 1958)] having a brief through-put time affecting many microzones over several regions of the cortex, any mossy fiber activity being represented over and over again simultaneously throughout the cortex at any particular moment. As discussed later, differences in cortical conduction times are probably quite important in establishing the timing of motor coordination.

5 Radial Organization of the Molecular Layer Afferents

One important feature regarding the organization of the mossy fiber/granule cell/parallel fiber system which has not been emphasized, is that, under appropriate conditions, given mossy fiber inputs may produce activation of neurons in a rather restricted region of the cerebellar cortex. The problem is the following. The parallel fibers extend over a rather wide area of the cerebellar cortex covering many millimeters (Ramon y Cajal 1909-1911) — in some cases (for instance, in the frog) the whole cerebellum. Furthermore, modern analysis of the problem (Mugnaini 1972; Brand et al. 1976) indicates that the parallel fibers have a lateral spread which may be as long as 6 mm. Throughout their length, the parallel fibers exercise an excitatory action on Purkinje cells (Eccles et al. 1966 a,b). Thus, from morphological considerations alone, it would be expected that activation of a local region of the granule cell layer would generate Purkinje cell activity along the whole length of the activated set of parallel fibers. The problem arises when comparing such expectations with the physiological results. Oscarsson and Sjölund (1977a,b) as well as Shambes et al. (1978) demonstrated that peripheral nerve or sensory stimulation will generate activity in rather restricted areas of the cerebellar cortex. Oscarsson's experiments indicate that the spatial distribution of Purkinje cell activity matches beautifully the spatial distribution of the mossy fiber afferent system into rostro-caudal bands, as described by Voogd (1969). An even more detailed description of the spatial distribution of mossy fibers in the granular layer has been determined by Shambes et al. (1978) by means of detailed electrical recording from granule and Purkunje cells. They have shown that the specific mossy fiber inputs activated by trigeminal stimulation produce very well localized activity in the granular layer. More important, however, such granule cell activity is translated into the exclusive activation of the Purkinje cells lying immediately above the area of activated granule cells. Indeed, Bower et al. (1980) demonstrated that such Purkinje cell activity does not exceed spatially the area of distribution of granule cell activity; that is, the maximal degree of Purkinje cell activity is related to the distribution of granule cell activity and not to the distribution of their parallel fibers.

One hypothesis that could explain this apparent discrepancy requires reconsideration of the basic anatomical organization of the molecular layer (Llinas 1979) (Fig. 4). Restricted activation could result from the synaptic contacts that granule cell axons make with Purkinje cells as they ascend through the molecular layer prior to their bifurcation. Thus, a given set of ascending granule cell axons would generate a statistically larger number of contacts with Purkinje cells lying immediately above than with Purkinje cells lying either to the left or right of the bifurcation point of their axons. In this case, the basic organization of the molecular layer would be such that the ascending axons of the granule cells would exert a greater effect on the excitability of Purkinje cells and interneurons than the horizontal axons of the granule cells, which may serve a more modulatory function.

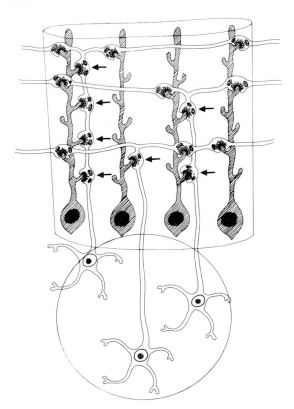

Fig. 4. Radial organization of the synaptic junctions between the ascending portion of the granule cell axons and Purkinje cell dendrites. The granule cells *(in circle)* generate ascending axons which penetrate the molecular layer of the cortex *(cylinder)*. Along their path, these axons make synaptic contacts *(arrows)* with Purkinje cell *(shaded)* dendritic spines as well as with the dendrites of the inhibitory interneurons of both granular and molecular layers. Because an ascending axon will contact a given Purkinje cell repeatedly, granule cell axons will have a more powerful synaptic action on the Purkinje cells located immediately above their cells of origin; thus, the radial organization of molecular layer input

Such an hypothesis does not de-emphasize the importance of the parallel fibers. It simply calls attention to the fact that the granule cell axons may have two distinct functions, one relating to their ascending portion which imparts the spatial specificity observed experimentally, and a more modulatory role related to their parallel fiber portion. This is essentially similar to the scheme proposed some years ago regarding horizontal and vertical integration of Purkinje cells (Llinás 1970). Vertical integration has a solid morphological basis, as clear examples of ascending parallel fibers synapsing on Purkinje cell dendrites have been illustrated by Mugnaini (1972) and by Palay and Chan-Palay (1974).

Recently, this hypothesis has been tested physiologically in guinea pig cerebellar slices (Llinás and Sugimori, unpublished observations). Thus, in the slice, local stimulation of the granular layer lying immediately under the Purkinje cell produces graded synaptic depolarization and firing of these large cells. These synaptic potentials are clearly distinguishable from the climbing fiber input and may be reversed by passing current through the recording electrode. Two types of data clearly indicate that the ascending axons of the parallel fibers must have a strong excitatory action on the Purkinje cells: (a) this depolarization is apparent only when the granule cells located immediately under the Purkinje cell are activated, and (b) because the slices are thin (50 μm) there is no lateral spread mediated by the parallel fibers.

The actual morphology of the granule cell/Purkinje cell system must be considered as a weighted input where the Purkinje cell located immediately above a set of granule cells receives a much more vigorous input than the cells located along the parallel fiber beam. In other words, the ascending axons of the granule cells have a more decisive role in Purkinje cell activity while their horizontal portion, the parallel fibers, have a more modulatory action on these cells' activity. This would be especially true of the more superficial granule cells where the ascending axon has a maximum chance to contact Purkinje cells before it bifurcates.

6 The Functional Significance of the Mossy Fiber/Parallel Fiber/Purkinje Cell System

Other than demonstrating its excitatory nature and demonstrating that different peripheral and central stimuli produce Purkinje cell activation by activation of this pathway, litte has been done relating to the true functional significance of this system.

At a more global level, Pellionisz and I have suggested that the mossy fiber input represents vector components of motor intention vectors which are transformed into coordination vectors by the parallel fiber/Purkinje cell junction (Pellionisz and Llinás 1980). In other words, the function (task) of the mossy fiber/parallel fiber/Purkinje cell system relates to putting the premotor command sequences, which are generated by the rest of the central nervous system, into the context of the functional state of the body. In order to "put movement into context", the nervous system requires a rather specialized and continuously upgraded description of both motor output and sensory input. This must be done in order to implement a continuous internal description of the status quo in which the premotor intentions must operate in order to be ultimately transformed into movement. The very connectivity alone and the neurological deficits following cerebellar trauma suggest quite eloquently that the cerebellum should be considered the place where motor intentions are transformed into coordinated motor patterns.

7 Present Status and Future Trends

From the above it can be surmised that I have a deep sense of optimism regarding the possibility of understanding the overall function of the cerebellum. It is true that an immense amount of work remains to be done in cerebellar research, both in its detailed operation and morphology as well as in its role as motor coordination. However, the issue of the presence of a basic cerebellar circuit continues to be one of the more exciting aspects of this particular region of the central nervous system. It seems that the cerebellum, more than any other part of the brain, has retained a certain basic organization and that this organization is, in almost every case, relatable to the organization of movement. This statement cannot be made about any other region of the CNS, where the detailed morphology and the electrophysiology may in fact change immensely during phylogeny. It is extraordinarily lucky for students of the cerebellum that although centrally located in the neuraxis and so richly endowed with inputs from all possible sources, its destruction produces no major deficits other than the inability to coordinate movement. This indicates most clearly that cerebellar function must be related to the proper weighting of the different sensory and motor components which ultimately generate organized movement. This "weighting" of the components has been formally treated by our tensorial network theory in which an attempt has been made to bring into a different context the enormous parallel nature of cerebellar computation with the equally enormous parallel nature of organized movement. Our point of view, that the main role of the cerebellum is that of converting covariant premotor intention vectors into contravariant effector vectors, must be considered the core of our view regarding cerebellar function. There remains, of course, as with any other hypothesis, the arduous job of finding its true value. The predictions suggested by the hypothesis are quite testable experimentally.

Indeed, the vestibular oculomotor system and its control by the cerebellum continue to be a choice paradigm. We would predict that those parameters of movement not requiring cerebellar function for their coordination (i.e. those surviving after cerebellar cortical lesion) would be related to the direction of the Eigen vector. In this respect, Pellionisz and I (1980) pointed out that in the case of eye movements, lesions of the vestibulo-cerebellum should have more serious effects on those eye movements which are further away from the Eigen direction of extra-oculomotor muscle activity. It is also clear that other aspects of coordinated motor performance do not require the cerebellum. For instance, rodents with cerebellar lesions have great difficulties performing the simplest of motor tasks; however, their grooming movements are absolutely precise in the absence of the cerebellar system. This suggests that only some aspects of coordinated motion require metric transformation. Other movements are so invariant and "noncomputational" as to be as hard wired as the most stubborn of our reflexes.

References

Albus JS (1958) A theory of cerebellar function. Math Biosci 10: 25-61

Armstrong DM (1974) Functional significance of the inferior olive. Physiol Rev 54: 358-417

Barmack NH (1979) Immediate and sustained influence of visual olivocerebellar activity on eye movement. In: Talbot RE, Humphrey DR (eds) Posture and movement: perspective for integration sensory and motor research on the mammalian nervous system. Raven Press, New York

Bell MM, Kawasaki R (1972) Relations among climbing fiber responses of nearby Purkinje cells. J Neurophysiol 35: 155-169

Benedetti F, Montarolo PG, Rabacchi S, Savio, T (1983a) Long-term functional changes in the Purkinje cell to climbing fibre deprivation. Neurosci lett Suppl (in press)

Benedetti F, Montarolo PG, Strata P, Tempia F (1983b) Inferior olive inactivation decreased the excitability of the intracerebellar and lateral vestibular nuclei in the rat. J Physiol 340: 195-208

Bloedel JR, Courville J (1981) A review of cerebellar afferent systems. In: Brooks VB (ed) Handbook of physiology, vol II. Motor control. Williams & Wilkins, Baltimore, pp 735-830

Bloedel JR, Ebner TJ, Yu QX (1983) Increased responsiveness of Purkinje cells associated with climbing fiber inputs to neighboring neurons. J Neurophysiol 50: 220-239

Bloedel JR, Roberts WJ (1971) Action of climbing fibers in cerebellar cortex of the cat. J Neurophysiol 34: 17-31

Bower J, Llinas R (1983) Simultaneous sampling of the responses of multiple, closely adacent, Purkinje cells responding to climbing fiber activation. Soc Neurosci Abstr 9: 607

Bower JM, Woolston DC, Gibson JM (1980) Congruence of spatial patterns of receptive field projections to Purkinje cell and granule cell layers in the cerebellar cortex of the rat. Soc Neurosci Abstr 6: 511

Braitenberg V, Atwood RP (1958) Morphological observations in the cerebellar cortex. J Comp Neurol 109: 1-34

Brand S, Dahl A-L, Mugnaini E (1976) The length of parallel fibers in the cat cerebellar cortex. An experimental light and elctron microscopic study. Exp Brain Res 26: 39-58

Brodal A, Hoivik B (1964) Site and termination of primary vestibulo cerebellar fibers in the cat: An experimental study with silver impregnation methods. Arch Ital Biol 102: 1-21

Bruggencate G ten, Teichmann R, Weller E (1972) Neuronal activity in the lateral vestibular nucleus of the cat. III. Inhibitory actions of cerebellar Purkinje cells evoked via mossy and climbing fibre afferents. Pflueger's Arch 337: 147-162

Crill WE (1970) Unitary multiple-spiked responses in cat inferior olive nucleus. J Neurophysiol 33: 199-209

Desclin JC, Escubi J (1974) Effects of 3-acetylpyridine on the central nervous system of the rat, as demonstrated by silver methods. Brain Res 77: 349-364

Dow RS (1939) Cerebellar action potentials in response to stimulation of various afferent connections. J Neurophysiol 2: 543-555

Ebner TJ, Bloedel JR (1981) Temporal patterning in simple spike discharge of Purkinje cells and its relationship to climbing fiber activity. J Neurophysiol 45: 933-947

Eccles JC, Llinás R, Sasaki K (1966a) The excitatory synaptic action of climbing fibres on the Purkinje cells of the cerebellum. J Physiol 182: 268-296

Eccles JC, Llinás R, Sasaki K (1966b) Parallel fibre stimulation and the responses induced thereby in the Purkinje cells of the cerebellum. Exp Brain Res 1: 17-39

Eccles JC, Ito M, Szentagothai J (1967) The cerebellum as a neuronal machine. Springer, Berlin Heidelberg New York

Faber D, Murphy J (1969) Axonal branching in the climbing fiber pathway to the cerebellum. Brain Res 15: 262-267

Hess R, Simpson JI (1978) Visual and somatosensory messages to the rabbit's cerebellar flocculus. Neurosci Lett Suppl 1: 146

Ito M, Simpson JI (1971) Discharges in Purkinje cell axons during climbing fiber activation. Brain Res 31: 215-219

Ito M, Orlov I, Shimoyama I (1978) Reduction of the cerebellar stimulus effect on rat Deiters' neurones after chemical destruction of the inferior olive. Exp Brain Res 33: 143-145

Ito M, Nisimaru N, Shibuki K (1979) Destruction of inferior olive induces rapid depression in synaptic action of cerebellar Purkinje cells. Nature (London) 227: 568-569

Ito M, Sakurai M, Tongroach P (1982) Climbing fibre induced depression of both mossy fibre responsiveness and glutamate sensitivity of cerebellar Purkinje cells. J Physiol 324: 113-134

King JS, Andrezik JA, Falls WM, Martin GF (1976) Synaptic organization of cerebello-olivary circuit. Exp Brain Res 26: 159-170

Leonard C, Simpson JI (1982) Effects of suspending climbing fiber activity on the discharge patterns of floccular Purkinje cells. Soc Neurosci Abstr. 8: 830

Llinás R (1969a) Functional aspects of interneuronal evolution in the cerebellar cortex. In: Brazier MAB (ed) The interneuron, UCLA Forum in Med Sci Vol XI. Univ Cal Press, Los Angeles, pp 329-347

Llinás R (1969b) Editor, Neurobiology of cerebellar evolution and development. Am Med Assoc (Chicago)

Llinás R (1970) Neuronal operations in cerebellar transactions. In: Schmitt FO (ed), The neurosciences: second study program, Rockefeller Univ Press, New York, pp 409-426

Llinás R (1974) 18th bowditch lecture: motor aspects of cerebellar control. Physiologist 17: 19-46

Llinás R (1979) The role of calcium in neuronal function. In: Schmitt FO, Worden FG (eds) The neurosciences: fourth study program, MIT Press, Cambridge, pp 555-571

Llinás R, Simpson JI (1981) Cerebellar control of movement. In: Towe A, Luschei E (eds) Handbook of behavioral neurobiology, Vol II. Plenum Press, New York, pp 171-195

Llinás R, Sugimori M (1980) Electrophysiological properties of in vitro Purkinje cell somata in mammalian cerebellar slices. J Physiol 305: 171-195

Llinás R, Sugimori M (1982) Functional significance of the climbing fiber input to Purkinje cells: An in vitro study in mammalian cerebellar slices. Exp Brain Res Suppl 6: 402-411

Llinás R, Volkind R (1973) The olivo-cerebellar system: functional properties as revealed by harmaline-induced tremor. Exp Brain Res 18: 69-87

Llinás R, Walton K (1977) Significance of the olivo-cerebellar system in compensation of ocular position following unilateral labyrinthectomy. In: Baker R, Berthoz A (eds) Control of gaze by brain stem neurons. Elsevier/North Holland Biomedical Press, Amsterdam, pp 399-408

Llinás R, Walton K (1979) The role of the olivo-cerebellar system in motor learning. In: Brazier MAB (ed) Brain mechanisms in memory and learning. Raven Press, New York, pp 17-36

Llinás R, Yarom Y (1980) Electrophysiological properties of mammalian inferior olivary cells in vitro. In: Courville J, Montigny de C, Lamarre Y (eds) The inferior olivary nucleus: anatomy and physiology. Raven Press New York, pp 379-388

Llinás R, Yarom Y (1981) Properties and distribution of ionic conductances generating electro-responsiveness of mammalian inferior olivary neurones in vitro. J Physiol 315: 569-584

Llinás R, Baker R, Sotelo C (1974) Electrotonic coupling between neurons in cat inferior olive. J Neurophysiol 37: 560-571

Llinás R, Walton K, Hillman DE, Sotelo C (1975) Inferior olive: Its role in motor learning. Science 190: 1230-1231

Maekawa K, Takeda T (1975) Mossy fiber responses evoked in the cerebellar flocculus of rabbits by stimulation of the optic pathway. Brain Res 98: 590-595

Marr D (1969) A theory of cerebellar cortex. J Physiol 202: 437-470

Marshall KC, Hendelman WJ (1982) Morphophysiological studies of a culture model of the cerebellum. Exp Brain Res Suppl 6: 69-74

Moatomed F (1966) Cell frequencies in the human inferior nuclear complex. J Comp Neurol 128: 109-116

Montarolo PG, Raschi F, Strata P (1981) Are the climbing fibres essential for the Purkinje cell inhibitory action? Exp Brain Res 42: 215-218

Montigny de C, Lamarre C 1973) Rhythmic activity induced by harmaline in the olivo-cerebello-bulbar system of the cat. Brain Res 53: 81-95

Mugnaini E (1972) The histology and cytology of the cerebellar cortex: In: Larsell O, Jahnsen J (eds), The comparative anatomy and histology of the cerebellum: human cerebellum, cerebellar connections and cerebellar cortex, Univ Minnesota Press, Minneapolis, pp 201-262

Oscarsson O (1980) Functional organization of olivary projection to the cerebellar anterior lobe. In: Courville J, Montigny de C, Lamarre Y (eds) The inferior olivary nucleus: anatomy and physiology, Raven Press New york, pp 279-289

Oscarsson O, Sjölund B (1977a) The ventral spino-olivocerebellar system in the cat. I. Identification of five paths and their termination in the cerebellar anterior lobe. Exp Brain Res 28: 469-486

Oscarsson O, Sjölund B (1977b) The ventral spino-olivocerebellar system in the cat. III. Functional characteristics of the five paths. Exp Brain Res 28: 505-520

Palay SL, Chan-Palay V (1974) Cerebellar cortex: cytology and organization. Springer Berlin Heidelberg New York

Palkovits M, Magyar P, Szentagothai J (1971) Quantitative histological analysis of the cerebellar cortex in the cat. II. Structural organization of the molecular layer. Brain Res 34: 1-18

Pellionisz A, Llinas R (1980) Tensorial approach to the geometry of brain function: Cerebellar coordination via metric tensor. Neuroscience 5: 1125-1136

Pellionisz A, Llinas R (1982) Space-time representation in the brain. The cerebellum as a predictive space-time metric tensor. Neuroscience 7: 2949-2970

Precht W (1978) Neuronal operations in the vestibular system. Springer Berlin Heidelberg New York

Precht W, Llinas R (1969) Comparative aspects of the vestibular input to the cerebellum. In: Llinas R (ed) Neurobiology of cerebellar evolution and development. Am Med Assoc (Chicago) pp 677-702

Ramón y Cajal S (1888) Estructura de los centros nerviosos de las aves. Rev Trimest Histol Norm Patol 1: 305-315

Ramón y Cajal S (1909-1911) Histologie du systeme nerveux de l'homme et des vertebres, vols I and II. Maloine, Paris

Schaeffer KP, Meyer DL (1973) Compensatory mechanisms following labyrinthine lesions in the guinea-pig. A simple model of learning. In: Zippel HZ (ed) Memory and transfer of information. Plenum Press New York, pp 203-232

Shambes GM, Gibson JM, Welker W (1978) Fractured somatotopy in granule cell tactile areas of rat cerebellar hemispheres revealed by micromapping. Brain Behav Evol 15: 94-140

Shinoda Y, Yoshida K (1975) Neural pathways form the vestibular labyrinths to the flocculus in the cat. Exp Brain Res 22: 97-111

Simpson JI, Precht W, Llinás R (1974) Sensory separation in climbing and mossy fiber inputs to cat vestibulocerebellum. Pflueger's Arch 351: 183-193

Sotelo C, Llinas R, Baker R (1974) Structural study of the inferior olivary nucleus of the cat: morphological correlates of electrotonic coupling. J Neurophysiol 37: 541-559

Voogd J (1969) The importance of fiber connections in the comparative anatomy of the mammalian cerebellum. In: Llinas R (ed) Neurobiology of cerebellar evolution and development. Am Med Assoc (Chicago) pp 493-514

Walton K (1980) Vestibular compensation in the rat. A model for motor learning. Doctoral Diss, New York Univ Med Ctr, NY

Wilson VJ, Maeda M, Franck JI (1975) Input from neck afferents to the cat flocculus. Brain Res 89: 133-138

Wilson WC, Magoun HW (1945) The functional significance of the inferior olive in the cat. J Comp Neurol 83: 69-77

Some Quantitative Aspects of Cerebellar Anatomy as a Guide to Speculation on Cerebellar Functions

M. Fahle and V. Braitenberg [1]

1 Introduction

Ever since it became fashionable to think of the nervous system in terms of computing machinery, the cerebellum has attracted speculators because of its limpid histology and well defined neuronal interactions (Braitenberg and Atwood 1958, Marr 1969). A re-evaluation of the old timing hypothesis 25 years later (Braitenberg 1984) in the light of the wave of electrophysiology inaugurated by Eccles (Eccles et al. 1967) and of the detailed mapping of the anterior lobe performed by Oscarsson and his school will be discussed later in this paper. We want to start with more macroscopical considerations, putting in the foreground the overall shape of the cerebellar cortex as it appears with remarkable constancy, and with equally remarkable quantitative variations, in all species of mammals investigated.

First a few general remarks. The cerebellar cortex is unique among other specialized regions of the brain in that it has a continuous weave throughout, which is not in any way interrupted where it cuts the median sagittal plane. It is common knowledge that most everything else in the brain comes in pairs, symmetrically housed in the two halves of the nervous system and discontinuous, or at least degenerate, in structure, on the midline. It is difficult to fathom the importance of this special feature of the cerebellar cortex. In most general terms it means that the cerebellum sees the problem of motor coordination in a perspective in which the symmetrical distribution of masses and muscles is abolished, while it also seems to ignore the balance between right and left sense organs which dominates perception in other contexts.

While it is homogeneous in structure, the cerebellar cortex is not isotropic: the stubborness with which in all larger cerebella (not only of mammals) the folds of the cortex run in one direction only is the macroscopic expression of the exclusive (transversal) orientation of parallel fibers, at right angles to the orientation of other components of the tissue (inhibitory axons, branches of the afferent fibers, Purkinje cell dendrites). Again, the interpretation is best given in most general terms: the cerebellar cortex as the sum of "beams" of parallel fibers, or as a set of sagittally oriented elongated "zones", is not truly a surface, not simply two-dimensional information space like the cerebral cortex or the optic tectum, but essentially one-dimensional machinery, repeated many times for reasons which are yet to be explained.

The third fundamental fact which is immediately apparent in the neuronal network of the cerebellar cortex is the local character of its operations. Not only is the sub-

---

[1] Tübingen, FRG

Cerebellar Functions
ed. by Bloedel et al.
© Springer-Verlag Berlin Heidelberg 1984

cortical white substance of the cerebellum exceedingly lean, consisting as it does only of afferent and efferent fibers without any of the corticocortical connections which make the telencephalic hemispheres so bulky, but the fibers within the cortex itself also span only short distances in either direction. Global modes of activity in the cerebellum, if they arise at all, can only be the effect of the sum of many short range interactions. General thoughts, which find such an abundant substrate in the system of long pyramidal cell axons in the telencephalon, do not seem to be the speciality of the cerebellum.

This short range computation, as far as can be inferred from comparative histology, is remarkably constant in different vertebrates. The length of parallel fibers is always a few millimeters to the right and to the left of the branching point, whether we look at the human cerebellum, which is very large compared to the length of the parallel fibers, or at the cerebellum of the frog, which is just about as wide as the parallel fibers are long. On one hand we are impressed by this constancy of the microcircuitry and are strongly driven to search for a corresponding functional principle, basic enough to be applicable to all the functional contexts in which the cerebellum might be involved. On the other hand we are justified in considering the macroscopical layout of the cerebellum separately from the problem of its microcircuitry. If the functional principle is the same in different animals but the overall shape of the cerebellum is so different, it should be possible to relate the different shapes in a systematic way to the different conditions in which the cerebellum operates. The shape of the cerebellar cortex may reflect the distribution of mass in the body of each animal, or the layout of the muscular system, or the complexity or the duration of movements, or a number of other things which our insufficient knowledge of sensorimotor coordination does not enable us to imagine. It was this sort of consideration that led us to the study of the macroscopical shape of the cerebellar cortex in different species.

2 Riley's Comparative Anatomy

In this effort we have eminent precursors, notably Riley (1928) who was dissatisfied with the anatomical subdivisions of the cerebellum which were in use at the time and proposed, rightly, to relate the terminology to a simple scheme inherent in the concept of the "folial chain". This goes back to an earlier book by Bolk (1906). The fact that there is a continuous succession of quasi parallel folia reaching from the anterior end of cerebellar cortex to its most posterior (anatomically, in most cases, really posteroventral) appendages introduces an unambiguous ordering principle. All we have to do is to number the folia on the vermis and use this vermal coordinate for the definition of the lateral portions of the cerebellum as well.

Riley's paper is one that should be periodically reconsidered as a test for any new theory of cerebellar function. The cerebella of 37 different species of mammals are described in great detail and illustrated with semi-schematic maps in which the overall order is made explicit by a common terminology. A brief description of the motor habits of the animals is also given, but the relation between the anatomical and behavioral pecularities is left for the most part to the reader's imagination. A few general propositions are suggested: the size of the cerebellum and the complexity of the folial pattern are dependent on the corporeal bulk of the animal. Aquatic mammals with degenerate extremities such as porpoises have an enormously large paraflocculus, whereas the manatee, whose flippers retain some of the mobility of ordinary legs does not. Ungulates show a special lateral extension of the posterior vermis, etc. The impression one gets is that the shape of the cerebellar cortex is not simply an image of the animal's body in any direct geometrical sense.

The main point we extract from Riley's (1928) paper is the constancy of the overall plan apparent in all mammalian cerebella. There is always (1) an anterior portion with folia thinning out laterally, (2) a central region in which the folial pattern is richer laterally than on the corresponding section of the vermis, (3) a paired extension toward the back, continuing on each side the rich folial pattern mentioned in (2), and (4) a median extension, the posterior vermis. In order to check this in a few species in a more quantitative way than was possible on the basis of Riley's illustrations (let alone his descriptions), the surface of the cerebellum of different species of animals was reconstructed by means of a computer program which was fed the outlines of the cerebellar cortex on serial histological preparations. Two examples will be shown here, referring to the white mouse and the guinea pig.

3 Computer Generated Maps

The sections were 20µm thick, the stain was Klüver-Barrera. Shrinkage of the tissue due to fixation and paraffine embedding amounted to approximately 20% (linear). Every 10th section was drawn on transparent sheets at a magnification of 1:30. Alignment of successive sections relied in part on markings deliberately applied to the specimen before sectioning, in part on the continuity of the folial pattern. The drawings were then fed into the computer (PDP 11/34) by means of a digitizing tablet. Programs were developed to handle the data and to calculate the surface area according to algorithms discussed in Fahle and Palm (1983).

It turned out that the main problem in charting the cerebellar cortex is that of the two-dimensional representation of a three-dimensional body with a curved surface, familiar from cartography. This is a trivial problem only in the case of surfaces which can be unrolled without stretching or tearing, such as the mantle of a cylinder or a cone. In all other cases it is impossible in principle to represent correctly surfaces, distances, angles, and neighbourhood relations on one and the same projection. The compromises which must be made have been standardized by geographers. If a sphere is sliced along circles which keep a constant distance from each other on the surface of the sphere (Fig. 1a), the pattern of cuts is that of Fig. 1b. These correspond to the parallels on the surface of the earth. The Mercator-Sanson projection transforms parallels and meridians into the pattern of Fig. 2. Distances along all parallels and along the one straight meridian are correctly represented. Areas are only approximately correct, and most angles of intersection deviate from the right angles which they represent on the surface of the sphere. Also, an artificial discontinuity is introduced: the extreme meridians on both sides of the diagram in reality coincide.

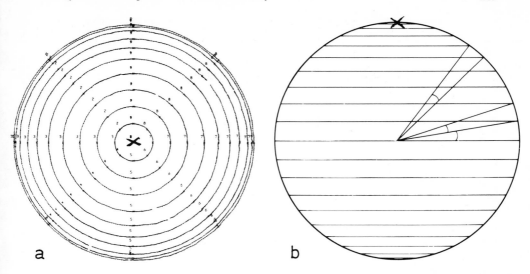

Fig. 1 a,b. A sphere is sliced along circles keeping a constant distance from each other on the surface of the sphere, similar to the parallels on the surface of the earth. **a** View in the plane of sectioning; **b** View perpendicularly to **a**

The parallels and meridians appear as a rectangular grid in the so-called Behrmann projection (Fig. 3), which represents angles and areas correctly but distorts distances (and makes lines out of the poles).

Serial sections (Fig. 4a) present a different situation. The pattern of the cuts is that of Fig. 4b. In the Mercator-Sanson projection they would appear as in Fig. 5, in the Behrmann projection as the regular grid of Fig. 6.

A complicated surface like that of the cerebellar cortex poses additional problems. The map of the mouse cortex shown in Fig. 7 is based on another principle, also re-

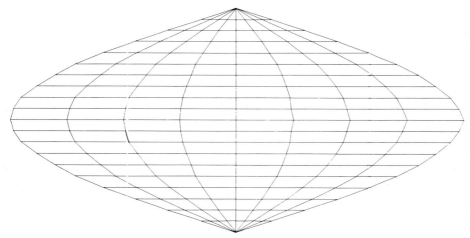

Fig. 2. The Mercator-Sanson projection of the geographers

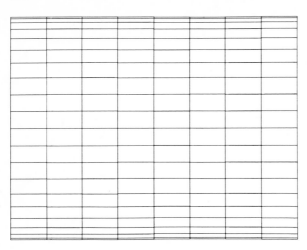

Fig. 3. The Behrmann projection

lated to one used in geography, that of isoelevation lines. The distances along the (sagittal) sections are represented by the number of marks in a row. Distances along the perpendicular (transversal) direction are only approximately correct. The outline of the map is that of an envelope covering the whole cerebellum without penetrating into the folds. The places where the marks are denser represent the sulci of the cerebellum.

Figure 8 is a map of the same cerebellum approximating the Mercator-Sanson projection of the cartographers. Figure 9 displays the same information in a form approximating a Behrmann projection. This introduces discontinuities but permits to keep all folia parallel to each other, a feature which might be particularly welcome in the cerebellum. Finally, Fig. 10 is a map of the guinea pig cerebellum constructed according to the same principle as Fig. 8.

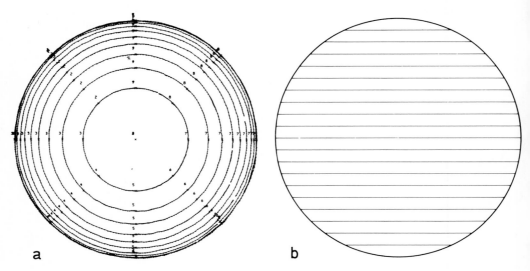

a   b

Fig. 4 a,b. A sphere is cut into slices of equal thickness. **a** View in the plane of sectioning. **b** View perpendicular to **a**

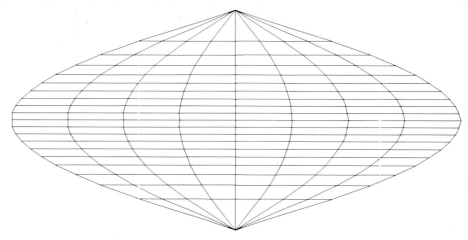

Fig. 5. A projection similar to the Mercator-Sanson projection (cf. Fig. 2). *Horizontal lines* do not, however, represent parallels but the circumferences of the sections indicated in Fig. 4

The computer generated maps confirm the validity of the general layout of the cerebellar cortical surface, with its various bulges (one anterior and two lateral) and tricuspid posterior margin, which we had already abstracted from Riley's illustrations.

We summarize the feeling which we gained from our survey of macroscopical shape of the cerebellum. Extraneous factors, such as the dimensions of the tentorial cavity or even developmental processes are hardly sufficient to explain the morphological variety. Nor is the variety exhausted by the simple rule which assigns larger cerebella to animals with a more highly developed muscular system. The quantitative relations between the various parts of the cerebellar cortical sheet obviously reflect different ways of coping with the problem of sensory-motor coordination, but not in any way that would make parts of the cerebellum clearly responsible for certain parts of the body, or even for certain well defined types of movements or perceptions. We must be careful

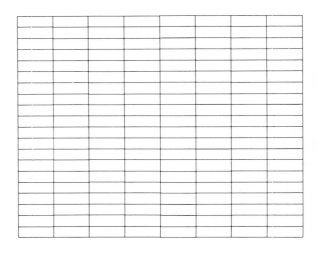

Fig. 6. A Behrmann-type projection of the serially sectioned sphere shown in Fig. 4

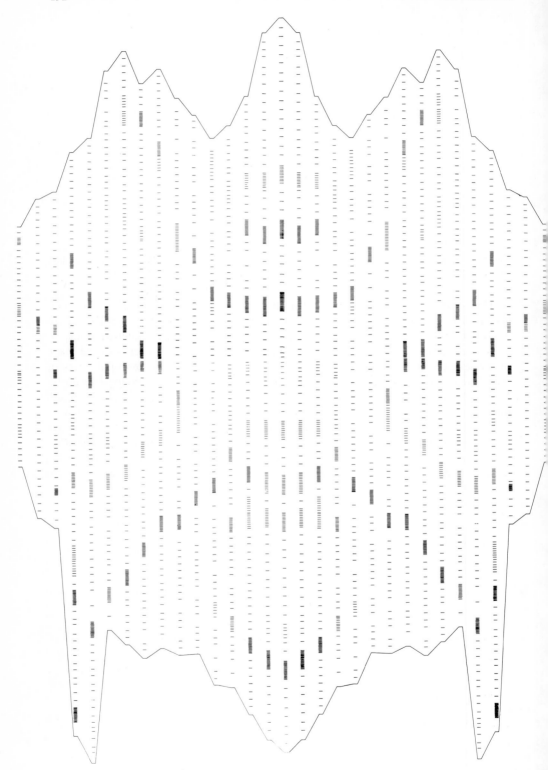

Fig. 7. An "isoelevation" map of the mouse cerebellum (cf. text)

Fig. 8. Mercator-Sanson type projection of the mouse cerebellum according to the principle of Fig. 5. The surface area is around 200 mm²

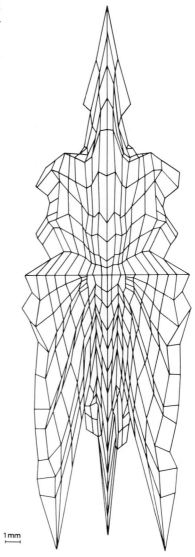

1 mm

with quantitative comparison. Quite apart from the difficulty of defining any measure of complexity in the tasks for which the cerebellum is held responsible, it would be wrong to compare the area (or the volume) of a piece of cerebellar cortex with the complexity which it deals with. In fact the area of the cortex reflects two entirely different measures which surely don't make much sense if they are simply multiplied: the length in the direction of the parallel fibers and the length at right angles to them. We must not forget that in one direction excitation spreads through the cortex, in the other direction inhibition. With this thought in mind we are not surprised to see that the different portions of the cerebellar cortex are not only different in size in various

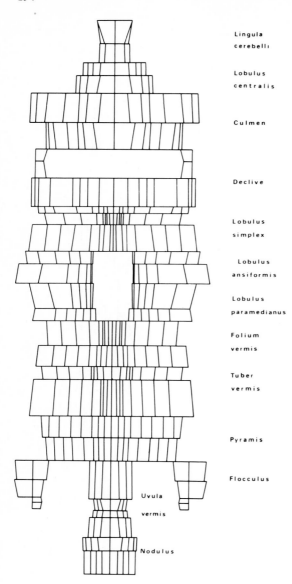

Lingula
cerebelli

Lobulus
centralis

Culmen

Declive

Lobulus
simplex

Lobulus
ansiformis

Lobulus
paramedianus

Folium
vermis

Tuber
vermis

Pyramis

Flocculus

Uvula

vermis

Nodulus

Fig. 9. Behrmann type projection
of the cerebellum shown in Fig. 8

species, but also different in shape: the vermis of the cat is so long that it must take a
S-shaped bend, the lateral-posterior extensions of the hemisphere (paramedian lobe
and paraflocculus) are narrow and long in the bear and in the giraffe (where they are
arranged in a number of second-order bends or loops), very wide and long in the porpoise, but wide and short in the apes. Evidently, enlargement in the direction of the
folia means one thing, increase in the number of folia another.

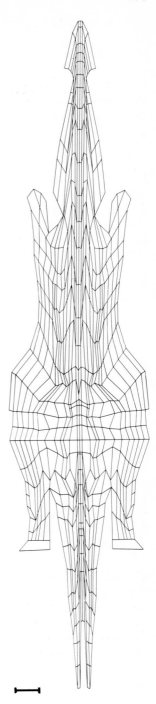

Fig. 10. Mercator-Sanson type projection of the guinea-pig cerebellum. The scale represents 3 mm. The surface area is approximately 600 mm²

4 Projection of the Input on the Anterior Lobe

We should be suspicious of homunculi drawn on the maps of the cerebellar surface, or at least, we should note very carefully how they are oriented. It is very likely that the internal computation of the cerebellar cortex deals with the information representing the homunculus in an entirely different way in the two orthogonal directions. The effect must be very different whether the excitatory influences are along the long axis of the homunculus and the inhibitory ones across, or vice versa. Already the old maps of Snider (1950) show homunculi cut lengthwise by parallel fibers and across by basket cell axons and others with the basket cell axons running head to tail and parallel fibers from side to side.

Modern research from Lund (Oscarsson 1980, Ekerot and Larson 1980, Andersson and Eriksson 1981, Ekerot and Larson 1982, Andersson and Nyquist 1983) provided examples of somatotopic mapping in the anterior lobe of the cat cerebellum with a resolution far superior to any of the previous maps. We shall not repeat these well known results here but rather extract some propositons related to the present discussion. In part these propositions are not explicitly stated by the authors, but are implicit in the maps.

The caveat that the cerebellar cortex is not to be treated as a homogeneous surface, but as a matrix in which two organizational principles are interwoven at right angles to each other receives additional support from the Lund papers. Sagittal zones no wider than about 1 mm but a few centimeters in length on the unfolded cerebellar map are revealed by anatomical techniques (Voogd 1964, 1969) as well as by an accurate phys-iological analysis (Oscarsson 1969, 1980, Ekerot and Larson 1980, 1982, Andersson and Nyquist 1983). Each of the zones is defined by special synaptic relations to dif-ferent cerebellar nuclei, to different parts of the olivary nucleus, and/or by different ways of input representation. Within each zone these properties are homogeneous for the whole length of it, providing a sort of identity for sagitally oriented lineararrays of cerebellar elements as far as their connections with extracerebellar (or extra cere-bello-cortical) regions are concerned. At right angles to the zones, the parallel fibers spanning several of the sagittal zones seem to disregard local pecularities of input-output mapping and define another sort of identity along the transversal direction. This is the identity or near identity of intracortical synaptic relations along a so-called beam of parallel fibers which distributes signals to a own of Purkinje and stellate cells.

On this background the varying orientation of somatotopy with respect to the axes of the cerebellar matrix becomes particularly important (Oscarsson 1980, Andersson and Eriksson 1981). On the schematic map of the cat's anterior lobe (Fig. 11), redrawn and simplified from Oscarsson (1980) we may ask the inverse question as to the mean-ing of the direction of parallel fibers in the various representations of the body on the anterior lobe which emerged from climbing fiber (and mossy fiber: Ekerot and Larson 1980) projection studies. We get the astonishing answer: (1) there are places on the anterior lobe (right and left a-zone on both sides of the midline) where the direction of parallel fibers corresponds to the transversal direction in the animal's body; (2) in other places (b-zone, also posteriorly between the a- and the c-zone) proceeding in the direc-tion of the parallel fibers the corresponding position in the body moves in an antero-posterior direction; (3) finally (between the c- and d-zone), the parallel fibers connect places which map proximal and distal parts of the limb. Thus, we may generalize, the

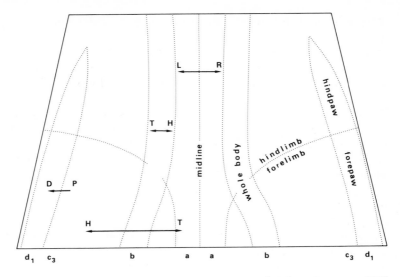

Fig. 11. Schematic map of the cat's anterior lobe, redrawn and modified from Oscarsson, 1980. *L* left, *R* right side of cat's body; *T* tail; *H* head; *D* distal; *P* proximal; *a, b, c, d* sagittal zones of the anterior lobe

three orthogonal axes of the cat's geometry (Fig. 12) are represented separately in different regions of the cerebellar cortex, each parallel to the direction of the folia. Apparently, the anterior lobe presents the information about the animal's body to the system of parallel fibers in such a fashion as to let them do their one-dimensional computation separately for all possible directions.

This strengthens our feeling that the cerebellar cortex in its logical structure is not really a two-dimensional surface, but the sum of many one-dimensional contrivances, coupled together by mechanisms of an entirely different kind.

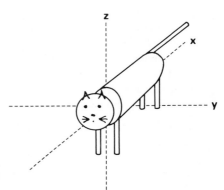

Fig. 12. Three orthogonal axes of the cat's body. These axes are represented separately in different regions of the cerebellar cortex

5 Functional Interpretation of Cerebellar Architecture

Before we embark on speculations about the nature of the computation in the parallel fiber system, we want to extract yet another fact from the map of Andersson and Oscarsson (1978); (cf. also Oscarsson 1980; Andersson and Eriksson 1981). The different representations of the cat's body on the cortex of the anterior lobe are at very different magnifications. There is a macroscopical order (evident in the d_3, c_2, c_1, x and a zones) in which the head-to-tail axis of the animal corresponds to a postero-lateral to antero-medial direction on the anterior lobe. In this macroscopical map the length of the cat corresponds to several centimeters in the cortex. In contrast, some of the zones, notably the b-zone, present a much finer topography within their own confines. In the b-zone Andersson and Eriksson (quoted in Oscarsson 1980) find a regular sequence of narrow "microzones" in which the parts of the cat's body from the snout to the tail are successively represented. The representation seems to be quite continuous, with the width of the microzones only reflecting the resolution of the experimental procedure. In this case the entire length of the cat occupies about one millimeter cortex in the direction of the parallel fibers. This observation provided the starting point for a new interpretation of the functional architecture in the cerebellar cortex (Braitenberg 1984). We shall give a brief summary here. Undoubtedly, parallel fibers sweep signals along the folia relaying them to rows of Purkinje cells. They are thin and long enough so that the conduction times cannot be entirely neglected. This, and the flat shape of Purkinje cell dendritic trees had suggested much earlier the importance of timing in the cerebellum (Braitenberg and Atwood 1958). The difficulty with the idea of parallel fibers as delay lines is that (with a conduction velocity of 0.3 to 0.5 m/s and a length of 3 to 5 mm on either side) they cannot generate delays of more than 10 ms, too short to be meaningful in motor coordination. Can we use conduction times in parallel fibers in some other sort of analogue computation?

With the whole cat represented on 1 mm in the b-zone, signals in the parallel fiber system run along the homunculus of the cat in about 2 to 3 ms, sequentially activating Purkinje cells related to the various portions of the body. The question is whether there are any situations in motor coordination that require such rapid sequencing. The length of the cat in 2 to 3 ms corresponds to velocities of 350 to 400 m/s. This is the order of magnitude of the propagation velocity of mechanical waves which of course depends on the material, on whether we are dealing with longitudinal or transversal waves etc. In spite of these uncertainties we venture the following hypothesis (Braitenberg 1984):

It is the task of the cerebellum to detect mechanical disturbances traversing the body and to adapt motor coordination to the passive mechanical propagation.

This requires some explanation. It is clear that the motor system could save much energy if in a sequence of innervations the subsequent ones respected the phases of the mechanical wave set up by the first muscular contraction. So the teleological argument works in favour of our hypothesis.

This effect could be achieved in two ways. Either the times of the innervations adapt to the mechanical wave, or, in the case of a fixed temporal pattern of movements, the elasticity of the system is adjusted so that the mechanical waves travel at the right velocity. The two actions of the cerebellum are familiar from old discussions: the timing and the tonic influences.

Fig. 13. Schematic diagram of the parallel fibre-Purkinje cell input to the cerebellum. Sequential activation of the input (t_1, t_2, t_3) at a velocity matching that of conduction in parallel fibers (v_0) produces maximal excitation of Purkinje cells. For abreviations, cf. text

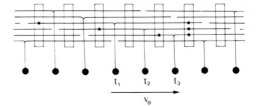

The cerebellum as a detector of movements is an unfamiliar thought, especially since it puts the cerebellum more on the sensory side. It is, however, a plausible idea in terms of the neuronal machinery (Fig. 13). If the input to a folium represents some portion of the body point to point, something moving through the body at a velocity v may produce a sequential activation of the input at times $t_1, t_2, t_3 \ldots$ If the velocity is that of conduction in parallel fibers, a sort of tidal wave will be set up in the molecular layers, since every new input adds to the wave travelling along the folium which was produced by the preceding input. Thus input moving at the right velocity excites the Purkinje cells (and the stellate cells) of the folium maximally, while higher or lower velocities have a lesser effect. This is a useful mechanism in a feedback designed to check on velocities. Note that in this case, when we ask about the duration of temporal sequences which the cerebellum may control, what counts is the length of the entire beam of parallel fibers, not the length of the individual fiber. The length of the folia in larger cerebella may be of the order of 100 mm. It takes signals a few tenths of a second to travel this at the speed of conduction of parallel fibers. Sequences of a similar duration may well play a role in motor coordination. The length of the folia e.g. in the paramedian lobes, which we have seen to vary a great deal on Riley's maps, can be interpreted as reflecting the various needs of longer or shorter epochs of motor coordination in the different species of animals.

We must learn much more about cerebellar maps and, generally, about the way the cerebellum is inserted in the rest of the nervous system before we can judge the validity of this idea.

References

Andersson G, Eriksson L (1981) Spinal, trigeminal, and cortical climbing fibre paths to the lateral vermis of the cerebellar anterior lobe in the cat. Exp Brain Res 44: 71-81

Andersson G, Nyquist J (1983) Origin and sagittal termination areas of cerebro-cerebellar climbing fibre paths in the cat. J Physiol 337: 257-285

Andersson G, Oscarsson O (1978) Projections to lateral vestibular nucleus from cerebellar climbing fibre zones. Exp Brain Res 32: 549-564

Bolk L (1906) Das Cerebellum der Säugetiere. Fischer, Jena

Braitenberg V (1984) The cerebellum revisited. J Theor Neurobiol 2: 237-241

Braitenberg V, Atwood RP (1958) Morphological observations on the cerebellar cortex. J Comp Neurol 109: 1-34

Eccles JC, Ito M, Szentagothai J (1967) The cerebellum as a neuronal machine. Springer, Berlin Heidelberg New York

Ekerot CF, Larson B (1980) Termination in overlapping sagittal zones in cerebellar anterior lobe of mossy and climbing fiber paths activated from dorsal funiculus. Exp Brain Res 38: 163-172

Ekerot CF, Larson B (1982) Branching of olivary axons to innervate pairs of sagittal zones in the cerebellar anterior lobe of the cat. Exp Brain Res 48: 185-198

Fahle M, Palm G (1983) Calculation of surface areas from serial sections. J Neurosci Meth 9: 75-85

Marr D (1969) A theory of cerebellar cortex. J Physiol 202: 437-470

Oscarsson O (1969) Termination and functional organization of the dorsal spino-olivocerebellar path. J Physiol 200: 129-149

Oscarsson O (1980) Functional organization of olivary projection to the cerebellar anterior lobe. In: Courville J et al. (eds) The inferior olivary nucleus:anatomy and physiology. Raven Press, New York, pp 279-289

Riley HA (1928) The mammalian cerebellum. A comparative study of the arbor vitae and folial pattern. Arch Neurol Psychiat 20: 895-1034

Snider RS (1950) Recent contributions to the anatomy and physiology of the cerebellum. Arch Neurol Psychiat 64: 196

Voogd J (1964) The cerebellum of the cat. Structure and fibre connexions. Thesis, Van Gorcum, Assen

Voogd J (1969) The importance of fiber connections in the comparative anatomy of the mammalian cerebellum. In: Llinas R (ed) Neurobiology of cerebellar evolution and development. Am Med Assoc (Chicago) pp 493-514

Tensorial Brain Theory in Cerebellar Modelling

A. J. PELLIONISZ[1]

1 The Goal: 3 · A Theory of the Cerebellum — Towards Understanding the Brain

1.1 A Challenge Posed by Cerebellar Research

For the last century and a half, the cerebellum (CB) has been known as the part of the brain that performs the most lucid global function: motor coordination (cf. classical treatises by Flourens, 1842; Sherrington, 1906; Holmes, 1939; Dow and Moruzzi, 1958; or recent review in Towe and Luschei, 1981). Experimentalists have also been enticed by the "crystalline" elegance of the microarchitecture of this remarkable neuronal circuitry (cf. pioneering studies by Purkinje, 1837; Golgi, 1874; Ramon y Cajal, 1911; and modern analyses by Palkovits et al., 1972; Oscarsson, 1973; Palay and Chan-Palay, 1974; Voogd and Bigare, 1980; and Hillman this volume). As a result, the CB has been studied by now in more detail than virtually any other part of the brain (cf. reviews in Eccles et al., 1967; Llinás, 1969a, 1981; Palay and Chan-Palay, 1982). Based on these pillars of general and detailed knowledge, attempts have also been made to erect a structure in order to show how knowledge of the functioning may be built into an understanding of neural function (cf. reviews in Szentagothai, 1968; Pellionisz, 1979a; Llinás and Simpson, 1981; Ito, 1984). Such understanding may ultimately be utilized in medicine (Mann, 1981; Dichgans this volume, Gilman this volume), as well as in novel applications, eg. in the construction of brain-like machines (Albus, 1981; Marr, 1982; Loeb, 1983; Pellionisz, 1983b).

Despite the extensive efforts above, whether there is a single theory that can be generally accepted as the "state of the art" explanation for the function of the CB, and one that makes the expected knowledge-understanding-utilization transfer possible, may remain an open question to the reader.

1.2 A Challenge Posed by Neuroscience

The main challenge is to undertake a long-overdue transfer from knowledge to understanding of the brain, but in a more global sense than in the specific case of the CB, where only motor coordination is to be explained. Indeed, since it has little to do with cognitive brain functions, the CB has always been a secondary target for both the

[1] Dept. of Physiology & Biophysics, New York University Medical Center, 550 First Ave, New York, NY 10016, USA

Cerebellar Functions
ed. by Bloedel et al.
© Springer-Verlag Berlin Heidelberg 1984

philosophers of "mental events" and the engineers of "brain-like machines". The prize is the neocortex, the presumed seat of consciousness and intelligence. The lack of a satisfactory understanding of how such a restricted brain function as motor coordination is implemented by the central nervous system (CNS) is, therefore, a good example of the neglect of the theoretical aspects of neurobiological research. While the aim of the conceptual thrust in brain research is not the modeling of any particular part of the CNS in itself, but the construction of general theories of CNS function, even partial integrative efforts are much needed since "what is conspicuously lacking is a broad framework of ideas within which to interpret all these different approaches... It is not that most neurobiologists do not have some general concept of what is going on. The trouble is that the concept is not precisely formulated" (Crick, 1979).

These issues are not only academic. Present-day technological needs of society already press for the next step, the understanding-utilization transfer. This, however is not possible before the interim goal, reaching an understanding, is accomplished. Since a full paper has been devoted to the key position of brain theory in connecting neuroscience to robotics (Pellionisz, 1983b), only some central issues are raised here. The challenge is explicit: can neuroscience provide a paradigm, phrased in a language suitable for engineering, to build (a) a mechanism that is capable of coordinated movements (providing a blueprint for a controller usable in present day robots), or (b) an advanced brain-like control system that integrates this basic design with sensorimotor functions (furnishing the organism with eg., robotic vision), and then one that is endowed with cognitive functions? While unified self-consistent formal theories are traditionally acclaimed in basic sciences, the looming industrial utilizations elevate these desirable features of theory into essential measures of practicality, since the success of system-engineering depends on the continuity and contiguity of global and local solutions.

For an assessment of the creditworthiness of brain research regarding these implied promises, cerebellar research is looked upon today as the test of the viability of an institutionalized transition in neuroscience at large, from the rich detailed knowledge to the elegant abstract understanding of brain function. From a broader perspective that is not limited to neuroscience, it is evident that society, especially when concentrating on short-term investments, expects all scientists not only to gather knowledge, but also to arrive at an understanding of phenomena and furthermore, to deliver socioeconomically useful results. Such expectations have amply been met, for instance, in physics. There, the knowledge of atomic particles was painstakingly transformed into an understanding of how energy relates to matter, leading to utilization in finding new sources of energy. Neuroscientists are confident that comparably profound relationships will, in time, be revealed between knowledge of neuronal networks and understanding of brain function.

While it is still debatable whether neuroscience and cerebellar research in its forefront have come to term for such delivery, this paper is designed at least to raise a voice regarding this hitherto silent question.

2 Problems With Cerebellar Theory

In a sense, cerebellar modeling and theory reaches back to classical Greek academia (cf. Table 1., updated from the reviews by Pellionisz (1979a) and Llinás (1981), where the reader can find a more detailed expostition of the listed concepts). An authoritative assessment of the early ideas was presented by Dow (1970). The modern concepts, regardless of whether they feature the cerebellum as a site of memory, as a timing device, or as a coordinator, all appear to be rooted in ancient conjectures. The plethora of modern interpretations, represented in the lower part of Table I., confronts one with some major controversies to be discussed in this section.

2.1 Fragmented Ideas, Concepts and Models, Versus a Unified Theory

Before hunting for the prized game of an explanation of cerebellar function, it is crucial to assess the dimensions of the vehicle that can take the quarry home. Equipped with increasingly potent instruments starting with an idea, then a concept, a model and finally a theory, one can aim at local features, subsystem theories and finally a general functional interpretation of the cerebellum.

Striving for a "crystal-clear" explanation of an increasingly complex entity, it may be enlightening to define some words, referring to representations, in geometrical terms. Knowledge is akin to finding points in a space, while an idea establishes a fundamental linkage between disparate sets of points. A concept lays down the fundamental local features of the geometry that governs the space, and a model is its elaboration in a limited domain. Thus, a general theory is an attempt to define the geometry as a whole, and understanding can be thought of as the geometry of the representation of reality. In these terms, utilization is analogous to a bidirectional interaction between the two geometries, that of the representation and that of reality. For this, either an idealized system of relationships is used as a guide for inducing modifications in the existing status (eg. in medicine), or the geometry revealed in a given organism is used as a guide for emulating the system (e.g., in machine intelligence).

A similar trend of using an increasing "radius of convergence" of the representation is a familiar feature in "Geo-metry", in the primary sense. Exploration there is done in order to generate charts, ultimately to allow navigation. The quality intrinsic to a set of maps can be rated according to the homogeneity, contiguity and self-consistency of the geometry that the maps express. Thus, ideally, a homomorphism of the real and model systems is attained when no domain is left unattached and no gaps or contradicting representations exist within the set of representation. Otherwise, the implied geometry is broken, and this renders a general utilization of such representations impossible.

The above considerations serve to underline the profound significance of the evolutionary trends in thinking about the cerebellum, sketched in Table 1, that begin with disparate ideas and evolve towards a homogeneous formal brain theory. There is also a necessity for such a gradually enlarging view on the function of CNS subsystems out of respect for the enormity of the efforts invested in ferreting out the available constructs. Thus, the truths and merits inherent in them must be preserved and their contribution acknowledged, even while embedding them into a broader structure. Given the existing array of theories and the timeliness of the goal to be accomplished through their inte-

Table 1. Chronological comparison of main ideas, concepts, models, and theories on cerebellar function

Author/Date	Function	Mechanism	Method
Poseidonious (1st cent. B.C.)	Memory		
Willis (1664)	Time activities		
Rolando (1823)	Motor activities		
Magendie (1825)	Equilibrium		
Flourens (1842)	Coordination		
Bernstein (1947)	Synergy control		Synergies
Boylls (1974)			
Arbib et al. (1974)			Cartesian
Boylls (1982)			vectoranalysis
Braitenberg and Atwood (1958)	Timing	Delays along PF	Intuition
Braitenberg (1967)			Algebra
Freeman (1969)			Electrophysiology
Kornhuber (1971)			Clinical observation
Szentágothai (1963)	Lateral inhibition	PC's flanked by basket cell inhibition	Intuition based on morphology
Brindley (1964)	Motor memory	Heterosynaptic	Intuition
Grossberg (1969)		unimodal alteration	Calculus
Marr (1969)		(e.g., facilitation)	Combinatorics
Albus (1971)		of PC/PF synapses	Cartesian vector
Gilbert &		by CF, as in	analysis
Thatch (1977)		Hebb (1949)	Electrophysiology
Fujita (1982)			Vector analysis
Eccles et al. (1967)	Interaction of	Read-out	Heuristics
Kado (unpublished)	PC/PF via CF,	Clearing	Heuristics
Pellionisz (1976)	in an active	Shaping the dynamism	Hodkin-Huxley model
Ito et al. (1982)	but non-Hebbian	Depression	Electrophysiology
Bloedel et al.(1983)	manner	Enhancement	Electrophysiology
Eccles (1969,1973)	Dynamic loops for evolving movements	Sculpting	Heuristics based on morphology and physiology
Oscarsson (1969,1973)	Comparator	Olivary intention- – execution comparison	Heuristics based on morphology
Llinás (1970)	Phasic control of ballistic acts	PF/CF time sharing on PC	Feedforward control. Electrophysiology Intuition
Ito (1970,1974)	Internal model representation	Model reference adaptive control	Feedback mechanisms System theory
Pellionisz and Llinás (1979,80,82a)	Tensorial Adaptive Coordination by geometric transformation of spacetime vectors	Essential network: covariant intention- contravar. execution IO: stores Eigenvectors of tensor ellipsoid CFs: adjust Eigenvalues	Multidimensional geometry:reference frame invariant tensor analysis of coordinates intrinsic in CNS

gration, it is no longer acceptable to introduce yet another detached effort; a critical synthesis of the available constructs is expected from brain theory.

Lateral Inhibition Model. Some attempts sampled in Table 1. were *ab ovo* narrowly focused on local features of the cerebellum, and thus it is only natural that they do not explain cerebellar function *per se.* A classic example of this is the Lateral Inhibition model (see Table 1.), which graphically synthesized the envisioned parallel action of a stack of hundreds or thousands of Purkinje cells (PCs), flanked by basket cell inhibition (Szentágothai, 1963). While this conjecture never claimed to elucidate how motor coordination emerges from such a local network phenomena, it did raise hopes. First, brain function appeared explicable in the intrinsic electrophysiological and morphological terms of the "neuronal machine" (Eccles et al., 1967). Second, as far as understanding is concerned, neuroscience started to move towards models of CNS function suitable to its parallel organization.

2.1.1 Assembly of Fragmented Features by Computer Modeling

In order to progress from intuitive phenomenology of such "parallel" models towards their quantitative analysis, computer models had to be constructed (Pellionisz, 1970; Mortimer, 1970; Calvert and Meno, 1972). Such *études* led to simulations of structuro-functional properties of "pieces" of CB networks (Pellionisz and Szentágothai, 1973, 1974). Integrative efforts were also undertaken in single cell computer modeling of CB neurons by the use of multicompartmental Hodgkin-Huxley models (Pellionisz and Llinás, 1977). Thus, explanations were offered, e.g., for the dynamism of generating simple and complex spikes of PCs and for the plastic characteristics of such firings (Pellionisz, 1976). While such computer models do not directly yield abstract understanding of motor coordination, they serve to increase the homogeneity of diverse sets of data arising at different levels of complexity, e.g., at membrane, single cell, and network levels. This kind of modeling (see review in Pellionisz, 1979b) provided us with the impetus for the development of a general brain theory (Pellionisz and Llinás, 1979, 1980, 1982a).

2.1.2 A Theoretical Focus: the Interaction of Climbing Fiber Activity With Ongoing Purkinje Cell Response

Sharply focused questions emerged at the single unit level of the PC, which is one of the most remarkable neurons in the CNS (cf. Ramon y Cajal, 1911; Hillman, 1979; Eccles et al., 1967; Llinás this Vol.). Indeed, one can easily become captivated by any aspect of this wondrous cell, especially by its widespread affair with the closely attached climbing fiber (CF). Finding an explanation for how a CF evokes the fancy waves of depolarization in a CF-evoked complex spike of the PC may consume years of computer modeling (Pellionisz and Llinás, 1977), without even questioning the functional impact of these wavelets or the significance of one complex spike in motor coordination. Yet an intensive PC/CF interaction or a lack of it has become a central issue, as evidenced by the convergence of several independent considerations on this possibility (see Motor Memory and Interaction Models in Table 1.). Since it is expected that an explanation that is satisfactory from all morphological, microphysiological and global functional viewpoints may unlock a central problem in cerebellar research, both theoretical and experimental investigations have focused on this issue, maybe overly so, overshadowing the question of motor coordination.

Heterosynaptic Interaction by Means of the Hebb-Synapse. Interpreted in the tradition set by Hebb (1949), a postulated CF-evoked PF (Parallel Fiber)/PC heterosynaptic interaction was used by Brindley (1964) and Grossberg (1969) as a cornerstone of the Motor Memory model, even in the absence of experimental support. The Hebb-postulate of synaptic modification (often interpreted as a "re-wiring" of CNS) utilizes the "record" that is built up in a PC by the preceeding PF-evoked excitation for imprinting such status into synaptic efficacies. However, this is not the only theoretical possibility. The other extreme to invoking a structural change is to assume, as below, that such a record has no bearing at all on the events occurring around a CF-evoked complex spike.

Time-sharing. Based on direct electrophysiological experience and global functional intuitions, Llinás (1969b, 1974) argued for the latter, passive interaction and against the active "re-wiring" of the cerebellum (see the Phasic Control model in Table 1.). The short-term, transient effect of eliciting a complex spike from the PC by the CF was emphasized, which was functionally interpreted as a "phasic control" mechanism. This would produce a quick and aggressive corrective jolt in the ballistic control of movements, via the output from PCs triggered by the interconnected CFs (it has been indicated, even at an electronmicroscopic level, that CFs are electrotonically coupled at the olivary neurons; Sotelo et al., 1974).

While such an independent "time-sharing" of the PF and CF systems on the PC requires no active PC/CF interaction (other than evoking a complex spike), theoretical studies pressed further into that direction, since data (eg. Bell and Grimm, 1969) did reveal some ambiguous effects of the CF on the PC.

Read-out. An active utilization of the "record" was proposed by postulating that it translates into the actual number of wavelets in a complex-spike (Eccles et al., 1967). An inverse "read-out" proposal was put forward by Gilbert (1974), suggesting that the various number of wavelets in the complex spike prints the frequency range, which is to be memorized, into the PC. Computer studies have quantitatively shown, however, that the complex spike, triggered by the massive depolarization of the PC by the CF, is far too robust to permit such a delicate variability in the number of wavelets (Pellionisz and Llinás, 1977).

Clearing. Representing yet another possibility, it was suggested that the "record" was neither printed into the structure of PC, nor functionally recalled from it, but "cleared" by the CF. Such an erase featured the "record", in a prodigal manner, as an existing but undesirable phenomenon (Kado, unpublished).

Shaping the PC Dynamism. More parsimoniously, the "record" of recent firings was proposed to be actively utilized in the shaping of the postsynaptic electroresponsive properties of the PC by the CF firing. Hodgkin-Huxley computer modeling has demonstrated (Pellionisz, 1976) that the excessive depolarizations of the PC membrane during the prolonged complex spike could be responsible (by means of altering the dynamism of potassium flux) for the known phasic-tonic differential properties of the PCs (Linás et al., 1971, Precht 1978). This possibility invokes the profound concept of modification of membrane electrical properties, leading to plasticity via Ca^{2+} ionic conductance modulation (Llinás 1979).

2.1.3 A Focus in Electrophysiology: Single Cell Studies of Purkinje Cell — Climbing Fiber Interaction

Research at the single neuron level has recently intensified to clarify which, if any, of the above variety of effects is actually implied in the facts.

Depression. Ito et al. (1982) have shown that activation of CF and PF inputs causes a sustained decrease of the excitation of the PC by PFs. This depression (which, to date, could not be confirmed eg. by the more sensitive intracellular methods; Llinás et al., 1981), is yet to be successfully interpreted in a broader conceptual framework in order to explain all major features of cerebellar function: coordination, timing and adaptation.

Enhancement. Bloedel et al. (1983), Ebner et al. (1983) and Bloedel and Ebner (in this volume) have shown an accentuation of the existing components of the simple spike response. This raises the primary question of how the two findings of depression and enhancement, arising from different experimental paradigms, relate to one another in describing the various underlying phenomena.

It is noteworthy, however, that all postulates and findings in the Interaction models in Table 1. absolutely require a conceptual interpretation in a broader framework, in order for them to be meaningful in an explanation of cerebellar motor coordination. Indeed, the complexity of these investigations calls for concentrating very closely on the cellular (sometimes even on synaptic and membrane) phenomena. Such proximity may prevent the attainment of perspective on these broader theoretical problems. Indeed, the required expertise and time investments are so specific and substantial that some investigators *ab ovo* forfeit claims for general interpretations and would release that responsibility to theoretical analysis, if that were easily available.

2.1.4 Morphological Investigations of the Pathways Involved

Similarly to how cellular properties inspired workers to postulate functional conclusions, the major neuronal paths taking part in cerebellar transactions have also led to profound insights into the mechanism underlying the functioning.

Dynamic Loop. This conjecture by Eccles (1969, 1973) emphasized the functional importance of "dynamic loops" found in cerebellar operations. Though the insights must be appreciated, how such reverberations subserve coordination was not elaborated much beyond the descriptive analysis that the movement "evolves" by means of such re-entry.

Intention-Execution Comparator. The comparator concept by Oscarsson (1969, 1973), inspired by the morphological connections to the inferior olive (IO), attributed the function to the IO of comparing the "intended movement" with the "movement actually performed". Again, such intuitions, precipitated from decades of devoted morphological analysis, await a conceptual and formal interpretation within a broader horizon (e.g., of how such comparison facilitates coordination) and in a more quantitative manner (e.g., of what type of mathematical operation is implied).

2.1.5 The Challenge of Integrating Cerebellar Models Into a Sensorimotor Theory

When synthesizing fragmented notions on the functioning into a coherent model of the function of the cerebellum, the process is not expected to stop at the boundaries of this subsystem. Indeed, a particularly serious challenge is to integrate disparate models on various subsystems of the CNS. For instance, modelists who have published papers on both the cerebellum and the optic tectum can realistically be expected to merge their models relating to motor coordination and the cerebellum with those relating to sensory centers (tectum), if the goal of a unified explanation of how the sensory input is transformed into the motor execution is to be upheld.

The possibility for integrating a cerebellar model into a sensorimotor theory including the optic tectum is not that remote, since excellent sets of morphological (e.g. Székely, 1973) and microphysiological data (e.g., Sparks and Pollack, 1977) are already available for this organ, whose investigation closely follows cerebellar research (see reviews Ingle and Sprague, 1975; Pellionisz, 1983a). Such synthesis is all the more important, since it is a paramount issue today (overshadowing motor coordination) to understand vision, both in the sense of how it is accomplished in natural organisms, and of how it can be implemented in man-made systems. Granted, a vast array of knowledge is available on the retina (e.g., Dowling, 1979), on the cytoarchitecture of the neocortex (cf. Mountcastle, 1979) and the microphysiology of the visual cortex (cf. Hubel and Wiesel, 1962). It is still an open question, however, whether this knowledge, together with a general concept of organization (e.g., Lashley, 1942), translates today into an understanding of the function of the visual cortex in particular, or of the neocortex in general (e.g., Edelman, 1979; or Eccles, 1982). Significant advances have already been made in the understanding of vision (cf. Marr, 1982), pattern recognition and associative memory (cf. Kohonen, 1977), self-organization (cf. von Malsburg and Cowan, 1982) and other cognitive functions (cf. Anderson et al., 1977). Is there an answer, however, to the question of when and how such knowledge yields a coherent understanding in a manner that such understanding is both accepted (1) in neuroscience as an account of the experimental facts, and (2) in engineering as a blueprint which is precise enough to put it into use?

2.2 Limited or Inappropriate Functional Identification of What is Known to be a Motor Coordinator

A special reminder of the conceptually fragmented nature of the explanations of a coordinator-function of the cerebellum is provided by the two notions of "timing" and "motor memory". Neither explains motor coordination per se and, in addition, they appear in the literature in a paradoxically antagonistic manner. Some constructs (timing models in Table 1.) feature the cerebellum only from the temporal point of view. The Motor Memory models do not incorporate the timing functional at all, but feature this organ as a site of motor memory. Conspicuously, these disparate characterizations have not been successfully reconciled, although attempted by Fujita (1982). Characterization of the cerebellum as a motor coordinator by means of synergies (synergy models in Table 1.) is not incompatible with accounting for temporal features, yet a corroboration of the two aspects at an axiomatic level has not been accomplished

by any of the above attempts. Since traditional views assumed that the CNS uses separate space and time reference frames, as in classical mechanics, such unification may
have been rendered impossible by the axioms implied in the methods. It has been pointed
out that such separation in the CNS is impossible for lack of a simultaneity agent; thus,
spatial and temporal coordination was explained in the tensor model as a unified function (Pellionisz and Llinás, 1982a).

Cerebellum as a Timing Device. The Bang-Bang timing model, introduced a quar-
ter of a century ago by Braitenberg and Atwood (1958), tied together local morphological features of the cerebellar circuitry, i.e., delays of propagation along the lengthy
and thin PFs, with the general functional property that is unquestionably inherent in
CB operations, the precise timing of fast motor actions (cf. Kornhuber, 1971). While
the timing model lacks a conceptual leverage on coordination itself, it was the first example of how a major aspect of cerebellar function may meet a theorist's explanation,
firmly based on the available structuro-functional knowledge. Also, it served as the first
model leading one to believe that (at some later date) useful applications might emerge
from such understanding. For the most recent version of the timing theory see Braitenberg (in this volume).

Cerebellum as the Site of Motor Memory. Throughout the last two decades, since
the promulgation of the idea by Brindley (1964) and Grossberg (1969) and its subsequent elaboration by Marr (1969) and Albus (1971), that the cerebellar cortex serves
as a motor memory (see in Table 1.), a great amount of effort has been spent concerning
this conjecture. The impetus for identifying cerebellar function with motor memory
has arisen from an obvious interpretation of a peculiar synaptic arrangement of the cerebellar cortex. It is well known that the CF and the MF-GC-PF systems represent the two
extremes in the specificity and dispersion of afferent projections to PCs (cf. Hámori and
Szentágothai 1966, Eccles et al. 1967). Therefore, it has been postulated that these two
types of synaptic arrangements subserve different functional purposes. This appeared
to fit the Hebb-postulate (1949) that the formation of synaptic strengths could serve
as a basis for adaptive features of the CNS. Thus, it was proposed that the CF with its
widespread synaptic contact of the dendritic tree of the PC plays the role of modifying,
by heterosynaptic facilitation, the synaptic efficacy of PF input to the PC. This alteration was suggested to last over a long enough period to provide a mechanism for the
memorization of motor patterns.

The motor memory model has served for more than a decade as a conjecture to
which many experimentalists related their findings, in the hope of meaningful interpretation. For example, Ito et al. (1970, 1982) attempted to corroborate his important findings with this paradigm, but the failure of the memory concept to account for the coordination and timing aspects of cerebellar function became increasingly obvious (Ito,
1970, 1980, 1984).

2.3 The Absence or Inadequacy of a Formalism Which Applies to Multidimensional Neuronal Systems

At times both the "radius of convergence" of the abstract representation and the functional identification of the system appear most adequate, yet shortcomings of the applied formalisms hinder the approach.

2.3.1 Cerebellum as a Synergy Control Device

Through the concept of "synergies", originated by Bernstein (1947), the cerebellum was envisioned as a parametric control device, acting on sets of actuators rather than on single effectors. Such a concept appears to be very appropriate for motor coordination. However, the mere descriptive notion of co-activated "synergistic" groups of muscles does not easily lend itself to formulation. Thus, even the strongly mathematically oriented Russian school in cerebellar research (cf. Orbeli, 1940; Gelfand et al., 1971; Smolyaninov, 1971; Dunin-Barkovsky, 1978) could not elevate this paradigm into suitable abstract analysis. However, a computer modeling approach by Boylls (1974) has recently led to a re-statement of the synergy concept in terms of vector analysis (Boylls 1982).

A particularly serious methodological problem is encountered when the formalism is in conflict with the fundamental properties of the system to which it is applied. An example for this is the use of vector analysis in neuroscience in general, and in cerebellar research (as in Synergy and Motor Memory models) in particular (for a detailed analysis of this issue see Pellionisz and Llinás, 1982b; and Pellionisz, 1983b). Suffice here to stress that while a Cartesian vector analysis can be applied for external description, an implication that the CNS uses orthogonal systems of coordinates in its inner workings would be profoundly mistaken.

Another major methodological limitation is assumed when treating the distributed and multidimensional CNS function by a formalism developed for spatially concentrated , single-variable systems (e.g. feedback-equipped amplifiers), e.g., by using a control system-theoretical approach. For instance, Ito (1970) translated his biological intuitions into an "internal representation model" to adequately accomodate his findings. However, for a quantitative treatment of e.g. the cerebellar-controlled gaze mechanisms, where an excellent paradigm of cerebellar influenced adaptation was ferreted out (Gonshor and Melvill-Jones, 1973), a suitable formalism was necessitated. Indeed, the application of control system theory (cf. Houk, 1980) was attempted for this purpose (cf. Ito, 1974; Robinson, 1968, 1975; Lisberger and Fuchs, 1978; Miles, 1980). The system-theoretical approach, albeit highly productive, for practical reasons limited the treatment to a single dimension until multidimensional methods were re-introduced into vestibulo-ocular research (cf. Pellionisz and Llinás, 1980; Robinson, 1982, see an analysis of this issue in Pellionisz, 1984b).

2.4 Inadequate Account for the Available Data

Since no theory ever accounts for reality in every aspect, a distinction is appropriate whether an inadequacy in the representation occurs because some data are (1) omitted intentionally, as they are assumed irrelevant, (2) missing, since the theory cannot account for them although they are deemed relevant, or (3) in conflict with the theoretical explanation. According to (1), *bona fide* subsystem theories (e.g., lateral inhibition, interaction, dynamic loop, comparator models) cannot be blamed for a lack of representation of data e.g. on motor coordination. However, if the timing and motor memory models are claimed as CB theories, then according to (2) they are at fault, because they do not account for basic clinical data, e.g., on CB dysmetria, that is central to motor coordination. Likewise, the merits of motor memory models are diminished for neglecting to account for temporal features. To the third category, where factual discrepancies can be found, belongs the attempt to attribute timing properties to the assumed cerebellar memory function by invoking the Golgi cell mechanisms (Fujita, 1982). This explanation runs counter to the facts that some cerebella (e.g. in amphibia) exhibit marked temporal dynamism (Freemann, 1969; Llinás et al., 1971), even though the Golgi cell interneuronal system is hardly found in these species (Hillman, 1969).

The possibility for such conflicts can be minimized if the hierarchy of the functional relevance of data is understood by the modelists in accordance with the intuitions of experimentalists, who acquired these through arduous interaction with reality. In return, theorists may satisfy the need felt by experimentalists that "it is essential to be guided by the insights that can be achieved by communication-theorists and cybernetists who have devoted themselves to a detailed study of CB structure and function" (Eccles et al., 1967). An example of such elementary guidance from experimentalists is the suggestion that the function of CB must be explained first for a network stripped of inhibitory interneuron system (leaving a "basic CB circuit", Llinás, 1969b), since the early evolutionary models contained only these MF-GC-PF-PC-NC-CF elements. An additional suggestion is made here, that the basic circuit without the CF system should be regarded as an "essential network", since cerebella deprived of CF system retain a rudimentary motor coordinator function (Llinás et al., 1975; Demer and Robinson, 1982).

3 Tensor Network Theory Featuring the Cerebellum as a Covariant Intention to Contravariant Execution Metric-Type Transformer, Acting in an Overcomplete Spacetime Manifold

Looking at the array of ten major concepts in Table 1. it would be difficult to maintain the position that presently no theories provide any explanation of cerebellar function. On the contrary, the diversity of the available constructs may represent the main problem. This relegates scientists either to carefully select their theory of choice, or "to compromise navigation by using a conflicting set of charts". It seems necessary, therefore, to look for a synthesis rather than to re-arrange fragmented ideas or to assign priorities to disparate explanations. A fundamental question is, however, how to base such an attempt at a unifying representation.

3.1 Basic Considerations of the Tensorial Approach to the Cerebellum

3.1.1 Tensor Network Theory of the CNS

As an explanation of cerebellar function must be primarily concerned with coordination it may be inevitable to interpret such function in terms of coordinates. Vectorial representations within the brain, however, are expressed in the CNS's own reference frames, intrinsic to the body, which are usually different from one another and in almost all cases are certainly different from the conventional extrinsic Cartesian frames. This fact necessitates a formalism that is sufficiently general to handle non-orthogonal systems of coordinates and, in addition, precise enough to define the reference frame invariant properties of such non-conventional vectorial transformations. This chain of logic led to the tensor network theory of the CNS and to its application to cerebellar modeling (Pellionisz and Llinás, 1979, 1980, 1982a). Since a summarized presentation was offered in Pellionisz and Llinás (1982b), the general features of the tensorial approach will not be reviewed in this paper. In additon, concise quantitative models using tensor theory are also available for both general and specific sensorimotor schemes (Pellionisz, 1984a,b, respectively) which provide a solution to the problem of coordination using the generalized inverse of the covariant metric.

3.1.2 Sensorimotor Systems: Expressing Physical Invariants by Covariant and Contravariant Vectors

The cerebellum is featured in Fig. 1 as a tensorial coordination device. It is shown in the context of a complete albeit greatly simplified sensorimotor system, since it is unlikely that an adequate explanation of CB function can be offered without regarding the CB as a subsystem of a larger CNS apparatus. Figure 1A depicts the vestibulo-collic compensation, raising the question of how sensory signals which detect a head movement are transformed into neck-muscle motor signals, which compensate for the occurred rotation. These multidimensional vectorial sensory r^j and motor e^n expressions are both assigned to the same rotation, with only a sign difference between the passive movement and its active compensation.

A "physical object", such as a head rotation, can be vectorially expressed in any system of coordinates. Mathematically speaking, the relation among different vectorial expressions is tensorial. While the conceptual identification of the tensorial function follows from the definition, the question of how particular neuronal networks in the CNS implement such transformations from sensory to motor systems of coordinates is very complex. The main difficulty is that the frames of reference intrinsic to a living organism are different from one another and are not restricted either in the number or direction of their axes to the three-dimensional orthogonal Cartesian systems. For instance, in Fig. 1A, the contractions of the α, β, and γ neck muscles generate a head-rotation around the corresponding axes. This is an obviously non-orthogonal arrangement, for the shown case with $\alpha = 210°$, $\beta = 185°$, and $\gamma = 173°$, and there is an overcomplete number of three axes in a two dimensional plane. Some other frames intrinsic to CNS function, while not visible, have also been found to be non-orthogonal, overcomplete, and even using non-classical mechanical (e.g., space-time) coordinates (Simpson et al., 1981; Goldberg et al., 1983). Such general frames of reference, e.g., non-orthogonal arrangements of the coordinate-axes, necessitate a fundamental distinction (well-known in mathematics, cf. Einstein, 1916; Levi-Civita, 1926; Synge and Schild, 1949; Coburn, 1970) between the two possible vectorial expressions belonging to one physical invariant in a general (e.g., oblique) system of coordinates. There is a profound difference between (a) the covariant decomposition of an invariant to independently established projection-type components that yield sensory-type analytical features, and (b) the contravariant assembly of an invariant from physical parallelogram-type components that are the motor-type elements of the function. For a particular example, compare the projection-components of i_k and the parallelogram-components of e^n in Fig. 1B and C, both vectors belonging to the same coordinate system invariant physical object of head rotation. For the mathematical basis of the covariant-contravariant distinction, the cornerstone of tensor network theory, see the original introduction, Fig. 3 in Pellionisz and Llinás (1980).

3.1.3 The Three-step Tensorial Scheme of Sensorimotor Coordination

The general question of how the CNS transforms vectorial expressions of an external physical invariant from one frame to another and from covariant expression to contra-variant ones is complicated by the additional fact that many motor systems may be of higher dimensionality, called overcomplete, compared to the sensory input. This increase in dimensionality is symbolically depicted in Fig. 1A in the simplest possible form, as a two dimensional vestibular sensory and a three dimensional collic motor system. The vestibulo-collic system, of course, is of much higher dimensionality — from six semicir-cular canals to a great number of neck muscles, even if only canals and muscles are count-ed. It has to be pointed out that, in neural terms, in the intrinsic expression of the CNS, any such frames are obviously of very high dimensionality. Nevertheless, the abstract problem, the need for a coordination among this more than necessary (overcomplete) number of elements in a single goal-oriented action, is evident even in the depicted symbolic scheme.

A solution to the question: "What solution does the CNS use to select a single execution vector from an infinitive number of possibilities?" was proposed in Fig. 4 of Pellionisz and Llinás (1980). The three-step scheme was later elaborated in Figs. 8-9 of Pellionisz and Llinás (1982a). This starts with covariant sensory reception, which is transformed in the first step by a sensory metric transformation into contravariant sensory perception. The second step is a covariant embedding procedure that implements a sensory to motor transformation, yielding a covariant motor intention. The third is the motor metric transformation, resulting in a contravariant motor execution vector. A qualitative solution, using the generalized inverse of the covariant metric tensor, which serves as a contravariant metric in overcomplete frames, was proposed by Pellionisz (1983a). More recently, it was quantitatively elaborated, concentrating on the theoret-ical problem of coordination in a general sensorimotor scheme and showing a particular solution for the specific system of the vestibulo-oculomotor reflex (Pellionisz, 1984a,b}.

As suggested in these papers, the cerebellum is the third and final step in the ten-sorial sensorimotor scheme: implementing the metric-type transformation of the covariant motor intention to contravariant execution. In order to be able to elaborate on this latter neuronal mechanism, the first two steps of the covariant sensory reception to covariant motor intention transformation are compressed into a single step in this paper.

3.2 Elaboration of the Essential Sensorimotor Transformation

It is stressed that for succinct exposition the complexity of the system shown in Fig. 1 is greatly reduced (and an even further simplified version of this diagram is provided in Llinás and Pellionisz, 1984). First, the dimensionality of an overcomplete transformation is kept at a minimum (from 2 to 3). Second, the vestibular frame is depicted as orthogo-

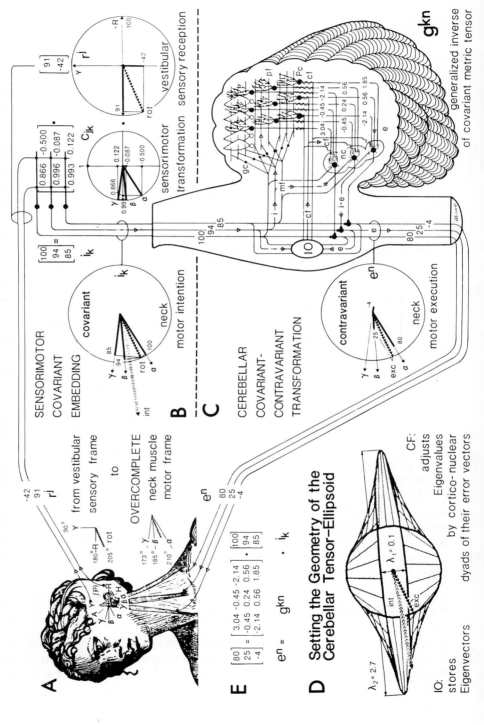

COORDINATION via the Cerebellum Acting as a Metric Tensor of the Motor Geometry

Fig. 1 A-D. *A concise explanation of tensor theory of the cerebellum in the context of a simplified but quantitative blueprint of the vestibulo-collic sensorimotor system.*

A Head-rotation *rot* as a coordinate-system-invariant physical object, and its different vectorial expressions in sensory and motor frames. The anterior A and horizontal H vestibular canals decompose the head rotation into roll and yaw vectorial components along R and X axes, respectively, yielding r^j *(Posterior canal P is rendered inactive in the situation depicted.)* The α, β, γ neck muscles, activated by the three-component execution vector e^n, rotate the head around respective axes, re-establishing the initial head position. Numerical expressions throughout the diagram quantitatively follow from the angles of sensory and motor axes shown in **A**. Note that the Y,R sensory- and the α, β, γ motor frames are different, not only in orientation, but also in the sense that the latter is of higher dimensionality; i.e., overcomplete.

B Sensorimotor transformation from two dimensional vestibular sensory vector r^j into a three-dimensional neck motor intention vector i_k via the sensorimotor covariant embedding procedure implemented by the transformation matrix c_{jk}. The sensory coordinates, to be embedded into the motor space, are shown in circle r^j, with vectorial components of the head rotation *rot* along R and Y axes. Note that the embedding, via c_{jk} matrix, whose components are the projections of motor axes into the sensory frame, can be executed from lower to higher dimensional spaces. However, it yields covariant vectorial expression in the form of orthogonal projection components i_k of the *rot* onto the α, β, γ motor axes. These covariant motor intention components do not physically add to yield the required physical object rotation *rot* but yield an ataxic performance; *dysmetric int,* with wrong, almost doubled, magnitude and with distorted direction.

C Cerebellar transformation of covariant intention i to contravariant execution e via the cerebellar neuronal network acting as the metric tensor g^{nk} of the motor space. With ablation of all cerebellar networks, the motor intention i descends the spinal cord to be directly executed, resulting in dysmetric performance. The essential network, consisting of mossy fibers *(mf)*, granule cells *(gc)*, Purkinje cells *(Pc)*, and cerebellar nuclear cells *(nc)* is comprised into a matrix g^{nk}, which acts as the covariant-contravariant transformer. Stacks of Purkinje cells, marked with open and full circles, represent "temporal lookahead modules". The execution vector e projects, via inhibitory Purkinje cells, to cerebellar nuclear cells nc. Together with excitatory mossy fiber collaterals, which carry the intention vector i, the signal that leaves the cerebellar nuclei is $i\text{-}e$, which in the brainstem nuclei may become the required execution vector $i\text{-}(i\text{-}e) = e$. This motor vector *exc* will provide the compensatory head rotation with a magnitude and direction that corresponds exactly to the initial rotation.

The system of the inferior olive *IO*, that gives rise to the climbing fibers *cf*, bases its function on receiving both the intention vector i and the execution vector e that is generated through the existing metric g^{nk}. This vector e generates a compensatory movement, that is measured by a consequent i' (after a reverberation). Assuming that the inferior olive stores the proper Eigenvectors of the motor system, it can provide the necessary climbing fiber vector *cf*, that projects both to the Purkinje cells and the cerebellar nuclear cells. Thus, on the nuclei, the dyadic product of the climbing fiber vector can be formed that is the matrix required to correct the metric in order to produce a zero error at the next performance.

D Geometrical representation of the covariant-contravariant cerebellar transformation. To every execution direction *(exc)* along a circle, there belongs a physical sum of the corresponding covariant intention components *(int)*. Not only is there an amplitude difference between intention and execution, but each of the infinite number of such distortions is different: about 2.7 (an Eigenvalue) along the bigger principal axis (Eigenvector) of the tensor ellipsoid, while about 0.2 along the other. In addition, there is a direction-deviation between intention and execution, except along the Eigenvectors of tensor ellipsoid. The geometry is set (1) by determining and storing in the olive the Eigenvectors of the tensor ellipsoid, and (2) by adjusting the Eigenvalues by *cf* signal, as indicated in **C**.

E Reference-frame independent tensorial expression, and particular vector-matrix representations of cerebellar transformations, to complete the set of the 2D pictograms, the network-implementation and the verbal description. The abstract notation defines the function of the cerebellum as a covariant to contravariant transformation (raising the lower covariant index into an upper contravariant one), no matter what particular motor frame is used. The numerical representation, different for each given frame, yields a particular quantitative description of the general function, in this case for the motor frame shown above in **A**

nal; thus the r^j sensory vector here is both covariant and contravariant (the covariant embedding is applicable to non-orthogonal frames as well; Pellionisz and Llinás, 1982a; Pellionisz, 1984b). However, in the latter case, if the sensory reference frame is oblique, an additional sensory metric transformation would also be required since the covariant embedding procedure requires a contravariant sensory vector for the transformation into a covariant motor intention. Since the sensory metric is elaborated elsewhere (Pellionisz and Llinás, 1982a; Pellionisz, 1983a,b, 1984b), it is omitted here by featuring the vestibulum as orthogonal, when the co-and contravariant expressions are identical.

A sensory to motor transformation, however, is an inevitable operation. Such a transfer is implemented by the network shown in Fig. 1B. This covariant embedding of the sensory space into a higher dimensional motor space allows the transformation of a sensory vector into even an overcomplete motor frame of reference (cf. Fig. 5 in Pellionisz, 1984b). However, the operation yields the covariant motor expression, denoted as intention, which is inappropriate for correct motor implementation (Pellionisz and Llinás, 1980). Thus, the sensorimotor coordinate-system change must be followed by a metric-type transformation implemented by the cerebellar network (Fig. 1C) that will convert the covariant motor intention vector into the physically implementable contravariant motor execution.

3.2.1 Sensory-motor Coordinate Transformation by Covariant Embedding

As for the first step, the physical invariant of a rotation (shown by solid triangles), its two dimensional vectorial sensory expression r^j is transformed via the c_{jk} transformation matrix into a three component motor vector expression i_k. The principle of the covariant embedding procedure is shown in Fig. 5 in Pellionisz (1984b). It demonstrates that a contravariant input vector, expressed in a sensory frame r^j, can be transformed into a covariant vector, expressed in a motor frame i_k, by multiplying the input vector by the matrix of the sensorimotor embedding c_{jk}. These matrix elements are the cosine projections of each motor unit vector (in the shown case 210°, 185°, and 173°), onto each of the sensory axes (180° and 90°). Establishing, by the investigator, the c_{jk} matrix in Fig. 1B, is as follows:

$$c_{jk}=\cos(\varphi_{jk})=\begin{pmatrix} \cos(210°-180°) & \cos(210°-90°) \\ \cos(185°-180°) & \cos(185°-90°) \\ \cos(173°-180°) & \cos(173°-90°) \end{pmatrix} = \begin{pmatrix} 0.866 & -0.500 \\ 0.996 & -0.087 \\ 0.993 & -0.122 \end{pmatrix}$$

To establish the sensorimotor transformation coefficients *by the CNS*, the following simple procedure is suitable. (a) Assume that each base of the intention-vector is generated by a unitary firing frequency of a premotor neuron. The cell bodies and dendritic trees for these neurons are shown symbolically by large dots and bars overlapping with the c_{jk} matrix in Fig. 1B. (b) Let the unitary firing of this single premotor neuron cycle through the entire sensorimotor system, producing a movement which is detected by the vestibular apparatus. (c) Set the synaptic efficacies on the dendritic tree of the same premotor neuron proportionately to the re-emerging r^j components (shown by small dots on the "dendritic tree" and by corresponding numbers). (d) By repeating this b-c procedure for each premotor neuron, the required covariant embedding c_{ik} matrix will arise. It is noteworthy, that these embedding coefficients can be established by the above procedure regardless of whether the cerebellum is totally involved or completely absent. The reason for this is that, for a motor base vector whose single non-zero component is a motor unit vector, the co- and contravariant expressions along this same basis are identical.

Once the c_{jk} embedding network is established, the r^j components of the rotation, multiplied through the c_{jk} matrix, will yield a covariant intention vector i_k. However, the physical resultant of the motor intention components would both be of the wrong magnitude and wrong direction as shown for the given neck muscle frame in Fig. 1B (dysmetric int). This feature of the sensorimotor transformation via covariant embedding necessitates a covariant motor intention to contravariant motor execution transformation, suggested to be implemented by the cerebellar circuitry, as shown in this paper in Fig. 1C.

3.2.2 Overall Tensorial Interpretation of the Function of Essential Cerebellar Network

The absolute functional minimum of the cerebellum consists of the essential network, consisting of only MF-GC-PF-PC-NC system. This is less than the so-called "basic cerebellar circuit " (Llinás, 1969b), since that contains the additional olivary-CF system. The first approximation of an explanation of cerebellar function, up to point 3.3, will based on this essential network.

Overall, the cerebellum is featured in Fig. 1C as an add-on system where a complete ablation of all circuits (cortical, nuclear and olivary) leaves only the spinal descending pathways that would carry the motor intention i_k to directly drive the motor apparatus. Indeed, even in the case of total cerebellar ablation motor execution function is still retained. However, this condition results in a dysmetric performance, yielding both a spatially and temporally erroneous decomposition of the formerly coordinated movement (Holmes, 1939). A computer model and its accompanying movie display showed (Pellionisz and Llinas, 1980) that the physical execution of covariant motor intention vectors results in such dysmetric performance where the errors, both in magnitude and in direction, depend on the orientation of the motor intention vector. This is in good agreement both with similar neurological observations (Holmes, 1939) and with the mathematical feature that the relationship of covariant and contravariant expressions in a given non-orthogonal frame depends on the orientation and their direction is identical only for special vetors, the so-called Eigenvectors. Paraphrased, the m number of Eigenvectors (E_m) are special input vectors to a matrix, for which the output will not be changed in "direction", only in "magnitude", which ratios are given by the corresponding Eigenvalues; λ_m (cf. Nering, 1963). The physical sums of the two vectorial versions are usually quite different and are only the same in their direction, by definition, if the motor intention and execution vectors are Eigenvectors of the motor metric (Pellionisz and Llinás, 1980).

This overall geometrical transformation by the cerebellum of the motor intention vector, which is deflected from the physical invariant both in magnitude and direction into a motor execution that is aligned with it, is visualized in Fig. 1D. All possible directions of a motor execution vector with a given magnitude *exc* constitute a circle. For the collic motor frame given in Fig. 1A the physical resultant of the covariant motor intention can be established by the parallelogram-rule for any particular rotation, e.g., for the one shown by solid triangles. For the depicted rotation *exc,* the physical execution of covariants yields a rotation vector *int.* Evidently, this deviates from *exc* both in its amplitude and direction, where the direction-difference, for a rotating *exc* resembles "phase". Such physical resultants of covariants-contravariants are connected by straight lines for 36 evenly spaced *exc* directions, thereby establishing the corresponding points of the ellipse and the circle. Physically executed intention vectors for all possible directions constitute an *ellipse*, the two dimensional version of the general tensor ellipsoid. A conceptual characterization of the transformation, implemented by the cerebellar neuronal network, can thus be stated as a geometrical deflection of the elliptic distortion of motor intentions into the desired circle of executions. Such shaping, intuitively described as attainable e.g., by a curved mirror, recalls the "mirror analogy" mentioned in Llinás (1974). An interpretation of cerebellar function in terms of multidimensional abstract geometry had also been voiced earlier by Greene (1972).

Adaptability is seen, as represented in Fig. 1D and elaborated in Section 3.3., not as the geometrical transformation function itself, but as a feature of the gradual realization of the proper function by setting of the geometry of this tensor ellipsoid, in order to accomplish a perfected motor coordination. While the cerebellum had been assumed to yield a single scalar-variable gain (Ito, 1974; Robinson, 1975b), the cerebellar tensor ellipsoid indicates that there is an infinite number of distortions that could be characterized only by an infinite number of "gains", at best. Since each such "gain" represents a multidimensional distortion of both amplitude and direction, the distortion is direction-dependent, and to each scalar magnification-factor there belongs a hitherto overlooked "refraction" angle (Pellionisz, 1983b). Thus, instead of studying the alteration of a single scalar "gain", both theoretical analyses and experimental studies, of the adjustments in a metric type function are warranted and now made possible.

The tensor ellipsoid, shown in Fig. 1D, is a visualization of the connection between co- and contravariant vectorial pairs. This fundamental relationship can also be expressed, in the language of tensor analysis, by the so-called fundamental tensor or metric tensor (Einstein, 1916). The mathematical device of covariant and contravariant metric tensors comprise the geometrical features of the given mathematical space (Levi-Civita, 1926). A general tensor of rank two can be expressed in a particular frame of reference, such as the neck muscle motor frame, in the form of a matrix. For instance, for the indicated motor frame, the matrix of the covariant metric tensor can be simply given as a table of the cosines of the angles among coordinate axes yielding.

$$g_{nk} = \cos(\varphi_{nk}) = \begin{pmatrix} 1.000 & 0.906 & 0.799 \\ 0.906 & 1.000 & 0.978 \\ 0.799 & 0.978 & 1.000 \end{pmatrix}$$

The contravariant metric tensor that is required for the transformation of a covariant vector into its contravariant counterpart, $e^n = g^{nk} \cdot i_k$ (see Fig. 1E), can be obtained in Riemannian spaces by the inverse of the above matrix. In the case of overcomplete motor hyperspace (as shown in Fig. 1) where the covariant metric is singular and hence the space is non-Riemannian, the generalized inverse of the covariant metric tensor that conserves the Eigenvectors yields a unique solution (see g^{nk} in Fig. 1E):

$$g^{nk} = (g_{nk})^+ = \sum_m (1/\lambda_m) \cdot E_m \!>\!<\! E_m; \text{ where, for the given frame}$$

$$E_1 = (\ \ 0.559 \ \ 0.597 \ \ 0.575)^T \text{ and } \lambda_1 = 2.791$$
$$E_2 = (-0.783 \ \ 0.153 \ \ 0.603)^T \text{ and } \lambda_2 = 0.209, \text{ thus}$$

$$g^{nk} = \begin{pmatrix} 3.04 & 0.45 & 2.14 \\ -0.45 & 0.24 & 0.56 \\ -2.14 & 0.56 & 1.85 \end{pmatrix}$$

where the superscript + denotes the Moore-Penrose generalized inverse, subscript m denotes the set of Eigenvectors-Eigenvalues, and superscript T denotes the transpose of a vector. The symbol $>\!<$ denotes the outer (dyadic matrix) product. The verbal expression is, therefore, that the generalized inverse is constructed as the sum of dyadic (outer) products of each Eigenvector with itself, weighted by the inverse of corresponding Eigenvalues. Thus, the same formula constitutes, via spectral representation, the Riemannian metric tensor if the manifold is complete, and generates the Moore-Penrose generalized inverse in non-Riemannian overcomplete manifolds. For the mathematics of the generalized inverse see Albert (1972), Ben-Israel und Greville (1980); for its applications in tensor theory of the CNS see Pellionisz (1983a,b, 1984a,b).

The matrix of the above covariant-contravariant transformer is suggested to be implemented *in toto* by the neuronal network from MF up to the cerebellar nuclei (see g^{nk} matrix in Fig. 1C, also shown in Fig. 1E). Thus, since MFs carry the covariant motor intention vector i_k, the cerebellar nuclei will receive the contravariant motor execution vector $g^{nk} \cdot i_k = e^n$. Given the two facts that a) the PCs are inhibitory (Ito et al., 1970) and, that b) the cerebellar nuclei receive excitatory MF collaterals (cf. Eccles et al., 1967), the output of the nuclear cells towards the brainstem nuclei will be the i_k-e^n vector. Assuming the the brainstem nuclear cells provide the vectorial difference of descending intention and cerebellar nucleofugal signals, the output driving the motor apparatus will be exactly the required contravariant execution vector $e^n = i_k - (i_k - e^n)$.

From the point of view of the result of the vector transformations, it is immaterial which part of the MF-GC-PF-PC chain implements a matrix component, e.g. a given to multiplication factor of 3.04 from a MF input to yield a particular PC output. It may be provided by the strength (number and synaptic efficacy) of MF endings, the number (or sensitivity) of GCs, or their synaptic efficacy to PCs, the electroresponsiveness of the PC itself, or a combination of the above. While such details will become important from the viewpoint of morphogenesis and functional modification of the metric, insufficient evidence is available at this time to establish the exact site of each numerical transformation. A similar interpretive issue may be raised concerning the actual spinal neuronal circuitry where the signals for the cerebellum and the motor cortex converge. The micromorphological and electrophysiological mechanisms of the brainstem nuclei, for instance, are not as well explored as those of the cerebellum (cf. Eccles et al., 1967). Nevertheless, the point of "neuronal schematics", as in Fig. 1C, is to demonstrate the ease with which the cerebellar-type neuronal networks may yield a matrix-transformation required from a conceptual point of view.

3.3 The Contribution of the Olivary-Climbing Fiber System to the Metric Function of the Essential Network

The essential cerebellar network was tensorially interpreted as a covariant-contravariant transformer. Such a function in itself explains what is required to construct a controller for coordinated movements (cf. the robot arm writing "OK" in Pellionisz and Llinás, 1979, 1980). This is in contrast to the Motor Memory models, in which case "even if the theory was correct, ... it did not, for example, tell one how to go about programming a mechanical arm" (Marr, 1982, p.15), yet hardware-implementations of the theory were attempted (Albus, 1981).

3.3.1 Identification of the Function of the Olivary-Climbing Fiber System

The consideration of the contribution of the olivary-CF system to cerebellar function evokes controversies both at the single cell level (PF/CF interaction on PC) and system level (adaptive feature of the cerebellum), as discussed earlier.

It has been proposed by the tensor theory that the CF system contributes to the essential cerebellar function by altering the metric tensor; in effect, changing the curvature of the motor hyperspace (Pellionisz and Llinás, 1980). An entire paper has been devoted to the subject of cerebellar function and the adaptive feature of the CNS (Llinás and Pellionisz, 1984) where these controversies were considered from a tensorial point of view. The conceptual core of the matter is that while a degree of plasticity probably cannot be excluded from any subsystem of the CNS (as a general means whereby the living organism becomes able to function), it may be improper, in a philosophical sense, to identify the becoming with the function (Pellionisz, 1983a).

Essentially, tensor theory features the function as a metric-type geometrical transformation via the cerebellar tensor ellipsoid. The role of the CF system is then to set the geometry of this tensor ellipsoid (see Fig. 1D), so that the covariant-contravariant transformation becomes a mathematically more perfect operation even in a curved space-time manifold where the metric must be position-dependent. In order to develop and perfect a metric transformation, the cerebellum as a system must be capable of plasticity, just like the rest of the CNS as shown in the forthcoming paper (on the Meta-organization of Geometries) of the tensor network theory series (Pellionisz and Llinás, 1979,1980,1982a). The most obvious reason for having to alter a metric is that since living organisms change their dimensions and proportions during development, the internal metric of the system must change in accordance with the change of reference frame, in order to perfect a coordinated functional state.

3.3.2 The Tensorial Basis of the Suggested Function of the CF System

As known from tensor theory, and as depicted in Fig. 1D, the geometry of the tensor-ellipsoid of the metric can be characterized by determining (a) the principal axes of the ellipsoid, ie. the Eigenvectors of the metric, and (b) the corresponding Eigenvalues.

It is proposed that whenever the existing metric is inadequately set, and thus an erroneous performance is detected by the olive, the CF system adjusts the lengths of the principal axes of the cerebellar tensor-ellipsoid, by trimming the Eigenvalues of the metric. In order to establish the necessary changes, the existing Eigenvectors must be available. It is proposed here that these are imprinted into the neuronal circuitry of the IO. It follows from the above postulates, that there are two distinctly different procedures for the setting of the geometry of the cerebellar tensor ellipsoid by the olivary CF system. One is a fine adjustment of the Eigenvalues, that can be implemented in a subtle manner along the principal directions (Eigenvectors), in a manner that possibly all Eigenvalues are altered by any single adjustment. This process is implemented by the CFs impinging both directly on PCs and via collaterals on the NCs, thus the matrix of the dyadic product of these two versions of CF vector can be impressed into the cortico-nuclear network. A more fundamental aspect of the setting the geometry of the transformation is the establishment (and re-establishment, in case of drastic inadequacy of the metric) of the principal directions (Eigenvectors) of the metric that fits the frame, and of the storage of them in the olive. As it will be elaborated in the Metaorganization of Geometries, the biologically all-important oscillatory reverberations may play a crucial role in this process, since the contravariant motor action, measured covariantly by proprioception not only implies the covariant metric (Pellionisz, 1983b) but by reverberating it as contravariant will establish the Eigenvectors, and thus can serve to construct the required general contravariant metric. As for the inferior olive, the oscillatory mechanisms of both the single cells (Llinás and Yarom, 1981a,b) and of the whole system (Llinás and Volkind, 1973) have already been extensively studied. Furthermore, an effect of Ca^{2+} ionic conductance modulation, enabling the possibility of a certain type of plasticity in the IO neurons, has been substantiated (cf. Llinás this volume).

3.3.3 Global Functional Characteristics of the Inferior Olive

Ever since the discovery of the olivary origin of the CF's (Szentagothai and Rajkovits, 1959) and the ensuing extensive research on the connections of the IO (cf. Armstrong, 1974), the functional interpretation of this subsystem presented a major challenge. The tensorial explanation is in accord with the original notion of Oscarsson (1969, 1973) that the inferior olive receives information both on the intended, as well as on the executed movements. This characterization was carried further by envisioning this organ as a comparator of the intended and actual performance in Pellionisz (1979a). Experimental evidence, also at the single PC level, has revealed that CF's carry an error signal (Maekawa and Simpson, 1973; Simpson and Alley, 1974), that was later found to be a vectorial expression in coordinates intrinsic to the CNS (Simpson, 1979). The interdependent multicomponental (vectorial) character of the CF system is also evident from the morphological and physiological findings that olivary neurons are electrotonically coupled (Sotelo et al., 1974) and from the existence of CF strips of Oscarsson (1969). Recently, direct evidence at the PC level showed that the IO is organized in such a way that clusters of CFs tend to fire in a close to synchronous manner (Bower and Llinás, 1982) and that such firing is produced by the electroresponsive properties of the IO neurons in conjunction with their electrotonic interactions (Llinás and Yarom, 1981a, b). Furthermore, the IO system has been shown to be activated by sensory stimuli such as retinal image slip, (Simpson and Alley, 1974) vestibular stimulation (Ferin et al. 1971), and neck afferent activation (Berthoz and Llinás, 1974). How these vectorial correction signals subserve motor coordination, however, has been an open question.

3.3.4 Detailed Mechanism of the Setting of the Cerebellar Geometry by the Olivary-CF System

The functioning of the IO-CF system can thus be elaborated as follows (cf. Fig. 1C). The IO that gives rise to the CFs bases its function on receiving both the motor intention vector i and the motor execution vector e that is generated through the existing metric g^{nk}. This vector e executes the movement and the physical invariant is measured, completing a reverberation through the whole sensorimotor system as performance vector p. Assuming that the IO stores the proper Eigenvectors of the motor system, it can measure, by their inner product with the e, i and p vectors, the Eigenvalues existing in the given metric: $E_m \oplus e / E_m \oplus i$, (symbol $\oplus$ denotes the inner product) and the Eigenvalues inherent in the external physical geometry: $E_m \oplus e / E_m \oplus p$. Since the metric can be constructed in its classical spectral representation as the sum of dyads of its Eigenvectors weighed by Eigenvalues, the difference of the existing and desired Eigenvalues can serve to correct the Eigenvalues of the existing metriy by adding the dyad of the correction vector c:

$$c = \sum_m E_m (E_m \oplus e / E_m \oplus p - E_m \oplus e / E_m \oplus i)^1 /_2$$

Thus, the dyadic product of the CF vector: $c >< c$ can be impressed on the corticonuclear network as a whole via CFs that project both to the PCs and the cerebellar nuclear cells. It can be verified that such a matrix provides not only the required perfection of the metric in order to produce a zero error in the next performance, but also by this correction the internal geometry becomes more homeometric with the external one; thus the CF system subserves a convergent process towards matching the physical geometry with its proper internal representation.

At a single neuron level (either on the PC's or on NC's), one component of the correction matrix may be either positive, negative or zero. Therefore, the required perturbation on one neuron should be expected as a bimodal effect, including the possibility of an undetectable zero action. Moreover, the correction in any matrix-component is a function of all vector elements. Thus, if only a single dimension is controlled by the experimental paradigm, as in conventional analyses, the prediction of a single component of the matrix may be impossible. Finally, any alteration is expected to be much more pronounced at the site of the dyadic convergence (at NC), as opposed to the site of the intensive search, the cerebellar cortex. These factors, plus a lack of a conceptual framework accounting for what is defined in this paper as the "cerebellar functional triad: Coordination, Timing and Adaptation", may explain the meager experimental results, despite dedicated efforts through one and a half decades, in an attempt to conclusively demonstrate an adaptive feature of the cerebellum at the PC level.

3.4 Tensorial Interpretation of the Use of General Intrinsic CNS Coordinates. The Total Cerebellar Network Acting as a Spacetime Metric

The description in point 3 of the tensorial model of the cerebellum was kept simple in order to provide a numerically traceable scheme of transforming covariant space coordinates into contravariant ones. However, the cerebellum appears to operate in a space-time manifold since a separation of space and time information within the CNS is impossible (Pellionisz and Llinás, 1982a).

An elaboration of the scheme shown in Fig. 1C (Pellionisz and Llinás, 1982a) unifies the "timing" and the "coordination" aspects of cerebellar function suggesting that the cerebellum serves as a metric of the space-time manifold. Such function is based on a temporal prediction of each contravariant component (for details of the "temporal lookahead module" see Fig. 1 in Pellionisz and Llinás, 1979). The principle of generating a prediction of the components in e^n requires that some PC's that are "in register" along a beam of PF's produce responses proportional not just to the MF input itself, but also to its first and second order time derivatives. Further, the numerical distribution of the Purkinje neurons taking such derivatives must conform with the requirements of a Taylor series expansion. In Fig. 1C such a "lookahead module" is symbolized by only outlining some PC's in a "stack". The spacetime feature of the tensor model incorporates, in the "lookahead modules" nontrivial morphological and physiological features of cerebellar neurons, and neuronal networks (cf. below) into a larger, yet coherent conceptual scheme. For instance, the electrophysiological observation that stacks of PC's exhibit different derivative-type dynamic features (Llinás et. al., 1971; Precht, 1978; and in this issue) led to the concept of "temporal lookahead modules" modeled morphologically in Pellionisz et al. (1977), and tensorially in Pellionisz and Llinás (1979). Consequently, the surrounding basket cell inhibition can be reinterpreted from the Lateral Inhibition model (Szentágothai, 1963) as a not absolutely essential but an advanced feature in local cortical networks; a protection and enhancement of the "lookahead-modules" (Pellionisz and Llinás, 1979).

There is a wide range of possible variations in the network depicted in Fig. 1 how the matrix-multiplication and temporal prediction can be achieved. An identical matrix component may be implemented either by the value of synaptic efficacy of PF-PC connections, the number of PCs executing the same function, postsynaptic electroresponsive properties of PC, or by a combination of the above. Likewise, the same quantitative effect may be achieved by the strength of the projection of a PC onto a NC. Finally, since the temporal differentiation is a distributive operation, the sum of the output of several PCs (yielding the same derivative) would be functionally equivalent to the output of a single PC taking a derivative of a summed input. The most timely questions in interpreting cerebellar function, however, concern not so much the difference between such possible variations, but the general principles of the solution that must be inherent in all variations of the scheme.

4 Outlook on Tensor Theory of the Cerebellum: Towards a "Solved Case" of "New Dimensions"

This essay concludes by emphasizing that since there is never a solved case in science, the proposed tensor model may only represent a stage in the evolution of theories on cerebellar function until a more advanced one, providing a broader perspective and more exact understanding, emerges.

Immediate tasks are, however, the further development of both the geometrical concept and formalism of the approach. It has already been considered for use in multidimensional analysis of the vestibulo-ocular mechanism (Robinson, 1982) and for outlining a multisensory-multimotor general sensorimotor theory (Pellionisz, 1983a). Since the formalism of tensor analysis is capable of providing implementable blueprints, a practical direction of development is the software and hardware realization of the cerebellar model, demonstrating an immediate possibility of an understanding-utilization transition in neuroscience (Pellionisz , 1983b).

As for general aspects of the theoretical advancement, it is basic knowledge that, once the boundaries of Newtonian mechanics were reached, instead of becoming a "completed science", physics was elevated into the new dimension of relativistic mechanics. Classical mechanics was not repealed — rather, its sphere of relevance was made apparent. Completion of mapping in one dimension often enhances conditions for a breakthrough, an opening of a new dimension. In this sense, featuring sensorimotor systems including the cerebellum, not by describing the system as a single dimensional mechanism, but by elevating the description into three-dimensions (Robinson, 1982) and further by formally treating their reference-frame invariant *multidimensional* character (Pellionisz and Llinås, 1980; Pellionisz, 1984b) fosters developments that may be interpreted more as an opening of new dimensions rather than as a closing of the case.

New dimensions enable us not only to look at existing "maps" from a higher perspective, thus revealing formerly unseen systems of relations among them, but they also provoke one to raise new types of questions. Elaboration of such problems is first the duty of theorists. For instance, beyond the explanation of the function by tensor transformation networks, it is important to elucidate how such networks arise in the CNS. Secondarily, based on a new approach, revealing experimental paradigms may be formulated. A most obvious idea to be forged into a practical paradigm is that the CF action should be investigated vectorially, along the Eigenvectors of the system.

The research on the cerebellum, as compared to the investigation of the rest of the CNS, has run a distinguished course through the past century. Its major stages were (a) classical physiological and morphological descriptions, (b) electrophysiological and electromicroscopical analysis, (c) contemporary quantitative, computer-aided data procurement, processing and phenomenological modeling, (d) functional interpretation by heuristic subsystem theories, (e) global explanation by unified theory and formalism, leading to (f) software and hardware applications of results of basic science in medicine and technology. Thus, although never yielding a "solved case", cerebellar research may, indeed, serve as a forerunner in neuroscience that represents the "state of the art" in the integration of experimental and theoretical aspects of unified brain research.

Abbreviations

CB: Cerebellum, CF: Climbing Fiber, CNS: Central Nervous System, GC: Granule Cell, IO: Inferior Olive, MF: Mossy Fiber, NC: Cerebellar Nuclear Cell, PC: Purkinje Cell

Acknowledgement. Research was supported by United Public Health Service grant NS13742 from the National Institute of Neurological and Communicative Disorders and Stroke.

References

Albert A (1972) Regression and the Moore-Penrose pseudoinverse. Academic Press, London New York

Albus J (1971) A theory of cerebellar function. Math Biosci 10:25-61

Albus JR (1981) Brains, behavior and robotics. McGraw-Hill, New York

Anderson JA, Silverstein JW, Ritz SA, Randall JA (1977) Distinctive features, categorical perception and probability learning: Some applications of a neural model. Psychol Rev 84:413-451

Arbib MA, Boylls CC, Dev P (1974) Neural models of spatial perception and the control of movement. In: Keidel WD, Handler W, Spreng M (eds) Cybernetics and bionics. Oldenbourg, Munich, pp 216-231

Armstrong DM (1974) Functional significance of connections of the inferior olive. Physiol Rev 54: 358-417

Bell CC, Grimm RJ (1969) Discharge properties of Purkinje cells recorded on single and double microelectrodes. J Neurophysiol 32:1044-1055

Ben-Israel A, Greville TNE (1980) Generalized inverses: theory and applications. Krieger Publ, New York

Bernstein NA (1947) O Postroyenii Dvizheniy (On the construction of movements). Medgiz., Moscow (English translation: The coordination and regulation of movements. Pergamon, New York 1967)

Berthoz A, Llinás R (1974) Afferent neck projection to the cat cerebellar cortex Exp Brain Res 20:385-401

Bloedel JR, Ebner TJ, Qi-Xiang Yu (1983) Increased responsiveness of Purkinje cell associated with climbing fiber inputs to neighboring neurons. J Neurophysiol 50:220-239

Bower J, Llinás R (1982) Simultaneous sampling and analysis of the activity of multiple, closely adjacent, cerebellar Purkinje cells. Soc Neurosci Abstr 8:830

Boylls CC Jr (1974) A theory of cerebellar function with applications to locomotion. PhD Thes, Stanford Univ

Boylls CC Jr (1982) Climbing fibers and the spatial reference frame for motor coordination. In: Proceedings of the workshop on visuomotor coordination in frog and toad: Models and experiments. COINS Tech Rep 82-16. Univ Mass, Amherst, pp 2-23.

Braitenberg V (1967) Is the cerebellar cortex a biological clock in the millisecond range? In: Fox CA, Snider RS (eds) Progress in brain research, vol 25. The cerebellum. Elsevier, Amsterdam, pp 334-346

Braitenberg V, Atwood RP (1958) Morphological observations in the cerebellar cortex. J Comp Neurol 109:1-34

Brindley GS (1964) The use made by the cerebellum of the information that it receives from sense organs. IBRO Bull 3:80

Calvert TW, Meno F (1972) Neural systems modelling applied to the cerebellum. IEEE Trans., vol SMC-2(3):363-374

Coburn N (1970) Vector and tensor analysis. Dover, New York

Crick FHC (1979) Thinking about the brain. Sci 241:219-232

Demer JL, Robinson DA (1982) Effects of reversible lesions and stimulation of olivocerebellar system on vestibuloocular reflex plasticity. J Neurophysiol 47:1084-1107

Dow RS (1970) Historical review of cerebellar investigation. In: Fields WS, Willis WD (eds) The cerebellum in health and disease, chap 1. Hilger, London, pp 5-38

Dow RS, Moruzzi G (1958) The physiology and pathology of the cerebellum. Univ Minnesota Press, Minneapolis

Dowling JE (1979) Information processing by local circuits: The vertebrate retina as a model system. In: Schmitt FO, Worden FG (eds) The neurosciences, IV study program. MIT Press, Cambridge, pp 163-182

Dunin-Barkovsky VL (1978) Information processing in neuronal structures. Nauka, Moscow (in Russian)

Ebner TJ, Qi-Xiang Yu, Bloedel JR (1983) Increase in Purkinje cell gain associated with naturally activated climbing fiber input. J Neurophysiol 50:205-219

Eccles JC (1969) The dynamic loop hypothesis of movement control. In: Leibovic KN (ed) Information processing in the central nervous system. Springer Berlin Heidelberg New York, pp 245-269

Eccles JC (1973) The cerebellum as a computer: Patterns in space and time. J Physiol 229: 1-32

Eccles JC (1982) The modular operation of the cerebral neocortex considered as the material basis of mental events. Neuroscience 6:1839-1856

Eccles JC, Ito M, Szentágothai J (1967) The cerebellum as a neuronal machine. Springer, Berlin Heidelberg New York

Edelmann GM (1979) Group selection and phasic reentrant signaling: A theory of higher brain function. In: Schmitt FO, Worden FG (eds) The neurosciences vol, IV: study program. MIT Press, Cambridge, pp 1115-1139

Einstein A (orig. 1916) The foundation of the general theory of relativity. In: Sommerfeld A (ed) The principle of relativity. (1952) Dover, New York, pp 111-164

Ferin M, Grigorian RA, Strata P (1971) Mossy and climbing fiber activation in the cat cerebellum by stimulation of the labyrinth. Exp Brain Res 12:1-17

Flourens P (1842) Recherches experimentales sur les proprietes et les fonctions du systeme nerveux dans les animaux vertebres, 2nd edn. Bailliere

Freeman JA (1969) The cerebellum as a timing device: An experimental study in the frog. In: Llinás R (ed) Neurobiology of cerebellar evolution and development. Am Med Assoc (Chicago) pp 397-420

Fujita M (1982) Adaptive filter model of the cerebellum. Biol Cybernet 45:195-206

Gelfand IM, Gurfinkel VS, Fomin SV, Tsetlin ML (1971) Models of the structural-functional organization of certain biological systems. MIT Press, Cambridge

Gilbert PFC (1974) A theory of memory that explains the function and structure of the cerebellum. Brain Res 70:1-18

Gilbert PFC, Thatch WT (1977) Purkinje cell activity during motor learning. Brain Res 128: 309-328

Goldberg J, Baker J, Hermann G, Peterson B (1983) Spatio-temporal convergence onto second order vestibular neurons. Abstr Soc Neurosci 9:316

Golgi C (1874) Sulla fine anatomia del cervelletto umano. Arch Ital Mal Nerv 1:90-107

Gonshor A, Melvill-Jones G (1973) Changes of human vestibulo-ocular response induced by vision-reversal during head rotation. J Physiol 234:102-103

Greene PH (1972) Problems of organization of motor system In: Rosen R, Snell FM (eds) Progr Theor Biol, vol II. Academic Press, London New York, pp 303-338

Grossberg S (1969) On learning of spatiotemporal patterns by networks with ordered sensory and motor components. 1. Excitatory components of the cerebellum. Studies Appl Math 48:105-132

Hámori J, Szentágothai J (1966) Identification under the electron microscope of climbing fiber and their synaptic contacts. Exp Brain Res 1:65-81

Hebb DO (1949) The organization of behaviour. John Wiley, New York

Hillman DE (1969) Neuronal organization of the cerebellar cortex in amphibia and reptilia. In: Llinás R (ed) Neurobiology of cerebellar evolution and development, Am Med Assoc (Chicago) pp 279-325

Hillman DE (1979) Neuronal shape parameters and substructures as a basis of neuronal form. In: Schmitt FO, Worden FG (eds) The neurosciences, IVth study program. MIT Press, Cambridge, pp 477-499

Holmes G (1939) The cerebellum in man. Brain 63:1

Houk JC (1980) Principles of system theory as applied to physiology: systems and models. In: Mountcastle VB (ed) Medical physiology, 14th edn, chapt 7. Mosby, St. Louis

Hubel DH, Wiesel T (1962) Receptive fields, binocular interaction and functional architecture in the cat's visual cortex. J Physiol 160:106-154

Ingle D, Sprague JM (1975) Sensorimotor function of the midbrain tectum. Neurosci Res Progr Bull 13 (2)

Ito M (1970) Neurophysiological aspects of the cerebellar motor control system. Int J Neurol 7: 162-176

Ito M (1974) The control mechanism of cerebellar motor system. In: Schmitt FO, Worden FG (eds) The neurosciences, IIIrd study program. MIT Press, Cambridge, pp 293-303

Ito M (1980) Experimental tests of constructive models of the cerebellum. In: Székely G, Lábos E, Damjanovich S (eds) Neural communication and control. Adv Physiol Sci, vol 30. Pergamon Press & Akadémiai Kiadó, New York

Ito M (1984) The cerebellum and neural control. Raven Press, New York

Ito M, Yoshida M, Obata K, Kawai N, Udo M (1970) Inhibitory control of intracerebellar nuclei by the Purkinje cell axons. Exp Brain Res 10:64-80

Ito M, Sakurai M, Tongroach P (1982) Climbing fibre induced depression of both mossy fibre responsiveness and glutamate sensitivity of cerebellar Purkinje cells. J Physiol 324:113-134

Kohonen T (1977) Associative memory. A system-theoretical approach. Springer, Berlin Heidelberg New York

Kornhuber HH (1971) Motor functions of cerebellum and basal ganglia: the cerebello-cortical saccadic (ballistic) clock, the cerebello-nuclear hold regulator, and the basal ganglia ramp (voluntary speed smooth movement) generator. Kybernetik 8:157-162

Lashley KS (1942) The problem of cerebral organization in vision. In: Kluever H (ed) Visual mechanisms. Biol Symp, vol VII. Jacques Cattel Press, Lancaster, pp 301-322

Levi-Civita T (1926) The absolute differential calculus (calculus of tensors) In: Persico E (ed) Dover, New York

Lisberger SG, Fuchs AF (1978) Role of primate flocculus during rapid behavioral modification of vestibuloocular reflex. I. Purkinje cell acting during visually guided horizontal smooth-pursuit eye movements and passive head rotation. J Neurophysiol 41:733-763

Llinás R (ed) (1969a) Neurobiology of cerebellar evolution and development, Am Med Assoc (Chicago)

Llinás R (1969b) Functional aspects of interneuronal evolution in the cerebellar cortex. In: Brazier MAB (ed) The interneuron. UCLA Forum Med, vol XI. Univ Cal Press, Los Angeles, pp 329-347

Llinás R (1970) Neuronal operations in cerebellar transactions. In: Schmitt FO, Worden FG (eds) The neurosciences, IInd study program. MIT Press, Cambridge, pp 409-426

Llinás R (1974) 18th Bowditch Lecture: Motor aspects of cerebellar control. Physiologist 17:19-46

Llinás R (1979) The role of calcium in neuronal function. In: Schmitt FO, Worden FG (eds) The neurociences, IVth study program. MIT Press, Cambridge, pp 555-571

Llinás R (1981) Electrophysiology of the cerebellum. In: Brooks VB (ed) Handbook of physiology, vol II. The nervous system, part II. Am Physiol Soc (Bethesda), pp 831-976

Llinás R (1983) Possible role of tremor in the organization of the nervous system. In: Capildeo Findlay, Int Neurol Symp Tremor, MacMillan, New York (in press)

Llinás R, Pellionisz A (1984) Cerebellar function and the adaptive feature of the central nervous system. In: Berthoz A, Melvill-Jones G (eds) Reviews of oculomotor research, vol I. Adaptive mechanisms in gaze control. Elsevier, Amsterdam

Llinás R, Simpson JI (1981) Cerebellar control of movement. In: Towe AL, Luschei ES (eds) Handbook of behavioral neurobiology, vol V. Motor coordination. Plenum Press, New York, pp 231-302

Llinás R, Volkind R (1973) The olivo-cerebellar system: Functional properties as revealed by harmaline-induced tremor. Exp Brain Res 18:69-87

Llinás R, Yarom Y (1981a) Electrophysiology of mammalian inferior olivary neurones in vitro. Different types of voltage-dependent ionic conductances. J Physiol 315:549-567

Llinás R, Yarom Y (1981b) Properties and distribution of ionic conductances generating electroresponsiveness of mammalian inferior olivary neurones in vitro. J Physiol 315:569-584

Llinás R, Precht w, Clarke M (1971) Cerebellar Purkinje cell responses to physiological stimulation of the vestibular system in the frog. Exp Brain Res 13:408-431

Llinás R, Walton K, Hillman DE, Sotelo C (1975) Inferior olive: Its role in motor learning. Science 190:1230-1231

Llinás R, Yarom Y, Sugimori M (1981) The isolated mammalian brain in vitro: A new technique for the analysis of the electrical activity of neuronal circuit function. Fed Proc 40:2240-2245

Loeb GE (1983) Finding common ground between robotics and physiology. Trends Neurosci 6:203-204

Maekawa K, Simpson JI (1973) Climbing fiber responses evoked in vestibulo-cerebellum of rabbit from visual system. J Neurophys 36:649-666

Magendie F (1825) Precis elementaire de physiologie. Meguiguon-Marvis (Paris): I-II.

Malsburg von C, Cowan JD (1982) Outline of a theory for the ontogenesis of iso-orientation domains in visual cortex. Biol Cybernet 45:49-56

Mann RW (1981) Cybernetic limb prosthesis. Ann Biomed Eng 9:1-43

Marr D (1969) A theory of cerebellar cortex. J Physiol 202:437-470

Marr D (1982) Vision. A computational investigation into the human representation and processing of visual information. Freeman, San Francisco

Miles FA (1980) Information processing at the cellular and systems levels in complex systems. Raven Press, New York

Mortimer JA (1970) A cellular model for mammalian cerebellar cortex. Tech Rep. Univ. Mich, Ann Arbor

Mountcastle V (1979) An organizing principle for cerebral function: The unit module and distributed system. In: Schmitt FO, Worden FG (eds) The neurosciences, IVth study program. MIT Press, Cambridge, pp 21-42

Nering ED (1963) Linear algebra and matrix theory. John Wiley, New York

Orbeli LA (1940) New notions on cerebellar functions. Usp Sovrem Biol 13:207-220

Oscarsson O (1969) The sagittal organization of the cerebellar anterior lobe as revealed by the projection patterns of the climbing fiber system. In: Llinás R (ed) Neurobiology of cerebellar evolution and development. Am Med Assoc (Chicago), pp 525-537

Oscarsson O (1973) Functional organization of spinocerebellar paths. In: Iggo A (ed) Handbook of sensory physiology, vol II. Springer, Berlin Heidelberg New York, pp 320-328

Palay SL, Chan-Palay V (1974) Cerebellar cortex: cytology and organization. Springer, Berlin Heidelberg New York

Palay SL, Chan-Palay V (eds) (1982) The cerebellum: New vistas. Springer, Berlin Heidelberg New York

Palkovits M, Magyar P, Szentágothai J (1972) Quantitative histological analysis of the cerebellar cortex in the cat: IV. Mossy fiber-Purkinje cell numerical transfer. Brain Res 45:15-29

Pellionisz A (1970) Computer simulation of the pattern transfer of large cerebellar neuronal fields. Acta Biochim Biophys Acad Sci Hung 5:71-79

Pellionisz A (1976) Proposal for shaping the dynamism of Purkinje cells by climbing fiber activation. Brain Theor Newslett 2:2-6

Pellionisz A (1979a) Cerebellar control theory. In: Lissák K (ed) Recent developments of neurobiology in Hungary, vol VIII. Akadémiai Kiadó, Budapest, pp 211-243

Pellionisz A (1979b) Modeling of neurons and neuronal networks. In: Schmitt FO, Worden FG (eds) The neurosciences, IVth study program. MIT Press, Cambridge, pp 525-550

Pellionisz A (1983a) Sensorimotor transformations of natural coordinates via neuronal networks: conceptual and formal unification of cerebellar and tectal models. In: Lara R, Arbib MA (eds) II. Workshop on visuomotor coordination in frog and toad (Mexico City, Nov 1982), COINS Tech Rep, Amherst

Pellionisz A (1983b) Brain theory: Connecting neurobiology to robotics. Tensor analysis: Utilizing intrinsic coordinates to describe, understand and engineer functional geometries of intelligent organisms. J Theor Neurobiol 2: 185-211

Pellionisz A (1984a) Coordination: A vector-matrix description of transformations of overcomplete CNS coordinates and a tensorial solution using the Moore-Penrose generalized inverse. J Theor Biol 101: (in press)

Pellionisz A (1984b) Tensorial aspects of the multidimensional approach to the vestibulo-oculomotor reflex and gaze. In: Berthoz A, Melvill-Jones G (eds) Reviews of oculomotor research, I. Adaptive mechanisms in gaze control. Elsevier, Amsterdam

Pellionisz A, Llinás R (1977) A computer model of the cerebellar Purkinje cells. Neuroscience 2: 37-48

Pellionisz A, Llinás R (1979) Brain modeling by tensor network theory and computer simulation. The cerebellum: Distributed processor for predictive coordination. Neuroscience 4:323-348

Pellionisz A, Llinás R (1980) Tensorial approach to the geometry of brain function. Cerebellar coordination via metric tensor. Neuroscience 5:1125-1136

Pellionisz A, Llinás R (1982a) Space-time representation in the brain. The cerebellum as a predictive space-time metric tensor. Neuroscience 7:2949-2970

Pellionisz A, Llinás R (1982b) Tensor theory of brain function. The cerebellum as a space-time metric. In: Arbib MA, Amari SI (eds) Competition and cooperation in neural nets. Proc US-Jpn Sem Kyoto. Lecture Notes Biomath, 45 Springer, Berlin Heidelberg New York, pp 394-417

Pellionisz A, Szentágothai J (1973) Dynamic single unit simulation of a realistic cerebellar network model. Brain Res 49:83-99

Pellionisz A, Szentágothai J (1974) Dynamic single unit simulation of a realistic cerebellar network model, II. Brain Res 68:19-40

Pellionisz A, Llinás R, Perkel D (1977) A computer model of the cerebellar cortex of the frog. Neuroscience 2:19-35

Precht W (1978) Neuronal operations in the vestibular system. Studies on brain function, vol II Springer, Berlin Heidelberg New York

Purkinje JE (1837) Bericht über die Versammlung deutscher Naturforscher und Ärzte in Prag, September 1837. 3. Sect. 5. Anat Physiol Verh, pp 177-180

Ramon y Cajal S (1911) Histologie du systeme nerveux de l'homme et des vertebres, vol 1-2. Maloine, Paris

Robinson DA (1968) The oculomotor control system: A review. Proc IEEE 56:1032-1049

Robinson DA (1975) How the oculomotor system repairs itself. Invest Ophthalmol 14:413-415

Robinson DA (1982) The use of matrices in analyzing the three-dimensional behavior of the vestibulo-ocular reflex. Biol Cybernet 46:53-66

Rolando L (1823) Experience sur les fonctions du systeme nerveux. J Physiol Exp 3:113-114

Sherrington C (1906) The integrative action of the nervous system. Scribner, New York

Simpson JI (1979) Erroneous zones of the cerebellar flocculus. Soc Neurosci Abstr 5:107

Simpson JI, Alley KE (1974) Visual climbing fiber input to rabbit vestibulo-cerebellum: A source of direction-specific information. Brain Res 82: 302-308

Simpson JI, Graf W, Leonard C (1981) The coordinate system of visual climbing fibers to the flocculus. In: Fuchs A, Becker WS (eds) Progress in oculomotor research. Elsevier/North Holland Biomedical Press, Amsterdam, pp 475-484

Smolyaninov VA (1971) Some special features of organization of the cerebellar cortex. In: Gelfand IM, Gurfinkel VS, Fomin SV, Tsetlin, ML (eds) Models of the structural-functional organization of certain biological systems. MIT Press, Cambridge, pp 251-325

Sotelo C, Llinás R, Baker R (1974) Structural study of inferior olivary nucleus of the morphological correlates of electrotonic oupling. J Neurophys 37:541-559

Sparks DL, Pollack JG (1977) The neural control of saccadic eye movements: the role of the superior colliculus. In: Brooks BA, Bajandas FJ (eds) Eye movements. Plenum Press, New York, pp 179-219

Synge JL, Schild A (1949) Tensor calculus. Dover, New York

Székely G (1973) Anatomy and synaptology of the tectum opticum. In: Jung R (ed) Handbook of sensory physiology, ud. VII. Springer, Berlin Heidelberg New York, pp 27-101

Szentágothai J (1963) Ujabb adatok a synapsis functionális anatómiájahoz. Magyar Tud Akad Biol Orv Oszt Közl 6:217-227

Szentágothai J (1968) Structuro-functional considerations of the cerebellar neuron network. Proc IEEE 56:960-968

Szentágothai J, Rajkovits KS (1959) Über den Ursprung der Kletterfasern des Kleinhirns. Z Anat Entwicklungsgesch 121:130-141

Towe AI, Luschei ES (eds) (1981) Handbook of behavioral neurobiology, vol V: Motor coordination. Plenum Press, New York

Voogd J, Bigare F (1980) Topographical distribution of olivary and cortico-nuclear fibers in the cerebellum. A review. In: Courville J, Montigny de C, Lamarre Y (eds) The inferior olivary nucleus. Anatomy and physiology. Raven Press, New York, pp 207-234

Willis T (1664) Cerebri anatomae; Cui accessit nervorum descriptio et usus. Schagen, Amsterdam

Inferior Olive: Functional Aspects

P. STRATA[1]

1 Introduction

The inferior olive nucleus is the source of climbing fibers to the cerebellar cortex (Szentágothai and Rajkovits 1959; Batini et al. 1976; Courville and Faraco-Cantin 1978; Montarolo et al. 1980; Campbell and Armstrong 1983). Much work has so far been devoted to understand its functional role in cerebellar operation and in motor control (see Armstrong 1974; 1978; Courville et al. 1980; Brooks and Thach 1981; Llinás 1981; Strata 1984). However, this problem is far from being solved. Several hypotheses have been proposed to explain the function of the climbing fiber input (see Thach 1980; Brooks and Thach 1981). I'm not going to review all of them here, but focus my attention on two theories which have been considered recently for experimental investigation in our laboratory.

2 The Trophic Theory

According to this theory the climbing fiber input is essential to maintain the Purkinje cells in their normal functional state. Morphological investigations have revealed that following an inferior olive lesion there is a remarkable remodelling of the Purkinje cell dendritic tree (Hámori 1973, 1981; Sotelo et al. 1975; Bradley and Berry 1976; Desclin and Colin 1980). These observations suggest a role of the climbing fibers in the mechanisms of plasticity. Desclin and Colin (1980) have described, however, additional morphological changes in the Purkinje cells following an inferior olive lesion by means of 3-acetylpyridine. A small amount of less than 1% of these cells degenerate after 4-6 weeks from the lesion. More interesting are the observations made in the Purkinje cell terminals. They were mainly of two types. (1) A swelling of the cisternae of the endoplasmic reticulum, giving rise in extreme cases to huge vacuoles. These alterations were prominent for several days in every second synaptic bulb and subsided gradually, but never disappeared even after six months. (2) A change in the pattern of distribution of the synaptic vesicles with a reduction in their number and size. This picture was prominent in the first four days from the lesion with a gradual recovery. Some alterations, however, were still present after three months. The morphological changes observed in the Purkinje cell terminals have been interpreted by the authors not to be of degenera-

---

[1] Istituto di Fisiologia Umana dell'Università, Corso Raffaello 30, 10125 Torino, Italy

Cerebellar Functions
ed. by Bloedel et al.
© Springer-Verlag Berlin Heidelberg 1984

tive nature, but rather the consequence of the hyperactivity observed at electrophysio-logical level (Colin et al. 1980).

From a functional point of view, it has been shown that following a lesion to the inferior olive, the Purkinje cell inhibitory action on the target neurons is strongly re-duced (Dufossé et al. 1978; Ito et al. 1978, 1979; Ito 1979). No such effect is observed, however, when the inferior olive electrical activity is selectively blocked by local appli-cation of tetrodotoxin (Ito et al. 1979). Therefore, the trophic action would be exerted by a substance carried along the olivocerebellar neuron by the axonal transport. The presence of these morphological and functional changes has suggested that the inferior olive exerts an important trophic action on the Purkinje cell. By this mechanism, the climbing fiber input may be able to induce long-term changes, which are the basis for the learning processes in the cerebellar cortex (Marr 1969; Albus 1971; Gilbert 1974; Ito 1982).

A series of experiments has been planned in our laboratory in order to better un-derstand the mechanisms of the possible climbing fiber trophic action. However, while we could detect a variety of morphological changes in the axons and synaptic terminals of early and long-term deafferented Purkinje cells (Rossi and Cantino 1984), we failed to confirm the basic experiment of a strong reduction of Purkinje cell inhibition follow-ing inferior olive lesions (Montarolo et al. 1981b).

2.1 Morphological Observations

As far as the morphological experiments are concerned, an attempt has been made to see whether alterations of Purkinje cell terminals, similar to those described by Desclin and Colin (1980), were present also when the inferior olive was destroyed in the rat by electrocoagulation, in order to exclude possible unspecific effects of the 3-acetylpyri-dine. Present observations on the cerebellar nuclei up to three months after the lesion showed in the Purkinje cells an early increase of the endoplasmic reticulum in preterm-inal segments and axon terminals, as well as the appearance of large vesicles and vacuo-les in axon terminals. These changes affect an increasing number of axons from 7 to 30 days after the lesion. In this period axon terminals exhibiting clusters of small vesicles and devoid of normal synaptic vesicles, as observed by Desclin and Colin (1980), appear. In addition, large membrane whorls become a prominent feature in a considerable number of synaptic terminals. At the end of the first month following an inferior olive le-sion, a large number of axon terminals filled with mitochondria, multivesicular bodies, and autophagic vacuoles including synaptic vesicles and endoplasmic reticulum could be detected (Rossi and Cantino 1984).

2.2 Electrophysiological Experiments

The electrophysiological experiments have been performed in Wistar rats, whose infer-ior olive was destroyed by means of 3-acetylpyridine (Desclin and Escubi 1974) three days to six months previously. A single electrical stimulus applied to the cerebellar cor-tex was effective in decreasing the spontaneous firing, for at least 20 ms, in 50.9% (27 out of 53 tested units) of the Deiters neurons, antidromically activated from the spinal cord. When the experiments were performed in intact rats, we have obtained similar re-

Table 1. Comparison of the number of Deiters neurons inhibited by cerebellar stimulation in intact (control) and lesioned rats. (Montarolo et al. 1981b)

	Control	Lesioned
Rats	3	5
Tested units inhibited (%)	43 23 (53.4)	64 34 (53.1)
Antidromically act. inhibited (%)	42 22 (52.3)	53 27 (50.9)

sults. The number of Deiters neurons inhibited by cerebellar stimulation was 52.3% (22 out of 42 tested units). Table 1 shows the results obtained on Deiters neurons identified either by spinal cord stimulation or by histological localization of the recording point.

In the same series of experiments, we have also shown that cerebellar stimulation is effective in depressing both the antidromic unitary activity and the antidromic field potential evoked in Deiters neurons by spinal cord stimulation. In addition, cerebellar stimulation was able to suppress the unitary orthodromic activity evoked in the Deiters neurons by vestibular nerve stimulation (Montarolo et al. 1981b).

In conclusion, our experiments show that the Purkinje cells maintain their ability to inhibit their target neurons also when they are deprived of their climbing fiber input. It is difficult to explain the discrepancy between our results and those by Ito et al. (1978), since the experiments were performed in similar conditions. However, some comments will follow in the discussion (Sect. 4).

In a further series of experiments, we have attempted to show whether a possible trophic action was exerted by the olivocerebellar pathway on other neurons of the cerebellar cortex. It is known that basket and Golgi cells receive collaterals of the climbing fiber input (Hámori and Szentágothai 1966; Eccles et al. 1967a; Chan-Palay and Palay 1971; Bloedel 1973; Palay and Chan-Palay 1974, Brodal 1981). The experiments were aimed at observing the size and the time course of the basket and Golgi cell inhibition in rats, following a lesion to the inferior olive. The basket cell inhibition was measured by the reduction in amplitude of the antidromic field (N_1 wave) elicited in the cerebellar cortex by stimulation of the underlying white matter, following parallel fiber stimulation (Eccles et al. 1966a). The Golgi cell inhibition, on the other hand, was measured by the reduction in the amplitude of the orthodromic positive field (P_2 wave) evoked in the granular layer by mossy fiber stimulation, following the activation of the Golgi cells by stimulation of the parallel fibers, either directly or through transfolial stimulation (Eccles et al. 1966b, 1967b). In both these types of experiments there was no significant reduction in the inhibitory properties of basket and Golgi cells, following a permanent inferior olive lesion performed by means of 3-acetylpyridine (Montarolo and Strata, unpublished observations, reported in Strata 1984).

On the basis of the experiments performed in our laboratory, we can state that in rats with a permanent lesion to the inferior olive, all three types of corticocerebellar neurons innervated by the olivocerebellar pathway maintain their full capability to inhibit their target neurons. On the other hand, it has been recently reported that in tissue

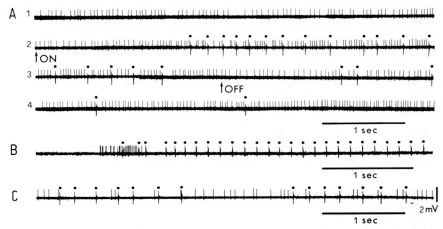

Fig. 1 A-C. Activation of Purkinje cells by caloric stimulation of the labyrinth. Complex spikes are marked with *dots*. A_1 to A_4 are continuous records. Warm Ringer at 52°C has been applied to the *left* labyrinth between the two *arrows (ON-OFF* period); **B** shows a different unit. Warm Ringer at 50°C has been applied to the *right* labyrinth starting 11 s before the appearance of the first complex spike and for a duration of 8 s. The complex spikes fire very regularly at about 8/s, with no simple spikes. In **C** another unit recorded after stimulation of the right labyrinth with warm Ringer at 52° C. When the complex spikes appear, the simple spikes are clearly suppressed. (Ferin et al. 1971)

cultures, the Purkinje cells can form functional inhibitory synapses on their target neurons, though in absence of climbing fibers (Marshall et al. 1980). In line with the hypothesis of Desclin and Colin (1980), the morphological alterations in the Purkinje cell terminals, observed also when the inferior olive is destroyed by electrocoagulation, are not to be considered as degenerative in nature, but likely the consequence of a cell hyperactivity.

3 The Tonic Theory

One of the most peculiar properties of the climbing fiber input is to fire at a rather low rate. At rest, the Purkinje cell activity due to the climbing fiber input, the so-called complex spike, has a discharge frequency near 1/s and during intense activation of peripheral receptors, it may reach at most 8/s (Ferin et al. 1971; see Strata 1976). In physiological conditions, slightly lower maximal values have been reported during motor phenomena of the sleep-waking cycle (Marchesi and Strata 1971) or during the performance of novel motor tasks (Gilbert and Thach 1977).

By observing the spontaneous firing of a Purkinje cell, one can see that after each complex spike there is a silence, which sometimes is followed by a short-lasting increased probability of firing, before the simple spikes reach again the control value. The olivocerebellar neurons, therefore, are able to induce in the Purkinje cells sequences of excitations and inhibitions. It has therefore been suggested that the climbing fiber input is a phasic system (Llinás et al. 1969). A support to this hypothesis is provided by studying the tremor induced by harmaline. Following injection of this drug, the complex spike activity may reach a frequency of 8/s, while a muscle tremor develops simultaneously at the same frequency (Lamarre and Mercier 1971; Lamarre and Weiss 1973; Llinás and Volkind 1973). These observations have suggested that climbing fibers have phasic properties by being able to trigger phasic motor activities. The concept of a phasic role of the climbing fiber input has been recently well supported by a series of papers by Bloedel and collaborators (see Bloedel this volume and Gilman et al. 1981).

The possibility that the olivocerebellar pathway may perform a tonic function has been suggested by Marchesi and Strata (1970, 1971). The idea was based on experiments where it was shown that complex spikes had a maintained higher average discharge frequency during the periods of paradoxical sleep with no phasic phenomena. Following caloric and galvanic stimulation of the labyrinth, it was shown that in most Purkinje cells the increase in complex spike firing rate is accompanied by a simple spike depression and viceversa (Ferin et al. 1970, 1971). In principle, a repetitive activation of the climbing fiber input could lead to a prolonged suppression of the simple spikes, whereas a suppression of the complex spike activity could lead to a prolonged release of the simple spike activity. Figure 1 shows the effect of caloric stimulation of the labyrinth on a Purkinje cell. A sequence of complex spikes (A_2 and C) tends to depress the activity of the simple spikes (Ferin et al. 1970, 1971). A reciprocal behavior in the simple and complex spike activity has been often observed (Ghelarducci et al. 1975; Gilbert and Thach 1977; Barmack 1979; Leonard and Simpson 1982). However, in all these experiments, it is not always easy to establish if the opposite behavior of the complex and simple spike activity is due only to a depressant effect of the climbing fibers or it is also due to opposite effects exerted on the two afferent channels to the cerebellar cortex by the same external or internal stimulus. To solve this problem it is necessary to inactivate selectively the inferior olive activity and to observe if there is any change in the spontaneous discharge of the simple spikes.

Before reporting on these results, it has to be mentioned that a tonic depression of the simple spike activity, consequent to an increased firing rate of the inferior olive neurons, has been postulated by Barmack and Simpson (1980). This problem will be discussed later (see Sect. 4).

3.1 Effect of Inferior Olive Inactivation on the Purkinje Cell Activity

Colin et al. (1980) were the first to investigate this problem. They performed a bilateral lesion of the inferior olive by means of 3-acetylpyridine and observed an increase in the background noise in the cerebellar cortex. In one Purkinje cell, they were able to see that at the time the Purkinje cell complex spike irreversibly disappeared, the simple spike frequency suddenly doubled for several minutes and was then maintained, although at a lower level, for the rest of the recording period of one hour. Repetitive stimulation of the still excitable inferior olive axons, showed in many units that the appearance of the evoked spikes had a prolonged depressant effect on the simple spike firing. The latter effect is also present with intact inferior olive stimulation (Rawson and Tilokskulchai 1981, 1982). Such a depressant effect has been attributed to the direct effect of the climbing fiber on the Purkinje cell. However, an action exerted through climbing fiber collaterals to corticocerebellar interneurons or to brain stem nuclei cannot be excluded.

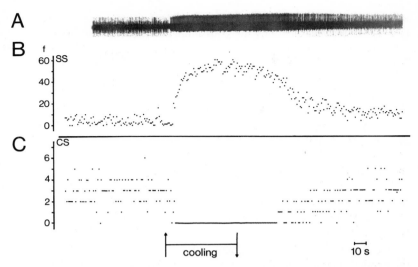

Fig. 2. A-C. Effect of cooling the left inferior olive on the Purkinje cell activity of the cerebellar cortex of the right side. **A** specimen of Purkinje cell activity. Simple spikes have a mainly upward (negative) direction and complex spikes a mainly downward direction; **B** the frequency *(f)* of the simple spikes has been counted every second on a specimen recorded at more expanded time base; **C** similar counts for the complex spikes. Period of cooling is indicated by the horizontal bar. (Montarolo et al. 1982)

The same problem has been studied also in our laboratory by using a different experimental approach. We have reversibly inactivated the inferior olive by applying a cooling probe to the ventral surface of the medulla (Montarolo et al. 1981a, 1982). The experiments were performed under barbiturate anaesthesia. Our main finding is presented in Fig. 2 which illustrates the effect of a reversible cooling of the left inferior olive on the Purkinje cell activity of the contralateral side. The frequency of the complex spikes decreases and they disappear in a few seconds. At the same time, one observes a remarkable increase of the simple spike frequency, which reaches a plateau level in about 10 s. Shortly after the end of the cooling, the simple spike activity gradually decreases together with the reappearance of the complex spikes. Both simple and complex spikes return to the control value.

The most remarkable fact of our experiments is that the above described increase in the simple spike frequency was a consistent phenomenon observed in all the Purkinje cells which showed a disappearance of the complex spikes. The average simple spike frequency of 22 Purkinje cells before inferior olive cooling was 28.02/s (± 13.7 SD). Following the disappearance of the complex spike, the frequency reached an average value of 57.62/s (± 11.9 SD).

That the observed effect is due specifically to inferior olive inactivation is shown by the following two experiments. (1) Two Purkinje cells were simultaneously recorded from each cerebellar hemicortex. Following cooling of the left inferior olive, only the Purkinje cell of the right side, where the complex spikes disappeared, showed the increase in simple spike frequency. (2) In a group of rats, the inferior olive was chronically destroyed by means of 3-acetylpyridine some weeks or months before. The resting simple spike discharge of the Purkinje cells showed a frequency similar to the intact rats (see later). However, cooling the same bulbar area at the level of the destroyed inferior olive was not followed by any significant variation in the simple spike discharge of the Purkinje cells in the contralateral side. These experiments show that the olivocerebellar pathway exerts a *tonic* inhibitory effect on the Purkinje cell activity. This inhibition may be due to the following mechanisms.

1. Each complex spike is accompanied by a prolonged increase of a calcium dependent potassium permeability (Llinás and Sugimori 1980a, b). A maintained complex spike discharge may be able to keep tonically activated this potassium permeability with the consequence of tonically decreasing the probability of simple spike firing.

2. It has been shown that calcium ions enter the Purkinje cell during the complex spike (Llinás and Sugimori 1980a, b) and that climbing fiber activity is associated with a decrease of calcium concentration in the Purkinje cell environment (Stöckle and ten Bruggencate 1980). A change in calcium concentration is likely present also during complex spike suppression and may influence both the synaptic transmission between the parallel fiber and the Purkinje cell and the excitability of the latter neurons.

3. The olivocerebellar neurons, in addition to a direct projection to the Purkinje cells, have collaterals which excite the corticocerebellar inhibitory interneurons — basket and Golgi cells. The Purkinje cells, therefore, receive both a direct excitation and an indirect inhibition from the inferior olive (Eccles et al. 1967a; Murphy and Sabah 1971; Bloedel and Roberts 1971; Latham and Paul 1971; Burg and Rubia 1972; Rubia et al. 1974). A maintained activity of the climbing fiber input is able to keep a tonic background activation of these interneurons and therefore a tonic inhibition on the Purkinje cells (Montarolo et al. 1982).

In conclusion, the inferior olive appears to be not only a structure capable of generating patterns of phasic excitation-inhibition sequences, but also a pathway which exerts a remarkable *tonic* inhibitory action on Purkinje cells.

The question is now how long does the simple spike frequency increase due to complex spike suppression last? In the experiments by Colin et al. (1980) the lesion to the inferior olive was irreversible, but an answer can be derived only for one unit recorded for 60 min. In this unit, the increase was present for the entire period of recording. In the experiments by Montarolo et al. (1982), the inferior olive was reversibly inactivated for durations up to 90 s. A careful answer to this question has been given by Benedetti et al. (1983a, 1984; see also this volume). Shortly, they have performed permanent lesions to the inferior olive by means of 3-acetylpyridine, by cryocoagulation and by electrocoagulation. The simple spike frequency was doubled during the first few days after the lesion. Then, there was a gradual recovery which was complete at the end of the first month.

A further question was addressed to the possibility for the simple spike frequency increase to be present only in the experimental conditions of barbiturate anesthesia. If so, the tonic theory would have little significance in cerebellar operation. It is known that GABA is the chemical transmitter of both basket and Golgi cells in the cerebellar cortex (Bisti et al. 1971). On the other hand, barbiturates enhance GABAergic inhibition (see Olsen 1982). Therefore, it is possible that under such an anesthesia there is an enhanced inhibitory tone exerted on the Purkinje cells by the corticocerebellar inter-neurons. Savio and Tempia (1983a, b; see also this volume) have shown that, although smaller, the tonic inhibition exerted on the Purkinje cells by the olivocerebellar path-way is significantly present also in unanesthetized rat and also under urethane anes-thesia, which is not known to affect GABAergic transmission. This fact suggests that such a tonic inhibition plays an important role also in physiological conditions.

3.2 Effect of Inferior Olive Inactivation on the Intracerebellar and Lateral Vestibular Nuclei

Granted that inferior olive inactivation leads consistently to an increased discharge rate of the Purkinje cells, it was interesting to investigate the behavior of the Purkinje cell target neurons in the intracerebellar and lateral vestibular nuclei (Benedetti et al. 1982, 1983b).

The average resting discharge of 20 cells recorded from fastigial and interpositus nuclei was 20.7/s (± 4.0 SD). Cooling of the contralateral inferior olive resulted in a complete suppression of activity in 17 out of 20 tested units.

In the Deiters neurons, the average resting discharge rate of 14 units was 11.7 (± 8.7 SD), whereas inferior olive cooling resulted in a complete suppression of the discharge in all units. In some units, cooling of the inferior olive suppressed also the unitary antidromic activity elicited in Deiters neurons by spinal cord stimulation. Such a suppression showed the same time course of the effect on the spontaneous ac-tivity and it has been attributed to a strong hyperpolarization of the Deiters unit, due mainly to the increased inhibitory drive from the Purkinje cells, but also to the suppres-sion of the excitatory drive exerted by the collaterals of the olivocerebellar fibers.

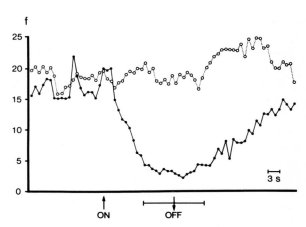

Fig. 3. A comparison between the activity of the neurons recorded from the intracerebellar and Deiters nuclei in intact (●) rats and (○) in rats whose inferior olive has been destroyed previously by 3-acetylpyridine. Each circle indicates the average frequency *(f)* of firing counted every second for all the units of the intact (thirty four units) and of the lesioned (thirty four units) rats which had a spontaneous discharge. In each unit the frequency computation started 20 s before the cool-ing. Cooling time varied from 7 to 40 s in different units. Its mean duration is indicated by the *downward arrow* and the standard deviation by the *horizontal line*. (Benedetti et al. 1983b)

A summary of the behavior of the 34 units recorded in the intracerebellar and Deiters nuclei in relation to cooling is displayed in Fig. 3 (filled circles). In another group of rats, the inferior olive was destroyed bilaterally some weeks before by means of 3-acetylpyridine. The average rate of discharge has now recovered and become similar to that of the intact rats, but cooling of the same bulbar region does not lead to any significant depression of activity in another set of 34 units (empty circles). This means that the difference in the pattern of response of the two groups of units is attributable to a specific effect of cooling of the inferior olive. A decreased activity of the neurons of the intracerebellar nuclei has been confirmed when the inferior olive was destroyed by means of 3-acetylpyridine (Bardin et al. 1982).

These experimental data suggest that the olivocerebellar pathway exerts an important tonic control on the excitability not only of the Purkinje cells, but also of their target neurons. Therefore, it is likely that also the postural activity and any information processed by subcerebellar structures is under the tonic control of the inferior olive. A support to this view is given in the next section.

3.3 Effect of Inactivation of the Inferior Olive on the Postural Activity

Although the proposal for a role of the inferior olive in control of postural activity was made by Marchesi and Strata (1970, 1971), more direct evidence was provided by Boylls (1978, 1980). He showed that repetitive stimulation of that area of the inferior olive which projects to zone A of the anterior lobe (Groenewegen and Voogd 1977) is able to increase or decrease the "tonic" activity levels within muscles for periods up to many tens of seconds.

The effect of inferior olive inactivation on postural activity was studied more recently (Batini et al. 1983, see also this volume). In intercollicular decerebrate cat with a well developed extensor tonus of the forelimb muscles, cooling of the caudal region of the left inferior olive resulted in a decrease of the electromyographic activity of the triceps muscle of the right forelimb, usually with no effect on the triceps of the right side. Following systemic administration of harmaline a well known tremor develops bilaterally. Cooling of the inferior olive of one side was very effective in suppressing the tremor with the associated postural activity only in the contralateral triceps.

A permanent lesion performed on the inferior olive of one side by means of kainic acid in the rat produced a clear-cut hypotonia on the contralateral side (Diana and Di Chiara, personal communication). This result has been confirmed in our laboratory (Rabacchi, Rocca, Rossi and Strata, unpublished observations).

It should be mentioned, however, that in other experiments where a unilateral kainic lesion of the inferior olive has been performed in intact cats, the animal developed a clear hypertonia in the contralateral limb (Pompeiano et al. 1981).

3.4 Inactivation of the Inferior Olive and the Metabolic Activity of the Cerebellar Nuclei

Batini et al. (1981) have shown that in rats with an irreversible bilateral lesion of the inferior olive performed by means of 3-acetylpyridine, there was an increased deoxyglucose uptake at the level of the intracerebellar and lateral vestibular nuclei. The increase was present up to one month from the time of the lesion. According to the trophic theory (see Section 2) this fact might be taken as evidence of a loss of inhibitory properties by the Purkinje cells and therefore as due to an increased electrical activity of the intracerebellar and Deiters nuclei.

We have therefore determined the deoxyglucose uptake at the level of the intracerebellar nuclei following inferior olive inactivation by cooling. In this condition, there is an increased activity of the Purkinje cell axons (Montarolo et al. 1982) and a remarkable depression of the cell activity of the intracerebellar nuclear cells (Benedetti et al. 1983b). Since the inferior olive inactivation lasted 45 min there is no time for a possible loss of inhibitory capabilities by the Purkinje cells (see Ito et al. 1979). The result was again an increased metabolic activity at the level of the intracerebellar nuclei (Batini et al. 1982, 1984). It is thus possible to reach the conclusion that the observed increase of metabolic activity is attributable to the presynaptic component of the nuclei, made by the Purkinje axon terminals and by the likely increase in metabolic activity required to maintain the intracellular chloride concentration below resting potential through a chloride pump (Lux 1971).

4 Discussion

Our findings will now be discussed in relation to the interpretation given to several experimental data reported in the literature. In some cases, they provide a direct experimental support to the given explanation, whereas in other instances they offer a different interpretation.

4.1 The Tonic Theory in Motor Control

Barmack and Simpson (1980) have observed a conjugate drift of the eyes toward the side contralateral to the lesion applied on the inferior olive of one side. On the basis of the results obtained by recording from and stimulating the dorsal cap of the inferior olive (Barmack and Hess 1980a, b) and by recording from Purkinje cells (Barmack 1979), they have given the following interpretation of their results: a lesion to the dorsal cap of the right inferior olive induces a net increase of discharge of the Purkinje cells of the left flocculus. Such an increase is then responsible for the depression of activity of the neurons of the medial vestibular nuclei of the left side. This depression has the effect of inducing a leftward drift of the eyes. Our experiments on the depression of activity of the Purkinje cell target neurons following inferior olive inactivation (Benedetti et al. 1983b), provide direct evidence for this explanation.

There is also evidence that an inferior olive lesion gives rise to a symptomatology which is similar to that due to cerebellectomy (Wilson and Magoun 1945, Carrea et al. 1947; Murphy and O'Leary 1971). Such similarity is in line with our experiments (Benedetti et al. 1983b). In fact, while cerebellectomy removes any influence of the cerebellar output, inferior olive lesion induces a silence in the cerebellar output, except for the fact that long axoned Purkinje cells are hyperactive.

It has been demonstrated that in cat and monkey a lesion to the inferior olive induces motor disabilities which are very similar to those due to lesion of the intracerebellar nuclei (Soechting et al. 1976; Kennedy et al. 1982). This similarity can now be explained with a tonic depression of the neurons of the intracerebellar nuclei following inferior olive inactivation (Montarolo et al. 1983b).

4.2 The Problem of the Plasticity

In the last decade several experimental evidences have suggested that the cerebellum is important for the adaptive modifications which occur in motor learning or in the phenomena of plasticity during the recovery from lesions. The inferior olive seems to play a basic role in these mechanisms (Ito 1979, 1982; Haddad et al. 1980; Harvey 1980; Llinás 1981; Andersen 1982; Demer and Robinson 1982; Ito et al. 1982). Among the supporting evidences, it is very attractive to speculate that one of the functions of the inferior olive is to exert a trophic action on the Purkinje cells by a substance carried along the neuron through the axonic transport (Ito et al. 1979). In principle, this substance could induce, in the postsynaptic neuron, long-term changes responsible for the phenomena of plasticity. However, we have seen above that the morphological changes observed in the Purkinje cells following climbing fiber deprivation cannot be taken as a sufficient proof in favor of the trophic theory, but they are likely the consequence of Purkinje cell hyperactivity. On the other hand, from a functional point of view, our experiments could not confirm the experiment of a loss or a significant reduction of the inhibitory properties of the Purkinje cells after an inferior olive lesion. However, in this respect, some considerations may help to understand the discrepancies.

1. First of all, it is possible that the apparent lack of Purkinje cell inhibition reported in the experiments of Ito et al. (1978) is due to the differences between intact and lesioned rats, specially when particular parameters of stimulation are used. In fact, in intact animals, stimulation of the cerebellar cortex, in addition to activating directly the Purkinje cells, activates also the climbing fiber terminals. Since the latter have several branches to different Purkinje cells, the same stimulus, particularly when weak, may result to irradiate more widely in intact than in the lesioned rats and to stimulate indirectly many more Purkinje cells. This explanation, however, seems to apply only to those experiments in which the Purkinje cell inhibition has been tested on the spontaneous firing or on the activity evoked in the Deiters neurons from the spinal cord or from the periphery (Dufossé et al. 1978; Ito et al. 1978, 1979; Montarolo et al. 1981b).

2. The same explanation does not apply, however, when the size of the monosynaptic inhibitory postsynaptic potential in Deiters neurons is measured following cerebellar cortex stimulation. In this case, the size is due only to the direct activation of the Purkinje neurons and not to indirect activation through climbing fiber terminals. Ito et al. (1978) have shown that the occurrence of an inhibitory postsynaptic potential in Deiters neurons following cerebellar stimulation is much smaller in the lesioned rat, compared to the intact one. In addition, also the size of this inhibitory potential is significantly smaller. This change has been taken as evidence of a loss or markedly reduced inhibitory properties by the Purkinje cell.

A different interpretation, however, may be given on the basis of the results reported in Sections 3.1 and 3.2. We have seen that following the suppression of the climbing fiber activity, the frequency of the simple spikes in the Purkinje cells undergoes a remarkable increase (Colin et al. 1980; Montarolo et al. 1981a, 1982), which lasts up to one month (Benedetti et al. 1983a, 1984). During this period of increased Purkinje cell activity the Deiters neurons are tonically hyperpolarized, as shown by their decreased spontaneous activity (Benedetti et al. 1982, 1983b). It is therefore likely that cerebellar stimulation may add little phasic inhibition to the background tonic inhibition already present in the Deiters neurons (Strata and Montarolo 1982; Strata 1984).

A more moderate loss of inhibition by the Purkinje cell, following climbing fiber deprivation, has been recently found, when a higher intensity of stimulation is applied to the cerebellum (Karachot and Ito 1984). In this condition, 30-38 days after the inferior olive lesion, the occurrence of the monosynaptic inhibitory postsynaptic potentials in Deiters neurons, following cerebellar white matter stimulation, was the same in the lesioned rat, compared to the intact one. However, the size of the inhibitory potentials was reduced by about 50%. According to this new finding, following climbing fiber deprivation, the Purkinje cell inhibitory properties are not totally or markedly reduced, but moderately affected (Karachot and Ito 1984).

The question remains open, however, whether the reduction of the inhibitory capability of the Purkinje cell shown by Karachot and Ito (1984), is due to a lack of a trophic action exerted by the climbing fibers or rather the consequence of the intense hyperactivity presented by the cell for over a month (Benedetti et al. 1984).

The trophic theory has also been invoked (Ito 1982) to explain the reduction in the gain of the horizontal vestibuloocular reflex, following inferior olive lesion in the rabbit (Ito and Miyashita 1975). Such a decrease was originally unexpected. As shown in Fig. 4, it has been assumed that in zone II of the flocculus, where there are the Purkinje cells related to the horizontal eye movements, the climbing fiber input is influenced by the visual and not by the vestibular input (Ghelarducci et al. 1975). Therefore, a lesion to the inferior olive should have been without any effect on the vestibuloocular reflex in dark. The actual decrease was thus later explained as due to the loss of inhibition by the Purkinje cells deprived of their climbing fibers. It should be here recalled that Purkinje neurons, during the vestibuloocular reflex, have an enhancing effect on the medial vestibular neurons, since, although they are inhibitory, they fire out of phase in respect to head rotation.

Fig. 4. A simplified scheme of vestibular and optic projections to zone II of the flocculus, according to Ito (1982). *VIII* vestibular nerve; *II* optic nerve; *Gr* granule cell; *MF* mossy fiber; *PC* Purkinje cell; *CF* climbing fiber; *IO* inferior olive; *MVN* medial vestibular nucleus; *M* ocular motoneuron

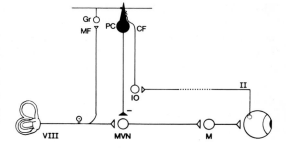

By contrast, a different interpretation for this experiment by Ito and Miyashita (1975) is offered by our findings, not only because they don't support the trophic theory. According to the tonic theory it is likely that when the inferior olive is destroyed, the hyperactivity of the Purkinje cells exerts a tonic depression of the medial vestibular neurons, with the consequence of reducing the gain of the vestibuloocular reflex.

The tonic theory may also be taken into account for the interpretation of some experiments on the role of the inferior olive and learning. It is still a matter of debate whether the cerebellar cortex is a site of learning (Ito et al. 1982) or whether the learning occurs at precerebellar level and appropriate informations are carried to the Purkinje cells through functional changes in the olivocerebellar fibers (see also Precht et al. this volume.

It has been proposed by Llinás et al. (1975) that learning occurs in the inferior olive itself. These authors have argued that if the learning is stored in the cerebellar cortex as a modification of the synapse made by the parallel fibers on the Purkinje cell, the removal of the inferior olive should abolish a new learning, but should not modify the learning already stored in the cerebellar cortex. In line with this view, Demer and Robinson (1982) have reversibly inactivated the inferior olive by means of a local anesthetic. They found that during the inactivation time, the adaptive modifications of the vestibuloocular reflex acquired by wearing visual reversing or magnifying lenses are no longer present. The conclusion was thus drawn that the plastic phenomena were not stored in the cerebellar cortex, but at precerebellar level.

Our experiments don't allow this conclusion. According to the tonic theory, inactivation of the inferior olive induces an increased firing in the Purkinje cells and a decreased firing in their target neurons. It is therefore unlikely that in the presence of such remarkable functional modifications, the animal is able to maintain the vestibuloocular reflex gain acquired during the adaptive modifications. The site of the learning process cannot be determined with this type of experiment.

On the other hand, though our experiments are not aimed at solving this problem, they suggest that the olivocerebellar pathway may be suited to carry a learning stored at precerebellar level. It is proposed by some investigators that the participation of the cerebellar cortex in learning may involve a modification in the processing of information at the level of the synapse between the parallel fiber and the Purkinje cell. In addition to assuming a change in the intrinsic property of this synapse (Ito et al. 1982), it is possible that a functionally maintained change of excitability may be induced by the climbing fibers. This input could in principle perform the latter function simply by changing its tonic firing rate. In other words, a learning stored at precerebellar level may be carried to the Purkinje cells by changing the complex spike firing and therefore by changing the performance of the cerebellar cortex.

Acknowledgement. Financial support for the experiments was provided by grants of Ministry of Education and of the Italian CNR. I thank Dr. R. Llinás for his helpful comments.

References

Albus JS (1971) A theory of cerebellar function. Math Biosci 10: 25-61

Andersen P (1982) Cerebellar synaptic plasticity – putting theories to the test. Trends Neurosci 5: 324-325

Armstrong DM (1974) Functional significance of connections of the inferior olive. Physiol Rev 54: 358-417

Armstrong DM (1978) The mammalian cerebellum and its contribution to movement control. Int Rev Physiol Neurophysiol 17: 239-294

Bardin JM, Batini C, Billard JM (1982) Disfacilitation cérébelleuse après destruction pharmacologique de l'olive inferieure. C R Acad Sci (Paris) 295: 391-393

Barmack NH (1979) Immediate and sustained influence of visual olivocerebellar activity on eye movement. In: Talbot RE, Humphrey DR (eds) Posture and movement: perspective for integrating sensory and motor research on the mammalian nervous system. Raven Press, New York, pp 123-168

Barmack NH, Hess DT (1980a) Multiple-unit activity evoked in dorsal cap of inferior olive of the rabbit by visual stimulation. J Neurophysiol 43: 151-163

Barmack NH, Hess DT (1980b) Eye movements evoked by microstimulation of dorsal cap of inferior olive in the rabbit. J Neurophysiol 43: 165-181

Barmack NH, Simpson JI (1980) Effects of microlesions of dorsal cap of inferior olive of rabbits on optokinetic and vestibuloocular reflexes. J Neurophysiol 43: 182-206

Batini C, Corvisier J, Destombes J, Gioanni H, Everett J (1976) The climbing fibers of the cerebellar cortex, their origin and pathways in cat. Exp Brain Res 26: 407-422

Batini C, Buisseret-Delmas C, Conrath-Verrier M, Corvaja N (1981) The effect of harmaline and 3-acetylpyridine on the olivo-cerebellar-nuclear system in rats studied with ^{14}C 2-deoxyglucose. In: Szentágothai J, Hámori J, Palkovits M (eds) Regulatory functions of CNS subsystems. Adv Physiol Sci, vol II. Pergamon Press & Akadémiai Kiadõ, Budapest, pp 145-149

Batini C, Benedetti F, Buisseret-Delmas C, Montarolo PG, Strata P (1982) Effect of local cooling of the inferior olive on the metabolic activity at the intracerebellar nuclei. Neurosci Lett Suppl 10: S61

Batini C, Bernard JF, Montarolo PG, Strata P (1983) The olivocerebellar pathway exerts a tonic control on the postural activity. Neurosci Lett Suppl 14: S20

Batini C, Benedetti F, Buisseret-Delmas C, Montarolo PG, Strata P (1984) Metabolic activity of intracerebellar nuclei in the rat: effects of inferior olive inactivation. Exp Brain Res 54: 259-265

Benedetti F, Montarolo PG, Strata P, Tempia F (1982) Effects of reversible inferior olive inactivation on the activity of cerebellar and vestibular nuclei. Neurosci Lett Suppl 10: S70

Benedetti F, Montarolo PG, Rabacchi S, Savio T (1983a) Long term functional changes in the Purkinje cell to climbing fibre deprivation. Neurosci Lett Suppl 14: S24

Benedetti F, Montarolo PG, Strata P, Tempia F (1983b) Inferior olive inactivation decreases the excitability of the intracerebellar and lateral vestibular nuclei in the rat. J Physiol 340: 195-208

Benedetti F, Montarolo PG, Rabacchi S (1984) Inferior olive lesion induces long-lasting functional modifications in the Purkinje cells. Exp Brain Res 55: 368-371

Bisti S, Iosif G, Marchesi GF, Strata P (1971) Pharmacological properties of the inhibitions in the cerebellar cortex. Exp Brain Res 14: 24-37

Bloedel JR (1973) Cerebellar afferent systems: a review. Prog Neurobiol 2: 1-68

Bloedel JR, Roberts WJ (1971) Action of climbing fibers in cerebellar cortex of the cat. J Neurophysiol 34: 17-31

Boylls CC (1978) Prolonged alterations of muscle activity induced in locomoting premamillary cats by microstimulation of the inferior olive. Brain Res 159: 445-450

Boylls CC (1980) Contributions to locomotor coordination of an olivo-cerebellar projection to the vermis in the cat: experimental results and theoretical proposals. In: Courville J, de Montigny C, Lamarre Y (eds) The inferior olivary nucleus: anatomy and physiology. Raven Press, New York, pp 321-348

Bradley PM, Berry M (1976) Quantitative effects of climbing fibre deafferentation on the adult Purkinje cell dendritic tree. Brain Res 112: 133-140

Brodal A (1981) Neurological anatomy in relation to clinical medicine. Oxford Univ Press, New York, Oxford

Brooks VB, Thach WT (1981) Cerebellar control of posture and movement. In: Brookhart JM, Mountcastle VB (eds) Handbook of physiology, section 1: The nervous system, vol II: Motor control. Am Physiol Soc (Bethesda), pp 877-946

Burg D, Rubia FJ (1972) Inhibition of cerebellar Purkinje cells by climbing fiber input. Pflüger's Arch 337: 367-372

Campbell NC, Armstrong DM (1983) The olivocerebellar projection in the rat: an autoradiographic study. Brain Res 275: 215-223

Carrea RME, Reissig M, Mettler FA (1947) The climbing fibres of the simian and feline cerebellum. Experimental inquiry into their origin by lesions of the inferior olive and deep cerebellar nuclei. J Comp Neurol 87: 321-365

Chan-Palay V, Palay SL (1971) Tendril and glomerular collaterals of climbing fibers in a granular layer of the rat's cerebellar cortex. Z Anat Entwicklungsgesch 133: 247-273

Colin F, Manil J, Desclin JC (1980) The olivocerebellar system. Delayed and slow inhibitory effects: an overlooked salient feature of the cerebellar climbing fibers. Brain Res 187: 3-27

Courville JL, Faraco-Cantin F (1978) On the origin of the climbing fibers of the cerebellum. An experimental study in the cat with an autoradiographic tracing method. Neuroscience 3: 797-809

Courville JL, Montigny de C, Lamarre Y (eds) (1980) The inferior olivary nucleus: anatomy and physiology. Raven Press, New York

Demer JL, Robinson DA (1982) Effects of reversible lesions and stimulation of olivocerebellar system on vestibuloocular reflex plasticity. J Neurophysiol 47: 1084-1107

Desclin JC, Colin F (1980) The olivocerebellar system. II. Some ultrastructural correlates of inferior olive destruction in the rat. Brain Res 187: 29-46

Desclin J, Escubi J (1974) Effects of 3-acetylpyridine on the central nervous system of the rat, as demonstrated by silver methods. Brain Res 77: 349-364

Dufossé M, Ito M, Miyashita Y (1978) Diminution and reversal of eye movements induced by local stimulation of rabbit cerebellar flocculus after partial destruction of the inferior olive. Exp Brain Res 33: 139-141

Eccles JC, Llinás R, Sasaki K (1966a) The action of antidromic impulses on the cerebellar Purkinje cells. J Physiol 182: 316-345

Eccles JC, Llinás R, Sasaki K (1966b) The mossy fibre-granule cell relay in the cerebellum and its inhibition by Golgi cells. Exp Brain Res 1: 82-101

Eccles JC, Ito M, Szentágothai J (1967a) The cerebellum as a neuronal machine. Springer, Berlin Heidelberg New York

Eccles JC, Sasaki K, Strata P (1967b) A comparison of the inhibitory actions of Golgi cells and of basket cells. Exp Brain Res 3: 81-94

Ferin M, Grigorian RA, Strata P (1970) Purkinje cell activation by stimulation of the labyrinth. Pflüger's Arch 321: 253-258

Ferin M, Grigorian RA, Strata P (1971) Mossy and climbing fiber activation in the cat cerebellum by stimulation of the labyrinth. Exp Brain Res 12: 1-71

Ghelarducci B, Ito M, Yagi N (1975) Impulse discharges from flocculus Purkinje cells of alert rabbit during visual stimulation combined with horizontal head rotation. Brain Res 87: 66-72

Gilbert PFC (1974) A theory of memory that explains the function and structure of the cerebellum. Brain Res 70: 1-18

Gilbert PFC, Thach WT (1977) Purkinje cell activity during motor learning. Brain Res 128: 309-328

Gilman S, Bloedel JR, Lechtenberg R (1981) Disorders of the cerebellum. Davis, Philadelphia

Groenewegen HI, Voogd J (1977) The parasagittal zonation within the olivocerebellar projection. 1. Climbing fiber distribution in the vermis of cat cerebellum. J Comp Neurol 174: 417-488

Haddad GM, Demer JL, Robinson DA (1980) The effect of lesion of the dorsal cap of the inferior olive on the vestibulo-ocular and optokinetic systems of the cat. Brain Res 185: 265-275

Hámori J (1973) Developmental morphology of dendritic postsynaptic specializations. Rec Dev Neurobiol Hung 5: 9-32

Hámori J (1981) Development of synaptic circuitry in the cerebellar cortex: role of mossy and climbing afferents. In: Szentágothai J, Hámori J, Palkovits M (eds) Regulatory functions of CNS subsystem. Adv Physiol Sci, vol II. Pergamon Press & Akadémiai Kiadö, Budapest, pp 117-131

Hámori J, Szentágothai J (1966) Identification under the electron microscope of climbing fibers and their synaptic contacts. Exp Brain Res 1: 65-81

Harvey R (1980) Cerebellar regulation in movement control. Trends Neurosci 3: 281-284

Ito M (1979) Is the cerebellum really a computer? Trends Neurosci 2: 122-126

Ito M (1982) Cerebellar control of the vestibulo-ocular reflex − around the flocculus hypothesis. Annu Rev Neurosci 5: 275-296

Ito M, Miyashita Y (1975) The effects of chronic destruction of the inferior olive upon visual modification of the horizontal vestibulo-ocular reflex of rabbits. Proc Jpn Acad 51: 716-720

Ito M, Orlov I, Shimoyama I (1978) Reduction of the cerebellar stimulus effect on rat Deiters neurones after chemical destruction of the inferior olive. Exp Brain Res 33: 143-145

Ito M, Nisimaru N, Shibuki K (1979) Destruction of inferior olive induces rapid depression in synaptic action of cerebellar Purkinje cells. Nature (London) 277: 568-569

Ito M, Sakurai M, Tongroach P (1982) Climbing fibre induced depression of both mossy fibre responsiveness and glutamate sensitivity of cerebellar Purkinje cells. J Physiol 324: 113-134

Karachot L, Ito M (1984) Confirmation of the remote depressant action of the 3-acetylpyridine deafferentation of climbing fibers on Purkinje cell inhibition of Deiters neurons. Neurosci Lett Suppl 17: 70

Kennedy PR, Ross H-G, Brooks VB (1982) Participation of the principal olivary nucleus in neocerebellar motor control. Exp Brain Res 47: 95-104

Lamarre Y, Mercier LA (1971) Neurophysiological studies of harmaline induced tremor in the cat. Can J Physiol Pharmacol 49: 1049-1058

Lamarre Y, Weiss M (1973) Harmaline-induced rhythmic activity of alpha and gamma motoneurones in the cat. Brain Res 63: 430-434

Latham A, Paul DH (1971) Spontaneous activity of Purkinje cells and responses to impulses in climbing fibres. J Physiol 213: 135-156

Leonard CS, Simpson JI (1982) Effects of suspending climbing fiber activity on the discharge patterns of floccular Purkinje cells. Soc Neurosci Abstr 8: 830

Llinás R (1981) Electrophysiology of the cerebellar networks. In: Brookhart JM, Mountcastle VB (eds) Handbook of physiology. Sect 1: The nervous system, vol II: Motor control. Am Physiol Soc (Bethesda), pp 831-876

Llinás R, Sugimori M (1980a) Electrophysiological properties of in vitro Purkinje cell somata in mammalian cerebellar slices. J Physiol 305: 171-195

Llinás R, Sugimori M (1980b) Electrophysiological properties of in vitro Purkinje cell dendrites in mammalian cerebellar slices. J Physiol 305: 197-213

Llinás R, Volkind RA (1973) The olivo-cerebellar system: functional properties as revealed by harmaline-induced tremor. Exp Brain Res 18: 69-87

Llinás R, Bloedel JR, Hillman DE (1969) Functional characterization of neuronal circuitry of frog cerebellar cortex. J Neurophysiol 32: 847-870

Llinás R, Walton K, Hillman DE, Sotelo C (1975) Inferior olive: its role in motor learning. Science 190: 1230-1231

Lux HD (1971) Ammonium and chloride extrusion: hyperpolarizing synaptic inhibition in spinal motoneurones. Science 173: 555-557

Marchesi GF, Strata P (1970) Climbing fibers of cat cerebellum: modulation of activity during sleep. Brain Res 17: 145-148

Marchesi GF, Strata P (1971) Mossy and climbing fiber activity during phasic and tonic phenomena of sleep. Pflüger's Arch 323: 219-240

Marr DA (1969) A theory of cerebellar cortex. J Physiol 202: 437-470

Marshall KC, Wojtowicz JM, Hendelman WJ (1980) Patterns of functional synaptic connections in organized cultures of cerebellum. Neuroscience 5: 1847-1857

Montarolo PG, Raschi F, Strata P (1980) On the origin of the climbing fibres of the cerebellar cortex. Pflüger's Arch 383: 136-142

Montarolo PG, Palestini M, Strata P (1981a) Effects of inferior olive cooling on the Purkinje cell activity. Neurosci Lett Suppl 7: S120

Montarolo PG, Raschi F, Strata P (1981b) Are the climbing fibres essential for the Purkinje cell inhibitory action? Exp Brain Res 42: 215-218

Montarolo PG, Palestini M, Strata P (1982) The inhibitory effect of the olivocerebellar input on the cerebellar Purkinje cells in the rat. J Physiol 332: 187-202

Murphy MG, O'Leary JL (1971) Neurological deficit in cats with lesions of the olivocerebellar system. Arch Neurol 24: 145-157

Murphy JT, Sabah NH (1971) Cerebellar Purkinje cell responses to afferent inputs. I. Climbing fiber activation. Brain Res 25: 449-467

Olsen RW (1982) Drug interactions at the GABA receptor-ionophore complex. Annu Rev Pharmacol Toxicol 22: 245-277

Palay SL, Chan-Palay V (1974) Cerebellar cortex: cytology and organization. Springer, Berlin Heidelberg New York

Pompeiano O, Santarcangelo E, Stampacchia G, Srivastava UC (1981) Changes in posture and reflex movements due to kainic acid lesions of the inferior olive. Arch Ital Biol 119: 279-313

Rawson JA, Tilokskulchai K (1981) Suppression of simple spike discharges of cerebellar Purkinje cells by impulses in climbing fibre afferents. Neurosci Lett 25: 125-130

Rawson JA, Tilokskulchai K (1982) Climbing fibre modification of cerebellar Purkinje cell responses to parallel fibre inputs. Brain Res 237: 492-497

Rossi F, Cantino D (1984) Ultrastructural changes in the cerebellar nuclei following electrolytic destruction of the inferior olivary nucleus. Neurosci Lett Suppl 18: S381

Rubia FJ, Höppener U, Langhof H (1974) Lateral inhibition of Purkinje cells through climbing fiber afferents. Brain Res 70: 153-156

Savio T, Tempia F (1983a) The inhibitory effect of the olivocerebellar fibres on the cerebellar Purkinje cells in the rat under urethane anaesthesia. Neurosci Lett Suppl 14: S327

Savio T, Tempia F (1983b) Inibizione tonica della via olivocerebellare sulle cellule di Purkinje nel ratto sveglio o sotto anestesia da uretano. Boll Soc Ital Biol Sperim 59: 9-18

Soechting J, Ranish, N, Palminteri R, Terzuolo C (1976) Changes in a motor pattern following cerebellar and olivary lesions in the squirrel monkey. Brain Res 105: 21-44

Sotelo C, Hillman DE, Zamora AJ, Llinás R (1975) Climbing fiber deafferentation: its action on Purkinje cell dendritic spines. Brain Res 98: 574-581

Stöckle H, Bruggencate ten G (1980) Fluctuation of extracellular potassium and calcium in the cerebellar cortex related to climbing fiber activity. Neuroscience 5: 893-901

Strata P (1976) A general review of the physiological function of the neuronal machine in the cerebellar cortex. Exp Brain Res Suppl 1: 103-112

Strata P (1984) Recent aspects on the function of the inferior olive. Exp Brain Res Suppl (in press)

Strata P, Montarolo PG (1982) Functional aspects of the inferior olive. Arch Ital Biol 120: 321-329

Szentágothai J, Rajkovits U (1959) Ueber den Ursprung der Kletterfasern des Kleinhirns. Z Anat Entwicklungsgesch 121: 130-141

Thach WT (1980) Complex spikes, the inferior olive, and natural behavior. In: Courville J, Montigny de C, Lamarre Y (eds) The inferior olivary nucleus: anatomy and physiology. Raven Press, New York, pp 349-360

Wilson WC, Magoun HW (1945) The functional significance of the inferior olive in the cat. J Comp Neurol 83: 69-77

Climbing Fiber Function: Regulation of Purkinje Cell Responsiveness

J.R. BLOEDEL[1] and T.J. EBNER[2]

1 Introduction

Since the intriguing theoretical paper by Marr (1969) on cerebellar cortical function, considerable attention has been directed towards the climbing fiber afferent system's role in motor learning. According to this hypothesis (see also Gilbert (1975) and Albus (1971)), climbing fiber afferent input produces a persistent modification in the strength of the parallel fiber synapses on Purkinje cell dendrites. Subsequently it was proposed that this mechanism mediated the adaptation of the vestibuloocular reflex (VOR) gain (Ito 1972, 1979, Ito and Mijshita 1975, Robinson 1976). Supporting experiments showed that the inhibitory action of Purkinje cells on vestibular neurons was dependent on the integrity of the olivocerebellar system (Ito et al. 1978, 1979). Since these initial observations there has been considerable controversy concerning the role of the climbing fiber system in modifying the plasticity of the VOR (Miles et al. 1980, Demer and Robinson 1982, Lisberger 1982) and the efficacy of Purkinje cell action on their target neurons (Montarolo et al. 1981, Benedetti et al. 1983).

Other views of the function of the climbing fiber system emphasized its role in ongoing real time processing in the cerebellar cortex without requiring that the climbing fiber afferents modify a Purkinje cell's response to mossy fiber inputs. In the 1960's and 1970's several hypotheses consistent with this concept were expressed. One hypothesis postulated that the climbing and mossy fiber systems use the same circuitry under different functional conditions (Llinas and Volkind, 1973). Another argued that the climbing fibers act by producing a "readout" of Purkinje cell excitability modulated by the mossy fiber-parallel fiber system (Eccles et al. 1967). Others theorized that the climbing fiber input stabilizes the cerebellar cortical circuitry (Bloedel and Roberts 1971).

Our studies were designed to examine the hypothesis that the climbing fiber system affects real time processing occurring in the cerebellar cortex, not by some independent effect on the cerebellar cortical output, but by producing a nonpersistent modification in the responsiveness of Purkinje cells to mossy fiber inputs. To evaluate this hypothesis a paradigm was sought which did not require the activation of climbing fiber inputs by electrical stimulation of either the inferior olive or the cerebellar white matter. This restriction was adopted for two reasons. First, electrical stimulation can activate mossy fiber inputs particularly within the cerebellar white matter. Secondly, electrical stimulation in either site is likely to activate a functionally inappropriate spatial pattern of

[1] Barrow Neurological Institute St. Joseph's Hospital and Medical Center 350 West Thomas Rd. Phoenix, Arizona 85013 USA
[2] Depts. of Neurosurgery and Physiology University of Minnesota, Minneapolis, MN 55455, USA

Cerebellar Functions
ed. by Bloedel et al.
© Springer-Verlag Berlin Heidelberg 1984

climbing fiber inputs to the cerebellar cortex. Electrical stimulation would activate a distribution of climbing fiber inputs based only on the distribution of stimulus current within the inferior olive. In contrast the distribution of naturally activated climbing fibers would reflect the spatial and temporal properties of neuronal interactions occurring within the nucleus. Therefore methods were devised to examine changes in the responsiveness of Purkinje cells to mossy fiber inputs using either spontaneous climbing fiber inputs or climbing fiber inputs evoked by natural peripheral stimuli.

2 Methods and Results

These experiments were carried out primarily in decerebrate, unanesthetized cats. However, most of the results obtained from data based on single Purkinje cells have been duplicated in awake unanesthetized animals. The details of the surgical preparation of the cerebellar cortex and recording techniques have been presented elsewhere (Ebner and Bloedel 1981a, Ebner et al. 1983).

Three stimulation-recording paradigms were employed in these studies. The initial experiments examined the change in the responsiveness of Purkinje cells to mossy fiber inputs activated at various times following the occurrence of a spontaneous climbing fiber input to the same Purkinje cell. In this paradigm the spontaneous simple and complex spike activity of a Purkinje cell are discriminated separately. The discrimination pulse triggered by the complex spike is used to trigger the application of a forepaw stimulus at specified delays following the occurrence of the complex spike. The discriminated complex spike is also used to trigger the poststimulus time histogram (PSTH) of the cell's simple spike response to the forepaw stimulus. The forepaw stimulus consists of a 1-3 mm dorsiflexion of the wrist joint produced by a tap to the dorsum of the forepaw. Complex spike histograms were also constructed to determine if any changes in simple spike responsiveness were related to the activation of climbing fiber inputs by the forepaw stimulus. In these experiments the Purkinje cells chosen for study exhibited minimal or no complex spike response to the peripheral stimulus.

An example of the results obtained with this initial climbing fiber conditioning paradigm is illustrated in Fig. 1. In A the forepaw stimulus was applied 300 ms following the occurrence of complex spikes in this Purkinje cell. The response consisted of a small initial decrease in impulse activity followed by a more marked increase in discharge rate. When the forepaw stimulus was timed to occur 30 ms following the spontaneous climbing fiber input (B), the amplitude of the excitatory component of the cell's response increased. The amplitude of the excitatory component returned to control values when the forepaw stimulus was again applied 300 ms following the spontaneous climbing fiber input to the neuron (C). In other cells an accentuation of inhibitory simple spike responses was observed. The time course of the increased responsiveness for both excitatory and inhibitory responses was generally about 100 ms, and usually did not persist longer than 200-300 ms (Ebner and Bloedel 1981a). Only a low percentage of cells (Ebner and Bloedel 1981a) demonstrated a persistent increased responsiveness in the control histograms constructed after the climbing fiber conditioning was discontinued. Simply stated, the interaction generally consisted of a short-lasting enhancement of an existing simple spike response component, independent of whether the response could

Fig. 1 A-C. The increased amplitude of a Purkinje cell's simple spike response evoked by a forepaw stimulus applied at short intervals following the occurrence of spontaneous climbing fiber inputs to the neuron. **A** The simple spike response of the Purkinje cell to a forepaw stimulus applied 300 ms following the occurrence of spontaneous climbing fiber inputs to the same neuron; **B** The increase in the excitatory component of the simple spike response evoked by a forepaw stimulus applied 30 ms after spontaneous climbing fiber inputs; **C** Return of the amplitude of the response to near control levels when the forepaw stimulus was again applied at an interval of 300 ms after spontaneous climbing fiber inputs. (Ebner and Bloedel, 1981a, with permission)

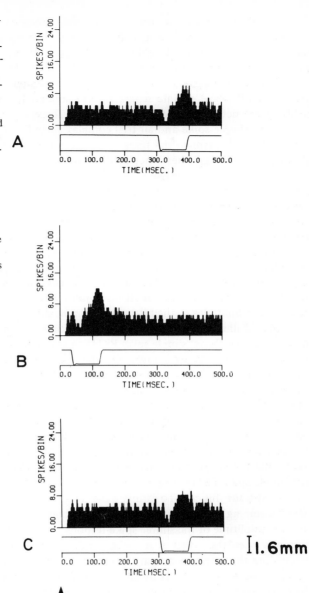

be characterized as inhibitory or excitatory. These results lead to the hypothesis that the climbing fiber activity produces a change in the gain of Purkinje cell responses to mossy fiber inputs, a concept referred to as the gain change hypothesis.

In order to argue that this increased responsiveness is important to information processing within the cerebellar cortex it was felt necessary to demonstrate a comparable accentuation of simple spike responses by climbing fiber inputs evoked by peripheral stimuli. This objective led to the development of a second methodology, the separation technique. As in the other method the simple and complex spike activity of the isolated Purkinje cell are separately discriminated, and simple and complex spike PSTHs constructed to the forepaw stimulus. These two histograms are referred to as the all trial simple spike and all trial complex spike histograms, respectively (C and D, Fig. 2). In this paradigm the forepaw stimulus is not coupled to the occurrence of a spontaneous climbing fiber input to the Purkinje cell but is applied randomly relative to this event. Based on a visual inspection of the complex spike post-stimulus time histogram, a time window is designated delimiting the period of the complex spike response (arrows below the base-line, Fig. 2). The data is then processed off line, and the original trials are separated into two groups from which two simple spike histograms are constructed. One histogram, the climbing fiber trial simple spike PSTH (B), is constructed from those trials in which a complex spike was evoked within the predetermined time window. The second simple spike histogram (nonclimbing fiber trial SS-PSTH) consists of those trials in which a complex spike was not evoked by the peripheral stimulus (A). The amplitude of all histograms was normalized to the number of trials, making the amplitudes of the histograms comparable.

Figure 2 illustrates the results from a Purkinje cell using the separation technique. In D and E the all trial simple spike PSTH and all trial climbing fiber PSTH are shown, respectively. The forepaw stimulus illustrated at the bottom evoked a small increase in the simple spike discharge of this neuron (D). Similarly an increased complex spike discharge was evoked by the stimulus (C), the arrows in C representing the time window chosen for the separation analysis. Comparing the climbing fiber (B) and nonclimbing fiber (A) trial simple spike PSTHs reveals that the amplitude of the excitatory response was greater in those trials in which the climbing fiber input was evoked.

To quantify the response amplitudes in the different conditions the bins encompassing the simple spike response were determined visually from the nonclimbing fiber trial simple spike PSTH. The vertical lines in A and B denote the first and last bin of the response for this cell. To estimate the relative change in the response amplitudes in the nonclimbing fiber trial SS-PSTH and the climbing fiber trial SS-PSTH histograms, first the amplitude of the simple spike response in A and B, demarcated by the vertical lines, was calculated relative to background. The gain change ratio, R, was calculated by dividing the response amplitude (present increase relative to background) in the climbing fiber trial SS-PSTH by the response amplitude in the nonclimbing fiber trial SS-PSTH, expressing this ratio as a percentage. In this cell the gain change ratio was 201%, indicating the simple spike discharge rate evoked by the peripheral stimulus was twice as great in those trials in which the peripheral stimulus also evoked a climbing fiber input. To illustrate that the excitability change in B was coupled to the time of occurrence of the climbing fiber input evoked by the peripheral stimulus, the climbing fiber trial aligned SS-PSTH (E) was calculated. In this PSTH the simple spikes in each trial were aligned on the occurrence of the complex spike. The bin chosen for the alignment was the first bin of the complex spike response window (arrow in E). The increased discharge rate was clearly associated with the time of occurrence of the climbing fiber input to this neuron.

Fig. 2 A-E. The use of the separation technique to demonstrate the accentuation of an excitatory response in trials in which the peripheral stimulus evoked a climbing fiber input to the Purkinje cell. The forepaw stimulus *(bottom)* evoked a small amplitude excitatory response across all of the trials **(D). C** is the complex spike histogram across the same trials. When the trials were sorted based on the occurrence of the complex spike response of the forepaw stimulus, the amplitude of the excitatory response was clearly larger in those trials in which the complex spikes were evoked **(B)** than in trials in which no climbing fiber input was activated **(A).** In **E** all trials were aligned on the time of occurrence of the climbing fiber input *(arrow)* evoked by the peripheral stimulus. R_E is the gain change ratio of this excitatory component. The number of trials from which each histogram is constructed is shown above each record in this and all successive figures. (Ebner et al. 1983, with permission)

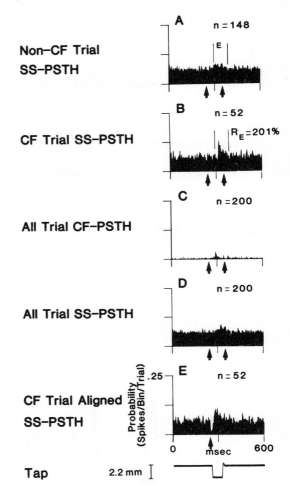

As observed in the climbing fiber conditioning paradigm both excitatory and inhibitory response components are accentuated by evoked climbing fiber inputs. This is illustrated in Fig. 3 for a Purkinje cell in which the peripheral stimulus evoked an initial increase followed by a decrease in simple spike activity (D). Gain change ratios were calculated separately for the excitatory (R_E) and inhibitory (R_I) response components. In the climbing fiber SS-PSTH the amplitudes of both the excitatory (R_E = 363%) and inhibitory response (R_I = 186%) were accentuated. The gain change ratios for inhibitory responses were calculated in a manner identical to the excitatory responses. Response amplitudes in both the nonclimbing fiber and the climbing fiber trial simple spike PSTH were calculated as percent decrease relative to background. The ratio of these response amplitudes were then used to calculate the gain change ratio. The climbing fiber trial aligned SS-PSTH (E) illustrates that both the enhanced excitatory as well as the inhibitory response components were temporally related to the occurrence of the evoked complex spikes.

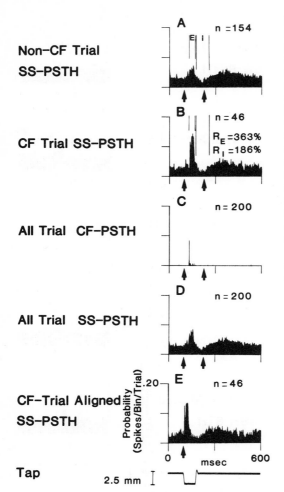

Fig. 3 A-E. Accentuation of both an excitatory and inhibitory response component in the same Purkinje cell. In this cell the forepaw stimulus evoked a very consistent complex spike response **(C)** and a simple spike response consisting of an initial increase followed by a decrease in impulse activity **(D)**. In those trials in which a complex spike was evoked by the peripheral stimulus **(B)** there was clearly an accentuation of both the excitatory and inhibitory component of the response when compared with the same response components in the non-climbing fiber trial SS-PSTH **(A)**. The response aligned on the occurrence of the climbing fiber inputs activated by the stimulus is shown in **E**. R_E and R_I refer to the gain change ratios for the excitatory *(E)* and inhibitory *(I)* response components, respectively. (Ebner et al. 1983, with permission)

The separation technique showed that both excitatory as well as inhibitory response components are enhanced in those trials in which the peripheral stimulus evokes concomitant climbing fiber input. Furthermore, the simple spike responses are time locked to the occurrence of the climbing fiber input to the Purkinje cell. Thus these data are consistent with the gain change hypothesis, indicating that an increased responsiveness of Purkinje cells can occur in association with climbing fiber inputs evoked by peripheral stimuli.

In an additional series of experiments the separation technique was used to study the relationship between the occurrence of a climbing fiber input to one Purkinje cell and the change in responsiveness of a neighboring neuron. In these studies two or three Purkinje cells were recorded simultaneously in the surface folium. Data shown in Fig. 4 were obtained from two neurons located 270 microns apart medial to the paravermal vein in lobule Vc. The results of separating the simple spike responses of cell 1 based on the evoked complex spikes of the same cell is shown in A-E. As in Fig. 3 the trials from which the all trial SS-PSTH (D) were constructed were separated based on whether

Fig. 4 A-J. Increase in the amplitude of simple spike responses in two Purkinje cells related to the occurrence of the climbing fiber input to one of the neurons. In this experiment the simple spike responses of cell 1 **(A-E)** and cell 2 **(F-J)** were sorted based on the occurrence of the climbing fiber input to cell 1. The complex spike responses of cell 1 are shown in **C** and **H**, and the simple spike responses of the two cells across all trials are shown in **D** and **I**. A comparison of the nonclimbing fiber *SS-PSTH* **(A)** and the climbing fiber trial *SS-PSTH* **(B)** indicates that the inhibitory response evoked in cell 1 by the peripheral stimulus is clearly greater (R_I = 789%) in those trials in which its climbing fiber input was evoked. Furthermore this inhibitory response was time locked to the occurrence of the climbing fiber input **(E)**. In F and G the simple spike responses of cell 2 were separated based on the activation of the climbing fiber input to cell 1.

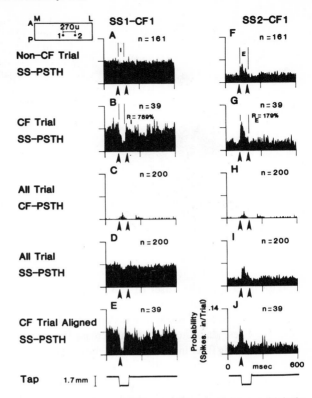

Notice that this neuron's excitatory response was enhanced **(G)** across the same trials in which the inhibitory response of cell 1 was enhanced **(B)**. Although the excitatory response of cell 2 was related to the occurrence of the climbing fiber input of cell 1 **(J)**, it was initiated slightly before the climbing fiber input to the neighboring neuron occurred. (Bloedel et al. 1983, with permission)

(B) or not **(A)** the peripheral stimulus evoked a concomitant complex spike in cell 1 within the time window shown by the two arrows in A-C. A small reduction in simple spike activity was evoked across all trials (D). The separation analysis reveals the inhibitory response was much greater when a complex spike was evoked (R_I = 798%).

In F-J the simple spike responses of the other neuron of the pair, cell 2, were sorted based on the occurrence of the same climbing fiber inputs, those activating cell 1. In contrast to cell 1, Purkinje cell 2 responded to the peripheral stimulus with an increase in simple spike activity (I). A comparison of F and G indicates the simple spike response of cell 2 was greater in those trials in which the climbing fiber input to cell 1 was evoked. Thus climbing fiber input to one Purkinje cell can be associated with an increase in the inhibitory response of the same neuron as well as an excitatory response of a neighboring cell. For both cell 1 and cell 2 an existing response component was enhanced (see Bloedel et al. 1983).

An examination of the climbing fiber aligned histogram of cell 2 in Fig. 4 reveals one additional feature. The excitatory response of this cell, although temporally coupled to the climbing fiber input to cell 1 (J), is initiated before the complex spike re-

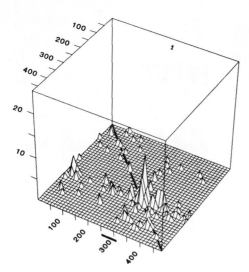

Fig. 5. Generalized cross-correlation function (GCCF) of the climbing fiber inputs to two neighboring Purkinje cells responding to a peripheral stimulus. The time course is indicated by the *heavy bar* below the time axis. (Bloedel et al. 1983, with permission)

sponse of cell 1. The onset of the excitatory response in J occurs before the arrow indicating the time of the complex spike. In contrast the inhibitory response of cell 1 is time locked to and follows the occurrence of the climbing fiber input to the same neuron (E). These data imply that an increased responsiveness in one cell can be associated with a climbing fiber input to an adjacent neuron even if that input occurs slightly after the onset of the simple spike response.

These observations prompted the hypothesis that the climbing fiber input evoked in neighboring neurons by the peripheral stimulus may be correlated although not necessarily synchronous. This possibility was examined using a generalized cross correlation analysis, as described by Ebner and Bloedel (1981b). This correlation analysis permitted examination of the correlation in two cell's complex discharge during the forepaw stimulus. The cross correlogram of the complex spike activity for one pair of neurons is shown in Fig. 5. The origin of the correlogram is at the rear left corner, and the bar below the time axis indicates the time course of the forepaw displacement. The higher peaks indicate a positive correlation between the climbing fiber inputs to cell 1 and to cell 2 evoked by the peripheral stimulus. Since the larger peaks representing the correlation occur slightly off of the diagonal (striped line) the two climbing fiber inputs, although highly correlated, were not evoked synchronously.

Before a general discussion of these findings, data obtained using a third method will be presented. This approach was developed to demonstrate that the interactions responsible for the increased responsiveness of Purkinje cells occur within the cerebellar cortex. In the initial conditioning paradigm (Fig. 1), the forepaw stimulus was timed to the occurrence of spontaneous climbing fiber inputs to a Purkinje cell. In this set of experiments a cerebellar surface stimulus which activated the parallel fiber input to the neuron was timed to occur at a set delay following spontaneous climbing fiber inputs to a Purkinje cell. The complex spike was also used to trigger the construction of the poststimulus time histograms as well as to determine the timing of the surface stimulus. Using this technique, it was possible to examine the change in a Purkinje cell's responsiveness to a surface stimulus applied at various intervals following a spontaneous climb-

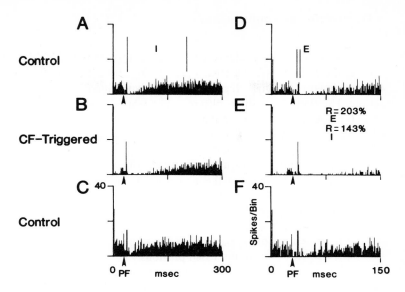

Fig. 6 A-F. The increased response of a Purkinje cell to a parallel fiber volley at short time intervals following the occurrence of spontaneous climbing fiber inputs to the same Purkinje cell. In this neuron the surface stimulus evoked a short-lasting excitatory response followed by a decreased impulse activity (**A** and **D**). When the response of the surface stimulus was conditioned at a short interval following the occurrence of spontaneous climbing fiber inputs to this neuron (**B** and **E**) both response components were enhanced. After the period of conditioning both response components returned to near control amplitudes (**C** and **F**)

ing fiber input to the cell. In these experiments the recording electrode was localized to a region of the cerebellar cortex in which the parallel fiber volley activated by the surface stimulus could be recorded. Purkinje cells were isolated in the surface folium below the parallel fiber volley.

One of these experiments is shown in Fig. 6. In the control trials the surface stimulus evoked a brief excitatory simple spike response followed by a longer decrease in the discharge rate (A and D) of this Purkinje cell. In B and E the surface stimulus was applied 30 ms following the occurrence of a spontaneous climbing fiber input to the Purkinje cell. Both the brief excitatory and subsequent inhibitory simple spike response components increased with the climbing fiber conditioning. The gain change ratio for the inhibitory component, R_I, was 143% and for the excitatory component, R_E, was 203%. A similar enhancement of response components evoked by surface stimuli was observed in 76% of the neurons tested. As has been the case for most neurons studied, the response amplitudes returned to near control values when the surface stimulus was no longer temporally coupled to the climbing fiber input (C and F).

There are many similarities between the increased simple spike responsiveness to the surface and peripheral stimuli applied following spontaneous climbing fiber inputs. In both paradigms excitatory as well as inhibitory response components are enhanced, and the interaction can be described as a short lasting increase in the amplitude of an existing response component. The surface stimulation studies support the hypothesis that the interactions responsible for the enhanced responsiveness of Purkinje cells by climbing fiber inputs occur within the cerebellar cortex.

3 Discussion and Implications

Two features of these findings are particularly pertinent to present hypotheses concerning the climbing fiber system's role in the cerebellar cortex: (1) the nature of the interaction with Purkinje cell simple spike activity, and (2) the time course of the interaction. The data from three different but related paradigms support the hypotheses that climbing fiber afferent input increases the responsiveness of Purkinje cells to mossy fiber inputs. This increased responsiveness consists primarily of an enhancement of existing simple spike responses and not merely an excitability change evoked by the climbing fiber input. This is supported by the observation that the same features of the response are enhanced when the separation technique is based on the occurrence of climbing fiber inputs to a neighboring Purkinje cell.

The time course of the gain change is best described as non-persistent, being observed in the trials in which the complex spike occurs. In the majority of the neurons studied in the conditioning paradigms, the response amplitudes returned to preconditioning levels. However, as discussed previously (see Ebner and Bloedel 1981a; Bloedel et al. 1983) occasionally a persistent change in responsiveness was observed. It must also be stressed that the presence of any progressive change in responsiveness occurring throughout the conditioning period has not been analyzed.

The enhanced responsiveness following climbing fiber inputs is also consistent with the data of Llinas and Sugimori (1980). These authors demonstrated that a Purkinje cell's response to intracellular current injection is increased after the occurrence of a climbing fiber input. They also showed that responses of this type were reduced at very short intervals following the complex spike. In our studies no observations were made on the changes in Purkinje cell responsiveness immediately following spontaneous climbing fiber inputs. The well-known inactivation period (Granit and Phillips 1956) and subsequent brief increase in the excitability of the Purkinje cell following the complex spike (McDevitt et al. 1982) would have made the interpretation of the results difficult. To avoid this problem only responses evoked at intervals greater than 20 ms after the climbing fiber inputs were routinely evaluated.

The time course and characteristics of the gain change observed in our experiments differ from those observed in tests of the conjunction hypothesis (Ito and Kano 1982; Ito et al. 1982). This theory (see also Ekerot this Vol.) contends that the simultaneous action of the climbing fiber input and a specific pattern of parallel fiber inputs to the Purkinje cell dendrites reduces the synaptic strength of the parallel fiber inputs. Furthermore this reduction persists, resulting in a smaller modulation of simple spike activity in response to the same pattern of parallel fiber inputs.

Differences in experimental protocol make direct comparisons between our studies and those supporting the conjunction theory difficult. In the conjunction experiments the reduction in the amplitude of simple spike responses occurs after electrically activating climbing fiber and mossy fiber inputs for several seconds. These studies did not specifically examine changes in the responses to parallel fiber inputs activated at short intervals after individual occurrences of climbing fiber inputs, as in our conditioning and separation paradigms. However, some observations from the conjunction studies do seem somewhat comparable to our data. During the period in which the olivary and vestibular nerve stimuli are applied the amplitude of the simple spike responses evoked by vestibular nerve stimulation is increased (Ito et al. 1982). A similar effect was observed for the response of Purkinje cells during the iontophoretic application of glutamate. The Purkinje cell's response to this agent appears to be enhanced during the period of olivary stimulation.

A major difference in these studies is that the conjunction protocol used electrical stimulation of olivocerebellar fibers rather than spontaneous or naturally evoked climbing fiber inputs. Furthermore these stimuli were applied at a rate (4 Hz) higher than either the evoked or spontaneously occurring climbing fiber inputs (approximately 0.3-1.0 Hz) used in our study. Both the method as well as the rate of climbing fiber activation differ in the two paradigms. These differences may also contribute to the difference in the time course of the changes in responsiveness observed in the two sets of experiments. Possibly the more persistent reduction in responsiveness in the conjunction studies is related to the activation of an unusually dense pool of olivocerebellar fibers or the comparatively high discharge rate of climbing fibers evoked by the electrical stimuli. Electrical activation of olivocerebellar fibers suppresses tonic simple spike discharge (Colin et al. 1980). Potentially the reduced response amplitude reflects a tonic change in the cerebellar circuitry with a time constant of a few minutes.

One of the intriguing features of the studies by Ekerot (this volume) is that the conjunction induced decrease in responsiveness of Purkinje cells occurs only for the parallel fiber inputs stimulated at the time the olivary stimuli are applied. A Purkinje cell's response to surface stimuli activating a different group of parallel fibers was not affected. Thus the conjunction interaction appears to be specific, affecting parallel fiber inputs activated coincidentally with the cell's climbing fiber input. However, even though this interaction is specific, it does depend on the activation of olivocerebellar fibers at frequencies as high as 4 Hz.

In our view, our data revealing the role of the climbing fiber in short term interactions is consistent with evidence on the role of the climbing fibers in the adaptation of the vestibuloocular reflex (VOR). In the studies of Demer and Robinson (1982) the temporary interruption of the olivocerebellar projection by a local anesthetic increased the gain of the adapted VOR. This suggests the climbing fiber input performs an ongoing role in maintaining the adapted gain and does not act as "teacher" during motor learning. If the latter were true, no change in the adaptive condition would be expected after the injection of local anesthetic, since the climbing fiber already would have performed its function in establishing the new VOR gain. The observed increase in VOR gain in the absence of the olivocerebellar system suggests the Purkinje cell modulation is actually less than is appropriate for maintaining the adaptive gain. In the absence of the climbing fiber input the increased VOR could reflect an inadequately low gain of the Purkinje cell to mossy fiber inputs, a possibility consistent with the gain change hypothesis.

In summary an increased responsiveness of Purkinje cells is associated with the occurrence of spontaneous or naturally evoked climbing fiber inputs to the cerebellar cortex. This increased responsiveness appears to be short lasting, occurs in the cerebellar cortex, and is present for both excitatory and inhibitory responses. These observations support the gain change hypothesis. According to this view, the climbing fiber input contributes to ongoing processing in the cerebellar cortex, not by encoding subtle properties about peripheral stimuli, but by initiating a specific short term operation, an increased responsiveness of Purkinje cells to mossy fiber inputs.

In the context of this hypothesis the overlapping, sagittal organization of the olivo-cerebellar and corticonuclear projections has some interesting functional implications. The mulit-unit data show the responsiveness of one Purkinje cell can be increased in association with the climbing fiber input to another neuron, and the climbing fiber input of neighboring neurons evoked by a peripheral stimulus can be temporally correlated. We propose that in the behaving animal a functionally specific group of olivocerebellar fibers is activated as specified by the convergence of olivary inputs and the cellular interactions within the inferior olive (Llinas et al. 1974; Llinas and Yarom, 1981). Based on our present understanding of the organization of spinal inputs to the inferior olive (Armstrong et al. 1982) and the organization of the olivocerebellar projection, the activated olivocerebellar fibers would be distributed as components of sagittal strips. These sagittal strips correspond to comparably organized sagittal zones of the cortico-nuclear projection (Bloedel and Courville 1981, for review). Due to the length of the parallel fibers (Mugnaini 1983) and the divergence of mossy fibers within the cerebellar cortex (Palay and Chan-Palay 1974), the Purkinje cells modulated by the activated mossy fiber inputs would likely be distributed across more than one of these sagittal zones. Because of the proposed relationship between the zones of the olivocerebellar and corticonuclear projections, the distribution of activated olivocerebellar fibers would determine which sagittal components of the corticonuclear projection are best modulated by the mossy fiber inputs to the cortex. It is further speculated that these interactions would determine the distribution of neurons in the cerebellar nuclei most modulated because of the precise distribution within these nuclei of the corticonuclear projections from each sagittal zone (Haines et al. 1982). The climbing fiber afferent system is seen as exercising ongoing gain control over the output of the cerebellar cortex and nuclei. Based on this view the contribution of the cerebellar cortex to the output of the cerebellar nuclei is highly dependent upon the spatio-temporal distribution of olivocerebellar fibers activated by the convergent patterns of inferior olivary afferents and by the integration of these inputs occurring within this nucleus.

Acknowledgement. We wish to acknowledge the help of Eunice Roberts in the experiments, Hamdy Makky in the preparation of the figures, and Linda Christensen in the preparation of the manuscript. These experiments were supported by NIH grants NS-81338 and NS-09447.

References

Albus JS (1971) A theory of cerebellar function. Math Biosci 10: 25-61

Armstrong DM, Campbell CN, Edgley A, Schild RF, Trott JR (1982) Investigations of the olivo-cerebellar and spino-olivary pathways. In: Palay SL, Chan-Palay V (eds) The cerebellum: new vistas. Springer, Berlin Heidelberg New York, pp 192-222

Benedetti F, Montarolo PG, Strata P, Tempia F (1983) Inferior olive inactivation decreases the excitability of the intracerebellar and lateral vestibular nuclei in the rat. J Physiol 340: 195-208

Bloedel JR, Courville J (1981) A review of cerebellar afferent systems. In: Brooks VB (ed) Handbook of physiology, vol II. Motor control. Williams & Wilkins, Baltimore, pp 735-830

Bloedel JR, Roberts WJ (1971) Action of climbing fibers in cerebellar cortex of the cat. J Neurophysiol 34: 17-31

Bloedel JR, Ebner TJ, Yu QX (1983) Increased responsiveness of Purkinje cells associated with climbing fiber inputs to neighboring neurons. J Neurophysiol 50: 220-239

Colin F, Manil J, Desclin JC (1980) The olivocerebellar system. I. Delayed and slow inhibitory effects: An overlooked salient feature of cerebellar climbing fibers. Brain 187: 3-27

Demer JL, Robinson DA (1982) Effects of reversible lesions and stimulation of olivocerebellar system on vestibuloocular reflex plasticity. J Neurophysiol 47: 1084-1107

Ebner TJ, Bloedel JR (1981a) Role of climbing fiber afferent input in determining responsiveness of Purkinje cells to mossy fiber inputs. J Neurophysiol 45: 962-971

Ebner TJ, Bloedel JR (1981b) Temporal patterning in simple spike discharge of Purkinje cells and its relationship to climbing fiber activity. J Neurophysiol 45: 933-947

Ebner TJ, Yu QX, Bloedel JR (1983) Increase in Purkinje cell gain associated with naturally activated climbing fiber input. J Neurophysiol 50: 205-219

Eccles JC, Ito M, Szentagothai J (1967) The cerebellum as a neuronal machine. Springer, Berlin Heidelberg New York

Gilbert P (1975) How the cerebellum could memorise movements. Nature (London) 254: 688-689

Granit R, Phillips CG (1956) Excitatory and inhibitory processes acting upon individual Purkinje cells of the cerebellum in cats. J Physiol 133: 520-547

Haines DE, Patrick GW, Satrulee P (1982) Organization of cerebellar corticonuclear fiber systems. In: Palay SL, Chan-Palay V (eds) The cerebellum: new vistas. Springer, Berlin Heidelberg New York, pp 320-371

Ito M (1972) Neural design of the cerebellar motor control system. Brain Res 40: 81-84

Ito M (1979) Neuroplasticity. Is the cerebellum really a computer? Trends Neurosci 2: 122-126

Ito M, Kano M (1982) Long-lasting depression of parallel fiber-Purkinje cell transmission induced by conjunctive stimulation of parallel fibers and climbing fibers in the cerebellar cortex. Neurosci Lett 33: 253-258

Ito M, Mijshita Y (1975) The effects of chronic destruction of the inferior olive upon visual modification of the horizontal vestibulo-ocular reflex of rabbits. Proc Jpn Acad 51: 716-720

Ito M, Orlov I, Shimoyama I (1978) Reduction of the cerebellar stimulus effect on rat Deiters neurons after chemical destruction of the inferior olive. Exp Brain Res 33: 143-145

Ito M, Nisimaru N, Shibuki K (1979) Destruction of inferior olive induces rapid depression in synaptic action of cerebellar Purkinje cells. Nature (London) 277: 568-569

Ito M, Sakurai M, Tongroach P (1982) Climbing fibre induced depression of both mossy fibre responsiveness and glutamate sensitivity of cerebellar Purkinje cells. J Physiol 324: 113-134

Lisberger SG (1982) Role of the cerebellum during motor learning in the vestibulo-ocular reflex. Trends Neurosci 5: 437-440

Llinás R, Sugimori M (1980) Electrophysiological properties of *in vitro* Purkinje cell dendrites in mammalian cerebellar slices. J Physiol 305: 197-213

Llinás R, Volkind RA (1973) The olivo-cerebellar system. Functional properties as revealed by harmaline-induced tremor. Exp Brain Res 18: 69-87

Llinás R, Yarom Y (1981) Electrophysiology of mammalian inferior olivary neurones *in vitro*. Different types of voltage-dependent ionic conductances. J Physiol 315: 549-567

Llinás R, Baker R, Sotelo C (1974) Electronic coupling between neurons in cat inferior olive. J Neurophysiol 37: 560-571

Marr D (1969) A theory of cerebellar cortex. J Physiol 202: 437-470

McDevitt CJ, Ebner TJ, Bloedel JR (1982) The changes in Purkinje cell simple spike activity following spontaneous climbing fiber inputs. Brain Res 237: 484-491

Miles FA, Braitman DJ, Dow BM (1980) Long-term adaptive changes in primate vestibuloocular reflex. IV. Electrophysiological observations in flocculus of adapted monkeys. J Neurophysiol 43: 1477-1493

Montarolo PG, Raschi F, Strata P (1981) Are the climbing fibres essential for the Purkinje cell inhibitory action? Exp Brain Res 42: 215-218

Mugnaini E (1983) The length of cerebellar parallel fibers in chicken and rhesus monkey. J Comp Neurol 220: 7-15

Palay SL, Chan-Palay V (1974) Cerebellar cortex. Cytology and organization. Springer, Berlin Heidelberg New York

Robinson DA (1976) Adaptive gain control of vestibuloocular reflex by the cerebellum. J Neurophysiol 39: 954-969

Rhythmic Properties of Climbing Fiber Afferent Responses to Peripheral Stimuli

T.J. EBNER[1] and J.R. BLOEDEL[2]

An intriguing property of inferior olivary neurons is their tendency to discharge rhythmically at frequencies from 5-12 Hz (Armstrong 1974, Llinas 1981). This report focuses on the rhythmicity in the responses of Purkinje cells to climbing fiber inputs evoked by natural forepaw stimuli. In decereberate, unanesthetized cats the complex spike (CS) activity of Purkinje cells evoked by a forepaw displacement was averaged in post-stimulus time histograms (PSTH), and the autocorrelogram of the PSTH was calculated. The surgical procedures, recording techniques and peripheral input are described elsewhere (Ebner and Bloedel 1981, Ebner et al. 1983, Bloedel and Ebner 1984). Rhythmicity was defined as a minimum of three equally spaced peaks of complex spike activity, observed either in the PSTH or autocorrelogram. In 220 Purkinje cells with a complex spike response to the forepaw tap, 105 responded with a periodic discharge, the majority exhibiting a periodicity ranging from 100 to 160 ms. In 10 of 25 pairs of simultaneously recorded Purkinje cells the forepaw stimulus evoked periodicity in the complex spike discharge at a similar frequency. For some cells exhibiting only two peaks of CS activity, altering the stimulus duration did not alter the timing of the second peak of CS response suggesting that the second peak of CS activity was due to a rhythmic activation of the climbing fiber afferent rather than a response to the "of" phase of the stimulus.

The relative independence of the periodic peaks of CS discharge in the PSTH was demonstrated using a separation technique (Ebner et al. 1983, Bloedel and Ebner 1984). As shown in the all trial PSTH in Fig. 1 (C, F, I) the cell's climbing fiber afferent discharged with a periodicity of 7.3 Hz. The occurrence of complex spikes within the time window demarcating the first peak (arrows in A-C), was used to separate all stimulus trials into two groups: trials in which a CS was evoked in the first peak (B) and trials in which no CS was evoked during this period (A). These PSTH's show that the trials in which a complex spike was evoked in the first peak (B) were relatively independent from the trials in which CS associated with the second and third were evoked (A). Almost all the CS contributing to the second and third peak occurred in the other trials (A). Analysis of the second (D-F) and third peak (G-I) shows a comparable independence of the trials in which the complex spikes associated with each peak of the rhythmic response were generated.

These results demonstrate the strong tendency of the inferior olive to discharge rhythmically to natural inputs. The inferior olive appears to behave as a population of coupled non-linear oscillators. Presumably, the forepaw input synchronizes a popula-

[1] Depts. of Neurosurgery & Physiology University of Minnesota, Minneapolis, MN 55455, USA
[2] Barrow Neurological Institute St.-Joseph's Hospital and Medical Center 350 West Thomas Rd. Phoenix, Arizona 85013 USA

Cerebellar Functions
ed. by Bloedel et al.
© Springer-Verlag Berlin Heidelberg 1984

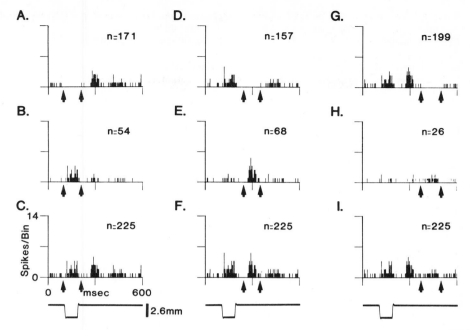

Fig. 1 A-I. Analysis of the independence of the periodic complex spike peaks evoked by the fore-paw stimulus. See text for details. (Bloedel and Ebner 1984)

tion of inferior olivary neurons, possibly by electrotonic coupling (Llinas 1981). Previous work in our laboratory has demonstrated the strong correlation in the complex spike discharge of nearby Purkinje cells to a similar forepaw displacement (Bloedel et al. 1983). The independence of the individual peaks comprising the rhythmicity suggests that an inferior olivary neuron's long refractory period (Llinas 1981) may prevent subsequent discharges. Although the forepaw stimulus results in a coupled rhythmic fluctuation in the excitability of a pool of inferior olivary neurons, it is postulated, that the long refractory period would greatly reduce the likelihood that an individual cell would discharge at more than a single peak in one trial.

Acknowledgement. This work was supported by NIH Grants NS 18338 and NS 09447.

References

Armstrong DM (1974) Functional significance of connections of the inferior olive. Physiol Rev 54: 358-417

Bloedel JR, Ebner TJ (1984) Rhythmic discharge of climbing fibre afferents in response to natural peripheral stimuli in the cat. J Physiol (in press)

Bloedel JR, Ebner TJ, Yu QX (1983) Increased responsiveness of Purkinje cells associated with climbing fiber inputs to neighboring neurons. J Neurophysiol 50: 220-239

Ebner TJ, Bloedel JR (1981) Role of climbing fiber afferent input in determining responsiveness of
    Purkinje cells to mossy fiber inputs. J Neurophysiol 45: 962-971
Ebner TJ, Yu QX, Bloedel JR (1983) Increase in Purkinje cell gain associated with naturally activated
    climbing fiber input. J Neurophysiol 50: 205-219
Llinás R (1981) Electrophysiology of the cerebellar networks. In: Brooks VB (ed) Handbook of
    physiology, vol II. Motor control. Williams & Wilkins, Baltimore, pp 831-877

Cerebellar Climbing Fibers Retrogradely Labeled With (³H)-D-Aspartate

L. WIKLUND[1], G. TOGGENBURGER[2], and M. CUENOD[2]

1 Introduction

Aspartate has been proposed as a transmitter of olivocerebellar climbing fibers, since pharmacologically induced degeneration of these afferents induces decreases of contents (Nadi et al. 1977; Rea et al. 1980) and in vitro release (Toggenburger et al. 1983) of aspartate from cerebellar tissue. Selective retrograde labeling with [³H]-D-aspartate ([³H]-D-asp) has recently been introduced as an autoradiographic method to identify connections with an excitatory amino acid, i.e. glutamate and/or aspartate, as transmitter (Streit 1980; Cuenod et al. 1982). Employing this technique in the cerebellum, we have found a strong retrograde labeling of the climbing fiber input with [³H]-D-asp (Wiklund et al. 1982), and the present communication describes the principal features of the labeling of the olivocerebellar system with this tracer.

2 Material and Methods

Female rats of the SIV strain (180-250 g body weight) were anaesthetized with Nembutal, 40 mg/kg i.p., and placed in a stereotaxic instrument. Microinjections of 50 nl containing 25 μCi [³H]-D-asp (D-[2, 3-³H] aspartic acid, 10-18 Ci/mmol, Amersham) in aq.dest were placed in various parts of cerebellar cortex. After 6-24 hr survival, the animals were reanaesthetized and fixed by perfusion: blood was rinsed out with 6% Rheomacrodex^R for circa 30 seconds, followed by 1200 ml 3.5% glutaraldehyde in 0.17 M phosphate buffer (pH = 7.4, room temp.) over 20 min. Dissected brains and spinal cords were stored in fixative for 1-2 days (4°C) before being transferred to 30% sucrose in the same buffer. After sinking, the specimens were sectioned on a freezing microtome at 30 μm thickness (additional sections 10 μm). Every fifth section was mounted on gelatinized slides, defatted through alcohols and xylene, dried, dipped in Kodak NTB-2 emulsion diluted 1:1 in aq.dest., and developed after 3 and 6 weeks exposure. After cresyl violet counterstaining, the specimens were investigated with bright and dark field microscopy.

[1]   Department of Histology, University of Lund, Biskopsgatan 5, S-223 62 Lund, Sweden
[2]   Brain Research Institute, University of Zurich, CH-8029 Zurich, Switzerland

Cerebellar Functions
ed. by Bloedel et al.
© Springer-Verlag Berlin Heidelberg 1984

3 Results

All injections of [³H]-D-asp into different parts of cerebellum resulted in strong retrograde labelling of the olivocerebellar climbing fiber system. Other cerebellar afferents from brain stem (Gould 1980) and spinal cord (Grant 1982) were never labelled by [³H]-D-asp. The diencephalon was, however, not included in the investigation, which is why it is unknown if the newly discovered hypothalamic afferents to cerebellum (Dietrichs 1984) were labeled.

As an example of [³H]-D-asp retrograde labeling, the results of an injection into lobulus simplex will be described (Figs. 1-6). Beneath a rather large injection site (Figs. 1, 2) which involved lobulus simplex, vermal lobulus VI, and medial crus I, labeled fibers appeared in the cerebellar white matter and could be traced into the restiform body, which they followed along the lateral aspect of the medulla oblongata (Fig. 1). Appearing below the trigeminal tract, the retrogradelly labeled fibers formed a broad bundle traversing the ventral medulla oblongata, passing the ipsilateral inferior olive, crossing the midline, and ending in the contralateral inferior olive where retrogradely labeled cell bodies appeared (Fig. 6). The labeled cells were distributed in distinct compartments of the principal, medial accessory and dorsal accessory olivary subnuclei (Fig. 1). Close examination of the olivary labeling revealed that labeled cell bodies were surrounded by spheres of somewhat lower grain density (Fig. 5), which was interpreted as migration of tracer out into the dendrites of retrogradely labeled cells.

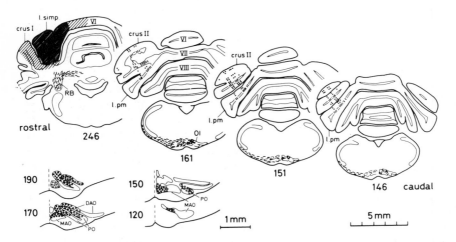

Fig. 1. Schematic representation of the results of an injection of [³H]-D-asp into lobulus simplex with spread into vermal lobule VI and crus I. *Wavy lines* indicate the course of labeled preterminal fibers through cerebellar white matter and brain stem. *Solid dots* in cerebellar cortex represent terminals of labeled climbing fiber collaterals. Sketches of the inferior olive at higher magnification give the distribution of well labeled *(filled dots)* and less labeled *(open dots)* cell bodies. Distance between sections is given by their numbers in a series of 30 μm sections. *DAO* dorsal accessory nucleus; *l. pm* lobulus paramedianus; *l. simp* lobulus simplex; *MAO* medial accessory nucleus; *OI* oliva inferior; *PO* principal nucleus; *RB* restiform body; *VI, VII, VIII* lobuli VI, VII, VIII of vermis. (Wiklund et al. 1984)

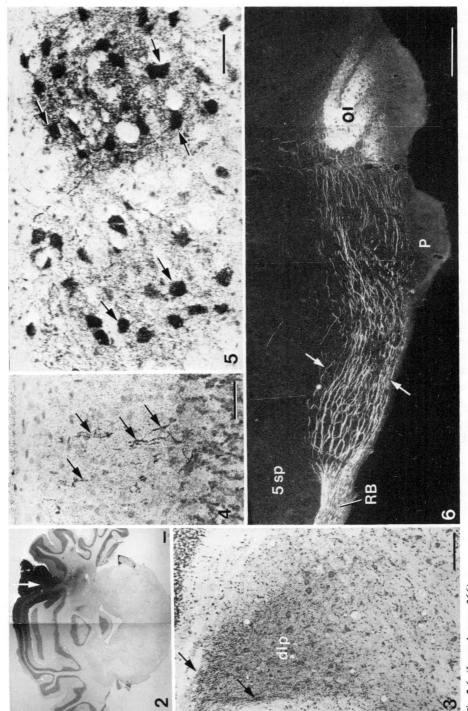

Fig. 2-6. (Legends see p 266)

Fig. 2. Low magnification view of injection into lobulus simples *(arrow)*. *Bar* 1 mm

Fig. 3. Labeled climbing fiber collaterals *(arrows)* appearing in the white matter overlying the dorso-lateral protuberance *(dlp)* of the medial cerebellar nucleus, where evidences of termination appears. *Bar* 200 μm

Fig. 4. Labeled climbing fiber collaterals *(arrows)* in the molecular layer of crus II after injection of [³H]-D-asp into lobulus simplex. *Bar* 50 μm

Fig. 5. Strongly labeled perikarya *(arrows)* in the ventral lamella of the principal olivary nucleus *(left)* and the dorsal accessory nucleus *(right)*. Note the "spheres" of silver grains surrounding the perikarya, which is interpreted as labeling of dendrites. Section thickness 10 μm. *Bar* 50 μm

Fig. 6. Dark field view of retrogradely labeled nerve fibers in the restiform body *(RB)* beneath the trigeminal tract and crossing the brain stem *(arrows)* from their origin in the contralateral inferior olive *(OI)*. *P* pyramidal tract; *5 sp* spinal trigeminal tract and nucleus. *Bar* 0.5 mm

---

Labeled nerve fibers were also observed in distant parts of cerebellum, which were not involved in the injection site (Fig. 1). Two or three bundles of fibers appeared in the white matter of crus II and lobulus paramedianus, and in the overlying molecular layer labeled terminals were found (Fig. 4). These fibers were, therefore, interpreted as collaterals of climbing fibers terminating within the injected area. After injections into other parts of cerebellum sagittally oriented bundles of labeled climbing fiber collaterals were demonstrated in different hemispheral and vermal areas (see, Wiklund et al. 1984). Also, the deep cerebellar and Deiters' nuclei demonstrated climbing fiber collateral labeling after different cortical cerebellar injections (Fig. 3).

4 Discussion

Retrograde labelling of inferior olivary neurons has been demonstrated after injections of [³H]-D-asp into cerebellum. Other afferents from the brain stem or spinal cord were not labeled. These observations are in line with suggestions that an excitatory amino acid, aspartate, may be a transmitter of the cerebellar climbing fibers (Nadi et al. 1977; Rea et al. 1980; Toggenburger et al. 1983).

The organization of the olivocerebellar system has been extensively investigated in the cat (for review, Brodal and Kawamura 1980). The present study was done in the rat, but the distribution of labeled olivary neurons after [³H]-D-asp injections into different parts of the cerebellum agreed very well with the topographical organization elucidated in the cat. The climbing fiber system is, therefore, similarly organized in these two species. Moreover, the numbers of retrogradely labeled olivary cells suggested that all neurons in every olivary compartment share this affinity for [³H]-D-asp. As far as this transmitter related parameter is concerned, they appear as a homogenous cell population.

All parts of the olivary neurons were labeled after cerebellar injection of [³H]-D-asp. The course of the retrogradely labeled climbing fibers could be followed through the cerebellar white matter and brain stem. In the olive, retrogradely labeled cell bodies appeared, but the tracer also migrated out into their dendritic trees. At axonal branching points some of the retrogradely migrating [³H]-D-asp was diverted in anterograde direction along the climbing fiber collateralizations. This collateral labeling confirmed the existence of climbing fiber collaterals to deep cerebellar and Deiters' nuclei (Andersson and Oscarsson 1978; Brodal and Kawamura 1980). Labeled climbing fiber collaterals were also demonstrated in cerebellar cortex, where they were organized in narrow sagittal bundles (cf. Armstrong et al. 1973). Due to the large size of [³H]-D-asp injections it was not possible to determine the olivary origin of the visualized zones of climbing fiber collaterals. Nevertheless, the outline of climbing fiber collateralizations with [³H]-D-asp should be of considerable aid in guiding retrograde double labeling experiments.

An extensive presentation of these experiments will appear elsewhere (Wiklund et al. 1984).

Acknowledgement. This study was supported by grants from the Swiss National Foundation (Nos. 3.506.79 and 3.505.79) and Swedish Medical Research Council (12X-06535).

References

Andersson G, Oscarsson O (1978) Projections to lateral vestibular nucleus from cerebellar climbing fiber zones. Exp Brain Res 32: 549-564

Armstrong DM, Harvey RJ, RF Schild (1973) The spatial organization of climbing fibre branching in the cat cerebellum. Exp Brain Res 18: 4-58

Brodal A, Kawamura K (1980) Olivocerebellar projection: A review. Adv Anat 64: 1-140

Cuenod M, Bagnoli P, Beaudet A, Rustioni A, Wiklund L, Streit P (1982) Transmitter specific retrograde labelling of neurons. In: Chan-Palay V, Palay SL (eds) Cytochemical methods in neuroanatomy. Liss, New York, pp 17-44

Dietrichs E (1984) Cerebellar autonomic function: direct hypothalamocerebellar pathway. Science 223: 591-593

Gould BB (1980) Organization of afferents from the brain stem nuclei to the cerebellar cortex in the cat. Adv Anat 62: 1-90

Grant G (1982) Spinocerebellar connections in the cat with particular emphasis on their cellular origin. In: Palay SL, Chan-Palay V (eds) Cerebellum: new vistas. Springer, Berlin Heidelberg New York, pp 466-475

Nadi NS, Kanter D, McBride WJ, Aprison MH (1977) Effects of 3-acetylpyridine on several putative neurotransmitter amino acids in the cerebellum and meduall of the rat. J Neurochem 28: 661-662

Rea MA, McBride WJ, Rohde BH (1980) Regional and synaptosomal levels of amino acid neurotransmitters in the 3-acetylpyridine deafferented rat cerebellum. J Neurochem 34: 1106-1108

Streit P (1980) Selective retrograde labeling indicating the transmitter of neuronal pathways. J Comp Neurol 191: 429-463

Toggenburger G, Wiklund L, Henke H, Cuenod M (1983) Release of endogenous and newly accumulated exogenous amino acids from slices of normal and climbing fibre-deprived rat cerebellar slices. J Neurochem 41: 1606-1613

Wiklund L, Toggenburger G, Cuenod M (1982) Aspartate: Possible neurotransmitter in cerebellar climbing fibers. Science 216: 78-80

Wiklund L, Toggenburger G, Cuenod M (1984) Selective retrograde labelling of rat olivocerebellar climbing fiber system with [³H]-D-aspartate. Neuroscience (in press)

Climbing Fibre Actions of Purkinje Cells — Plateau Potentials and Long-Lasting Depression of Parallel Fibre Responses

C.-F. EKEROT[1]

Understanding of the information processing occurring in the cerebellar cortex requires knowledge about the properties and specific functions of the two major kinds of afferents received by the Purkinje cells, the parallel fibres and the climbing fibres. The synapses between these two kinds of afferents and the Purkinje cells are both excitatory but have otherwise an entirely different organization. Each Purkinje cell receives about 100,000 parallel fibres which make synapses on the distal dendrites, but only one climbing fibre which makes an extraordinarily powerful synaptic contact on more proximal dendrites. Activity in parallel fibres is, at least partly, responsible for the background activity of Purkinje cells which is usually between 20 and 100 Hz. A climbing fibre impulse causes a discharge of the Purkinje cell, which extracellularly is recorded as a "complex spike" from the soma. The complex spike consists of an initial action potential followed by one or a few abortive spikes. Although some of the abortive spikes may be conducted down the Purkinje cell axon (Ito and Simpson, 1971) the overall contribution of climbing fibres to the output activity of Purkinje cells must be small because of the low discharge rate of climbing fibres, usually 1-2 Hz.

The unique one-to-one relationship between climbing fibres and Purkinje cells, together with the powerful synaptic responses generated in the Purkinje cells, suggest a highly specific function for this input. In the learning theories advanced by Marr (1969), Albus (1971) and Ito (1972, 1982), the mossy fibres and climbing fibres have entirely different functions (see Fig. 1). Impulses in mossy fibres are largely responsible for the output of the Purkinje cells which controls the execution of motor acts. It has been suggested that the inferior olive evaluates the motor performance (Miller and Oscarsson, 1970) and errors are signalled through the climbing fibres to the Purkinje cells and result, according to Albus (1971), in a heterosynaptic depression of those parallel fibre synapses which have just been active and therefore partly responsible for the misperformance. Repetition of these events increases the suppression of the transmission with, finally, elimination of the erroneous movement. These theories have received support from experimental work, particularly from studies on adaptation of the vestibulo-ocular reflex (for references see Ito, 1982). The results from these investigations show that Purkinje cell responses to vestibular mossy fibre-parallel fibre input change during adaptation of the reflex in a manner predicted by the hypothesis (Dufosse, Ito, Jastreboff and Miyashita, 1978; Watanabe, 1984). More direct support for the hypothesis was recently presented by Ito et al. (1982), who showed that conjunctive stimulation of a vestibular nerve and climbing fibres resulted in a long-lasting depression of the

[1]   Institute of Physiology, University of Lund, Sölvegatan 19, S223 62 Lund, Sweden

Cerebellar Functions
ed. by Bloedel et al.
© Springer-Verlag Berlin Heidelberg 1984

Cerebellar cortex

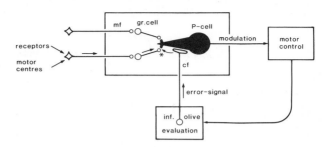

* error–signal depresses transmission

Fig. 1. The "learning" theory of cerebellar cortex. Impulses in mossy fibres *(mf)* largely determine the output form the Purkinje cells, which in turn modifies the execution of motor acts. The correctness of the motor acts is evaluated by the inferior olive and errors in motor performance are signalled through the climbing fibres *(cf)* to the Purkinje cells and result in heterosynaptic suppression of those parallel fibre synapses which have just been active and therefore partly responsible for the misperformance. Abbreviations: *gr. cell* granule cell; *P-cell* Purkinje cell. See text

parallel fibre responses evoked in Purkinje cells by stimulation of the nerve, whereas the responses evoked from the vestibular nerve on the other side were unchanged.

What is the mechanism responsible for the climbing fibre induced, heterosynaptic depression of parallel fibre synapses? Since the parallel fibre synapses and the climbing fibre synapses are located on different regions of the Purkinje cell dendrites there must exist a mechanism by which information about climbing fibre activity is transferred to the parallel fibre synapses. An explanation is offered by the recent discovery of Ekerot and Oscarsson (1980, 1981) that climbing fibre impulses evoke not only the complex spikes in Purkinje cell somata but also prolonged plateau-like depolarizations in Purkinje cell dendrites. Such plateau potentials are, under physiological conditions, evoked exclusively by the large EPSP's generated by impulses in climbing fibres (Campbell, Ekerot, Hesslow and Oscarsson, 1983). The plateau potentials are set up at the climbing fibre synapses and spread actively to the distal dendrites. The plateau potentials in proximal and distal dendrites have different properties. In proximal dendrites, which are readily studied by intracellular recording, the climbing fibre response consists of an initial spike-like potential followed by a plateau potential of an almost constant amplitude and with a relatively fixed duration, usually about 100 ms (Fig. 2A). Intracellular recordings are difficult to obtain from distal dendrites, but climbing fibre responses can be recorded extracellularly as prolonged negative unitary potentials resembling mirror images of the intracellularly recorded plateau potentials (Fig. 2B). The plateau potentials recorded from distal dendrites differ from those of proximal dendrites in that their duration varies considerably, from some ten to several hundreds of milliseconds (Fig. 2C). The possibility that the duration of plateau potentials is influenced by the membrane potential was examined in experiments in which Purkinje cells were hyperpolarized by inhibition. The inhibitory potentials were evoked by stimulation of parallel fibres "off beam" to activate stellate and basket cells which make inhibitory synapses on the Purkinje cells (Eccles, Ito and Szentagothai, 1967). An extracellular recording from a distal Purkinje cell dendrite is illustrated in Fig. 3. When the climbing

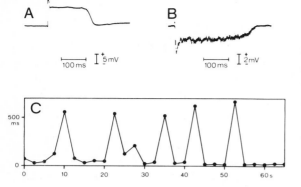

Fig. 2 A-C. Plateau potentials evoked in Purkinje cell dendrites by impulses in climbing fibres. **A** Intracellular recording from proximal dendrite; **B** Extracellular recording from distal dendrite; **C** Variation in duration of consecutive plateau potentials evoked at intervals of 2.5 s and recorded extracellularly from distal dendrite. *Ordinate* duration of response in ms. *Abscissa* time of consecutive responses in s. The observations were made on cats under pentobarbitone anesthesia

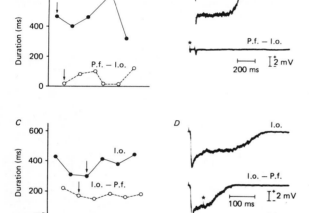

Fig. 3 A-D. Effect of preceding **(A, B)** and following **(C, D)** parallel fibre *(P.f.)* volley on extracellularly recorded climbing fibre responses from distal Purkinje cell dendrite. Parallel fibre stimulus preceded stimulus to inferior olive *(I.o.)* by 45 ms in A and B *P.f.-I.o.)* and followd it by 55 ms in **C** and **D** *(I.o.-P.f.)*. **A** and **C** duration of consecutively recorded unconditioned *(filled circles)* and conditioned *(open circles)* climbing fibre responses. *Horizontal arrow* in **C** indicates interval between I.o. and P.f. stimuli. **B** and **D** sample records corresponding to points indicated by *vertical arrows* in **A** and **C** (From Campbell et al. 1983a)

fibre response is preceded by the "off beam" stimulus the plateau potential has a much reduced duration or is completely abolished (Fig. 3 A and B). The effect of the "off beam" stimulus during an already established plateau potential is less prominent but causes a considerable reduction of the duration (Fig. 3 C and D). These findings indicate that the duration of plateau potentials in distal dendrites is influenced by the membrane potential and suggest that the marked fluctuations in duration of plateau potentials in distal dendrites may depend on fluctuations in the membrane potential mediated by the local parallel fibre activity and that individual dendritic branches may thus act as independent integrators of mossy fibre and climbing fibre information (Campbell, Ekerot and Hesslow, 1983).

If the climbing fibre-induced depression of parallel fibre synapses depends on dendritic plateau potentials, what step connects the plateau potentials with the plastic changes of parallel fibre synapses? The plateau potentials are probably generated by a calcium conductance increase (Llinas and Sugimori, 1980) and would give rise to an increased intradendritic calcium concentration. The calcium ions might represent a second

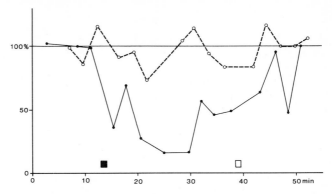

Fig. 4. Depression of parallel fibre-evoked responses in Purkinje cell induced by conjunctive stimulation of climbing fibres and parallel fibres. *Continuous line* responsiveness to parallel fibre beam stimulated conjunctively with climbing fibres for 1 min at 4 Hz and with an interval of 50 ms between the climbing fibre and parallel fibre stimulus. *Filled rectangle* period of conjunctive stimulation. *Interrupted line* responsiveness to unstimulated control parallel fibre beam. *Open rectangle* stimulation of control parallel fibre beam alone for 1 min at 4 Hz. *Ordinate* responsiveness in percent of mean responsiveness before conjunctive stimulation. See text

messenger responsible for reducing the sensitivity of the recently activated synaptic receptors for the transmitter in the parallel fibres. A similar action of intracellular calcium has been reported for the muscle endplate, where an increased concentration of calcium in the muscle fibre is supposed to enhance the desensitization of acetylcholine receptors (Miledi, 1980).

To investigate if the climbing fibre-evoked plateau potentials are responsible for the heterosynaptic depression of parallel fibre synapses, a detailed study of the effect of climbing fibre activity on parallel fibre responses in Purkinje cells was performed by Ekerot and Kano (1983). In these experiments activity from single Purkinje cells in the paraflocculus was recorded from unanesthetized decerebrated rabbits. Both climbing fibres and parallel fibres were activated by direct electrical stimulation, climbing fibres by an electrode in the contralateral inferior olive and parallel fibres by two microelectrodes inserted into the molecular layer. The two microelectrodes were positioned to activate two separate parallel fibre beams converging onto the investigated Purkinje cell. The responsiveness of the Purkinje cell to stimulation of the parallel fibre beams was determined from peristimulus time histograms consisting of 60 stimulations. One of the parallel fibre beams was selected for conjunctive stimulation with climbing fibres. During conjunctive stimulation climbing fibres and parallel fibres were activated by single stimuli using a fixed interval between the climbing fibre and parallel fibre stimulus. The unstimulated parallel fibre beam was used as a control to exclude that changes of responsiveness following conjunctive stimulation depended on general changes in excitability of the Purkinje cell. Fig. 4 shows the effect of conjunctive stimulation at 4 Hz for 1 min. The responsiveness of the parallel fibre beam used for conjunctive stimulation with climbing fibres is shown as a continuous line, and that of the unstimulated beam as an interrupted line. The short period of conjunctive stimulation (indicated by a filled rectangle) resulted in a strong, long-lasting depression of the responses evoked from the conjunctively stimulated beam whereas the responses from the unstimulated

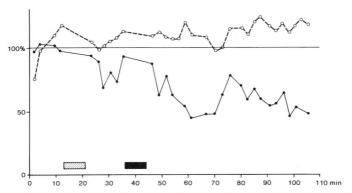

Fig. 5. Effect of "off beam"stimulation of parallel fibres on climbing fibre-induced depression of parallel fibre-evoked responses in Purkinje cell. *Continuous line* Purkinje cell responsiveness to parallel fibre beam stimulated conjunctively with climbing fibres and interrupted line responsiveness to unstimulated control beam. *Rectangles* indicate 8 min conjunctive stimulation at 2 Hz and with an interval of 20 ms between the climbing fibre and parallel fibre stimulus. *Hatched rectangle* conjunctive stimulation with "off beam" stimulus preceding the climbing fibre stimulus by 50 ms; *filled rectangle* conjunctive stimulation without "off beam" stimulation. *Ordinate* responsiveness in percent of mean responsiveness before conjunctive stimulation. See text

beam were unchanged. In most units the duration of the depression was between 1 and 2 h. To exclude that parallel fibre stimulation per se results in a depression the control beam was later stimulated at this frequency for 1 min. (open rectangle). This did not change the Purkinje cell responses.

If the climbing fibre induced depression of parallel fibre responses is mediated by the climbing fibre-elicited plateau potentials, it would be expected that the depression of parallel fibre responses following conjunctive stimulation with climbing fibres is influenced by the interval between the climbing fibre and parallel fibre stimulus. After conjunctive stimulation of climbing fibres and parallel fibres at 2 Hz for 8 min a significant depression of parallel fibre responses occurred in 67% of the Purkinje cells tested at an interval of 20 ms, in 50% of the cells tested at intervals of 125 and 250 ms and only in 29% of the cells tested at 375 ms interval. These results support the hypothesis that the climbing fibre-evoked plateau potentials are mediators of the heterosynaptic depression of parallel fibre responses since the length of the effective interval is similar to the duration of plateau potentials in distal Purkinje cell dendrites (Ekerot and Oscarsson, 1981).

More decisive evidence in support of the plateau potentials as mediators of the climbing fibre-induced depression of parallel fibre responses was obtained in studies on the effect of inhibition during conjunctive stimulation of climbing and parallel fibres. The climbing fibre-evoked plateau potentials are shortened or abolished by inhibition preceding the climbing fibre response (see Fig. 3A, B) (Campbell et al., 1983a). If the plateau potentials mediate the depression of parallel fibre responses it would be expected that inhibition during conjunctive stimulation of climbing and parallel fibres would prevent the development of a depression or reduce its size. This was tested in experiments in which disynaptic inhibition was evoked in Purkinje cells from stellate and basket cells activated by a third parallel fibre stimulation electrode positioned "off beam" to avoid excitation of the Purkinje cell (cf. Eccles et al., 1967). The stimulus consisted of a train of 3 pulses delivered at 100 Hz and preceding the climbing fibre stimulus by 50 ms during conjunctive stimulation. The stimulation strength was set to inhibit the spontaneous activity of the Purkinje cells for at least 100 ms. Figure 5 illustrates the effect of inhibition during conjunctive stimulation. As seen in the graphs conjunctive stimulation preceded by inhibition (hatched rectangle) resulted in a short-lasting and relatively weak depression of the responses evoked form the stimulated parallel fibre beam compared to the depression seen after conjunctive stimulation without inhibition (filled rectangle).

These findings strongly suggest that the climbing fibre evoked plateau potentials mediate the heterosynaptic depression of parallel fibre synapses. They also suggest that the depressive effect of climbing fibre impulses on simultaneously active parallel fibre synapses is graded and depends on the local membrane potential. Synapses located on dendrites receiving a strong net excitatory input will be most affected, whereas synapses located on hyperpolarized dendrites will be little or not at all influenced by a climbing fibre impulse. This mode of functioning would be expected to increase the cerebellar learning capacity compared to previous hypotheses on cerebellar learning which postulate the same change in effectiveness of all active parallel fibre synapses on a Purkinje cell regardless of the membrane potential.

Acknowledgement. This work was supported by grants form the Medical Faculty, University of Lund, Sweden and the Swedish Medical Research Council (Project 1013).

References

Albus JS (1971) A theory of cerebellar function. Math Biosci 10: 25-61

Campbell NC, Ekerot C-F, Hesslow G (1983a) Interaction between responses in Purkinje cell evoked by climbing fibre impulses and parallel fibre volleys in the cat. J Physiol (Lond) 340: 225-238

Campbell NC, Ekerot C-F, Hesslow G, Oscarsson O (1983a) Dendritic plateau potentials evoked in Purkinje cells by parallel fibre volleys in the cat. J Physiol (Lond) 340: 209-223

Dufosse M, Ito M, Jastreboff PJ, Miyashita Y (1978) A neuronal correlate in rabbit's cerebellum to adaptive modification of the vestibulo-ocular reflex. Brain Res 150: 611-616

Eccles JC, Ito M, Szentágothai J (1967) The Cerebellum as a Neuronal Machine. Springer Verlag, Berlin-Heidelberg-New York

Ekerot C-F, Kano M (1983) Climbing fibre induced depression of Purkinje cell responses to parallel fibre stimulation. Proc Int Union Physiol Sci, vol XV. Sydney, p 393

Ekerot C-F, Oscarsson O (1980) Prolonged dendritic depolarizations evoked in Purkinje cells by climbing fibre impulses. Brain Res 192: 272-275

Ekerot C-F, Oscarsson O (1981) Prolonged dendritic depolarizations elicited in Purkinje cell dendrites by climbing fibre impulses in the cat. J Physiol (Lond) 318: 207-221

Ito M (1972) Neural design of the cerebellar motor control system. Brain Res 40: 81-84

Ito M (1982) Cerebellar control of the vestibulo-ocular reflex — around the flocculus hypothesis. Ann Rev Neurosci 5: 275-296

Ito M, Sakurai M, Tongroach P (1982) Climbing fibre induced depression of both mossy fibre responsiveness and glutamate sensitivity of cerebellar Purkinje cells. J Physiol (Lond) 324: 113-134

Ito M, Simpson JI (1971) Discharges in Purkinje cell axons during climbing fibre activation. Brain Res 31: 215-219

Llinás R, Sugimori M (1980) Electrophysiological properties of in vitro Purkinje cell dendrites in mammalian cerebellar slices. J Physiol (Lond) 305: 197-213

Marr D (1969) A theory of cerebellar cortex. J Physiol (Lond) 202: 437-470

Miledi R (1980) Intracellular calcium and desensitization of acetylcholine receptors. Proc R Soc B 209: 447-452

Miller S, Oscarsson O (1970) Termination and functional organization of spino-olivary cerebellar paths. In: The Cerebellum in Health and Disease. Eds Field WS, & Willis Jr, WD. Warren H. Green, Inc. Publisher, St. Louis, Missouri, USA, p 172-220

Watanabe E (1984) Neuronal events correlated with long-term adaptation of the horizontal vestibulo-ocular reflex in the primate flocculus. Brain Res. 297: 169-174

Functional Changes of the Purkinje Cell Following Climbing Fiber Deafferentation

F. BENEDETTI, P.G. MONTAROLO, and S. RABACCHI[1]

By destroying or inactivating in a reversible manner the inferior olivary nucleus, the source of climbing fibers to the cerebellar cortex, it has been shown that, beside the disappearance of the Purkinje cell complex spikes, a parallel increase in the frequency of discharge of the simple spikes occurs (Colin et al. 1980, Montarolo et al. 1982). Such a phenomenon has been studied so far in acute experiments in the order of time of minutes; therefore, it is interesting to investigate how long the simple spikes firing increase lasts, in the case of an irreversible lesion.

The experiments have been performed on 83 adult Wistar rats with the inferior olivary nucleus destroyed by means of cryocoagulation (6 rats), electrocoagulation (10 rats) and 3-acetylpyridine (70 mg/kg i.p. 67 rats). Recording of unitary activity was done up to 12 hr from the lesion in the rats treated with the first two methods, whereas in the 3-acetylpyridine treated rats unitary recording was performed from 27 hr to 1 month after the lesion, in order to avoid possible acute side effects.

The analysis of the spontaneous activity of 679 Purkinje cells recorded from the homonymous layer, identified through the typical alternate high and low background activity of the cerebellar cortex (Montarolo et al. 1980), showed that the average simple spike frequency increase in the first 5 days was to $52.7/s$ (± 22.6 S.D.); the simple spike frequency gradually decreased, as shown in Fig. 1, to reach the value of $24.2/s$ (± 12.1 S.D.) at the end of the first month after the lesion. The simple spike frequency increase is statistically significant with respect to the control value of $22.6/s$ (± 13.7 S.D.), obtained from 45 Purkinje cells of 17 intact rats (Mann-Whitney U test, $P < 0.001$ for the first 3 columns of Fig. 1 and $P < 0.05$ for the 4th one).

These results confirm that, when the spontaneous activity of the inferior olive is abolished, there is a marked increase of activity of the Purkinje cells (Colin et al. 1980, Montarolo et al. 1982); in addition, they show that such an increase gradually diminishes to disappear at the end of the first month (33.5 days considering the regression line of Fig. 1).

By employing the radioactive labeling techniques, with ^{14}C-2 deoxyglucose, Batini et al. (1981) have observed an increased metabolism at the level of the intracerebellar and lateral vestibular nuclei, following a lesion to the inferior olive. Further experiments have demonstrated that the metabolic increase is due to the presynaptic component of the nuclei, namely, to the axon terminals of the Purkinje cells (Batini et al. 1982, 1984). Bardin et al. (1983) showed that such an increased metabolism gradually decreases to reach a normal value at the end of the first month. There is thus an excel-

[1]   Istituto di Fisiologia Umana dell'Università, Corso Raffaello 30, 10125 Torino, Italy

Cerebellar Functions
ed. by Bloedel et al.
© Springer-Verlag Berlin Heidelberg 1984

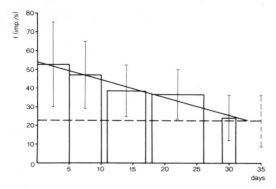

Fig. 1. Time course of the simple spike frequency of the Purkinje cells following the lesion of the inferior olivary nucleus. The columns represent the mean frequencies of discharge of all the cells recorded in the same time interval (396 in the 1st column, 128 in the 2nd, 70 in the 3rd, 49 in the 4th and 36 in the 5th), with their standard deviations. The simple spike mean firing rate of control is shown by the *broken line*. The regression line, calculated from five values of simple spike rate of discharge of all the Purkinje cells recorded in five different days (15 the 3rd day, 30 the 7th, 13 the 15th, 18 the 23rd, 18 the 30th), is also shown: it crosses the *broken line* of control at the value of 33.5 days

lent agreement in measurements of the Purkinje cell activity at both the metabolic and electrophysiological levels.

The persisting increase in frequency of Purkinje cells discharge (Montarolo et al. 1982) and the consequent strong inhibition of the nuclear neurons (Benedetti et al. 1983) could explain the neurobehavioral data showing severe motor disorders with hypotonia and ataxia after inferior olive lesion (Llinás et al. 1975), suggesting that the inferior olivary nucleus would play an important role in the maintenance of tonus. The recent observation of Batini et al. (1983) who described a decrease of forelimb extensor tonus in the decerebrate cat, following reversible inferior olive inactivation, supports this view.

References

Bardin JM, Batini C, Billard JM, Buisseret-Delmas C, Conrath-Verrier M, Corvaja N (1983) Cerebellar output regulation by the climbing and mossy fibers with and without the inferior olive. J Comp Neurol 213: 464-472

Batini C, Buisseret-Delmas C, Conrath-Verrier M, Corvaja N (1981) The effect of harmaline and 3-acetylpyridine on the olivocerebellar-nuclear system in rats studied with [14] C 2-Deoxyglucose. In: Szentágothai J, Hámori J, Palkovits M (eds) Regulatory functions of CNS subsystem, vol II. Adv Physiol Sci, Budapest, Akadémiai Kiadò, pp 145-149

Batini C, Benedetti F, Buisseret-Delmas C, Montarolo PG, Strata P (1982) Effect of local cooling of the inferior olive on the metabolic activity of the intracerebellar nuclei. Neurosci Lett Suppl 10: S61

Batini C, Bernard JF, Montarolo PG, Strata P (1983) The olivocerebellar pathway exerts a tonic control on the postural activity. Neurosci Lett Suppl 14: S20

Batini C, Benedetti F, Buisseret-Delmas C, Montarolo PG, Strata P (1984) Metabolic activity of intracerebellar nulcei in the rat: effects of inferior olive inactivation. Exp Brain Res 54: 259-265

Benedetti F, Montarolo PG, Strata P, Tempia F (1983) Inferior olive inactivation decreases the excitability of the intracerebellar and lateral vestibular nuclei in the rat. J Physiol 340: 195-208

Colin F, Manil J, Desclin JC (1980) The olivocerebellar system. I. Delayed and slow inhibitory effects: an overlooked salient-feature of cerebellar climbing fibers. Brain Res 187: 3-27

Llinâs R, Walton K, Hillman DE, Sotelo C (1975) Inferior olive: its role in motor learning. Science 190: 1230-1231

Montarolo PG, Raschi F, Strata P (1980) On the origin of the climbing fibres of the cerebellar cortex. Pflueger's Arch 383: 137-142

Montarolo PG, Palestini M, Strata P (1982) The inhibitory effect of the olivocerebellar input on the cerebellar Purkinje cells in the rat. J Physiol 332: 187-202

Inferior Olive: Its Tonic Inhibitory Effect on the Cerebellar Purkinje Cells in the Rat Without Anesthesia

T. SAVIO and F. TEMPIA [1]

In rats under barbiturate anesthesia, following a reversible inactivation of the inferior olivary nucleus (IO) by cooling, the Purkinje cell (PC) shows, together with the disappearance of the complex spikes (CS), a remarkable increase of the frequency of the simple spikes (SS) (Montarolo et al. 1982). This tonic inhibitory effect of the olivocerebellar pathway on the PC has been attributed in part to the activation of the corticocerebellar interneurons by collaterals of the climbing fibers (CF). It is known that these interneurons are GABAergic (Bisti et al. 1972) and that barbiturates enhance GABA action (Olsen 1982). Therefore, it is possible that the SS frequency increase might be due to the removal of a background inhibition which is present only or mainly under barbiturate anesthesia. If so, the tonic inhibitory action of the olivocerebellar pathway on the PC would have little physiological significance. The aim of the present experiments is to show that the SS frequency increase due to the inactivation of the CF input does not depend on the presence of an anesthetic agent which interferes with GABA inhibition.

In six Wistar rats the IO has been destroyed bilaterally by means of 3-acetylpyridine (3–AP) 3-5 days before recording the PC activity. During the recording session, the rats head was held to a bar through a nut fixed to the skull by means of dental cement under halothane anesthesia. The cerebellum was then exposed and the general anesthesia discontinued, while lidocaine was applied to the wound. At least 1 h later we started recording the unitary activity. The average spontaneous SS frequency of discharge of 31 PC's recorded from six intact rats similarly prepared was 36.44/s (± 17.1 SD), and that of the CS was 0.54/s (± 0.3 SD). The SS frequency recorded from 25 PC's of the lesioned rats was 53.37/s (± 25.6 SD). The difference of the SS frequency of discharge in the two groups of animals is statistically significant (Mann-Whitney U-test; $p < 0.01$).

In order to confirm on the same PC the data obtained by comparing two different neuronal populations, we have performed a series of experiments on another six rats by recording the activity of each PC before and during IO cooling, as already described (Montarolo et al. 1982). However, the rats were under urethane anesthesia. It is known that this anesthetic does not affect GABAergic inhibition (Roberts et al. 1978; Carrer and Ferreyra 1980). The results have been obtained by recording the activity of 18 PC's. Before cooling the average SS frequency of discharge was 16.21/s (± 15.1 SD), whereas that of the CS was 0.59/s (± 0.5 SD). In 15 of these units the average SS frequency of discharge increased during cooling to 24.25/s (± 12.2 SD). The difference is statistically significant ($p < 0.01$).

---

[1]   Istituto di Fisiologia Umana dell'Università, Corso Raffaello 30, 10125 Torino, Italy

Cerebellar Functions
ed. by Bloedel et al.
© Springer-Verlag Berlin Heidelberg 1984

Fig. 1. Average simple spike frequency of discharge of Purkinje cells recorded in three different experimental conditions. The data relative to the barbiturate anesthesia are taken from the paper by Montarolo et al. (1982). In each condition, *left column* refers to the intact rats and the *right column* to rats with IO inactivation or lesion. *IO* inferior olive; *f* frequency expressed as number of simple spikes in 1 s

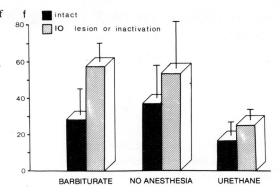

Figure 1 shows the results obtained in our experiments in comparison with those obtained previously under barbiturate anesthesia by Montarolo et al. (1982). It should be noted that the spontaneous SS frequency in the intact unanesthetized rat is higher than in the rat under barbiturate anesthesia. In contrast after IO lesion the two values are similar. This fact indicates that the tonic inhibitory action of the olivocerebellar input on the PC is increased by the barbiturate. This result is in line with the current concept that this anesthetic potentiates GABA action.

Our results show that the reversible inactivation or the lesion of the IO induces a SS frequency increase of the PC also in the unanesthetized animals. This fact suggests that the tonic inhibitory action exerted by the IO on the PC operates also in pyhsiological conditions.

References

Bisti S, Iosif G, Marchesi GF, Strata P (1972) Pharmacological properties of the inhibition in the cerebellar cortex. Exp Brain Res 14: 24-37

Carrer HF, Ferreyra H (1980) Anaesthetic dependent excitability changes in the hypothalamic ventromedial nucleus of the rat. Exp Neurol 67: 524-538

Montarolo PG, Palestini M, Strata P (1982) The inhibitory effect of the olivocerebellar input on the cerebellar Purkinje cells in the rat. J Physiol 332: 187-202

Olsen RW (1982) Drugs interactions at the GABA receptor-ionophore complex. Annu Rev Pharmacol Toxicol 22: 245-277

Roberts F, Taubern PV, Hill RG (1978) The effect of 3-mercaptopropionate, an inhibitor of glutamate decarboxylase, on the levels of GABA and other aminoacids, and on presynaptic inhibition in the rat cuneate nucleus. Neuropharmacology 17: 715-720

Tonic Influence of the Climbing Fiber System on the Postural Activity

C. BATINI[2], J.F. BERNARD[2], P.G. MONTAROLO[1], and P. STRATA[1]

Recent electrophysiological experiments performed by means of reversible inferior olive (IO) cooling (Montarolo et al. 1982; Benedetti et al. 1983) have shown that the climbing fibers (CF), besides inducing phasic patterns of exitation-inhibition sequences, exert a powerful tonic influence on the cerebellar Purkinje cells (PC) and consequently on the intracerebellar nuclei. The net result of suppression of the CF discharge is an increased cortico-nuclear inhibitory effect. It has been suggested (Marchesi and Strata 1971) that the olivo-cerebellar system may be involved in control of postural activity. This "tonic hypothesis" has received further support (Boylls 1978, 1980; Barmack and Hess 1980; Barmack and Simpson 1980; Colin et al. 1980), in addition to the previously mentioned cooling experiments.

It is well known from the literature (see Dow and Moruzzi 1958) that stimulation of the vermis of the cerebellar anterior lobe induces a drastic reduction of the decerebrate rigidity through the inhibition of the vestibulo-spinal and fastigio-reticulo-spinal pathways. On the basis of our experiments (Montarolo et al. 1982; Benedetti et al. 1983), we made the hypothesis that the inactivation of the IO region which projects to the anterior lobe could induce a reduction of the decerebrate extensor tonus.

In order to test this proposal we have used nine cats decerebrated at intercollicular level under fluothane anesthesia. The ventral surface of the medulla overlaying the left inferior olivary region was exposed; a couple of needles was inserted in each forelimb triceps muscle in order to record the electromyographic activity. By means of a cooling probe (1.5 mm diameter tip) we could selectively inactivate the caudal part of the IO. Figure 1 shows that cooling of this part of the IO induces an almost complete disappearance of the electromyographic activity of the contralateral extensor muscle and almost no modification in the ipsilateral one. In 20 out of 37 trials we have obtained similar results. In the remaining 14 trials and when nearby medullary areas were cooled no significant changes were observed in both forelimbs. In three cats a single dose of harmaline was given (15 mg/kg i.v.). After the appearence of the typical tremor, we repeated the cooling trials. In 14 out of 16 tests, inactivation of the caudal IO of one side induced the disappearance of both the tremor and the electromyographic activity only in the contralateral side. No changes were present in the other trials.

From our experiments it seems clear that the tonic effect exerted by the IO on the cerebellar cortex and the intracerebellar nuclei appears to have a powerful influence on the postural activity. Therefore it is reasonable to assume that, in physiological conditions, the informations processed by the cerebellum can also be controlled by the change in the level of the complex spike activity.

[1] Istituto di Fisiologia Umana dell'Università, Corso Raffaello 30, I-10125 Torino, Italy
[2] Laboratoire de Neurophysologie Pharmacologique de l'INSERM (U. 161) 2 rue d'Alesia, F-75014 Paris, France

Cerebellar Functions
ed. by Bloedel et al.
© Springer-Verlag Berlin Heidelberg 1984

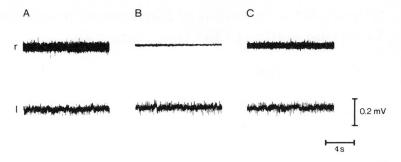

Fig. 1 A-C. Effect of reversible cooling of the left caudal olivary region on the extensor tonus of the forelimbs. The electromyographic records of the left *(l)* and right *(r)* triceps muscles are illustrated. The cooling for 28 s has been applied between **A** (control) and **B. B** and C are taken, respectively, immediately and 48 s after the end of the cooling

Acknowledgement. The experiments have been supported in part by a grant for international collaboration of National Research Council (Italy).

References

Barmack NH, Hess DT (1980) Eye movements evoked by microstimulation of dorsal cap of inferior olive in the rabbit. J Neurophysiol 43: 165-181

Barmack NH, Simpson JI (1980) Effects of microlesions of dorsal cap of inferior olive of rabbits on optokinetic and vestibuloocular reflexes. J Neurophysiol 43: 182-206

Benedetti F, Montarolo PG, Strata P, Tempia F (1983) Inferior olive inactivation decreases the excitability of the intracerebellar and lateral vestibular nuclei in the rat. J Physiol 340: 195-208

Boylls CC (1978) Prolonged alterations of muscle activity induced in locomoting premammilary cats by microstimulation of the inferior olive. Brain Res 159: 445-450

Boylls CC (1980) Contribution to locomotor coordination of an olivo-cerebellar projection to the vermis in the cat: experimental results and theoretical proposals. In: Courville J, Montigny de C, Lamarre Y (eds) The inferior olivary nucleus – anatomy and physiology. Raven Press, New York, pp 321-348

Colin F, Manil J, Desclin JC (1980) The olivocerebellar system. Delayed and slow inhibitory effects: an overlooked salient feature of the cerebellar climbing fibers. Brain Res 187: 3-27

Dow RS, Moruzzi G (1958) The physiology and pathology of the cerebellum. Univ Minnesota Press, Minneapolis

Marchesi GF, Strata P (1971) Mossy and climbing fiber activity during phasic and tonic phenomena of sleep. Pflueger's Arch 223: 219-240

Montarolo PG, Palestini M, Strata P (1982) The inhibitory effect of the olivocerebellar input on the cerebellar Purkinje cells in the rat. J Physiol 332: 187-202

Sensory Representation of Movement Parameters in the Cerebellar Cortex of the Decerebrate Cat

F.P. KOLB and F.J. RUBIA [1]

1 Introduction

Each organism interacts with the environment in two ways: (1) Information from the 3-dimensional external space, considered as the reference frame, is transmitted as the sensory input to the n-dimensional internal space. (2) Information from the internal space, transmitted as the motor output, has to be adjusted to the external space.

If one accepts this mathematical concept, described in detail by Pellionisz and Llinás (1980, 1982), then parts of the central nervous system can be interpreted as a n-dimensional system, or, mathematically expressed, as a n-dimensional hyperspace, which is endowed with data processing facilities. An intended movement does not necessarily depend on external geometrical properties. Therefore the intention can be regarded as an internal activity vector, which is invariant to the reference frame. On the other hand, the sum of physical stimuli can be seen as an external vector, which is independent of the internal space. Thus, one of the tasks of biological networks is the coordination of these two vectors. This coordination will be accomplished by different nervous structures. The cerebellum seems to be predominantly involved in these problems, since its intermediate part receives the sensory feedback information as well as the motor output signal from the motor cortex.

One of our aims was to investigate the sensory feedback information, which is evoked by passive limb movements. Responses to hand manipulations (Thach, 1967), to limb positions, or to squeezing and touching (Konorski and Tarnecki, 1970; Tarnecki and Konorski, 1970) have been described qualitatively. With reproducible movements these results were supported by Rushmer et al. (1976), Rubia and Kolb (1978), Kolb and Rubia (1980), Ebner and Bloedel (1981b, c), Ebner et al. (1983) and Bloedel et al. (1983). On the other hand, Armstrong et al. (1973) reported no specific relationship between cerebellar Purkinje cell firing and to limb position.

The results presented here deal with the representation of movement parameters up to their second derivative in the cerebellar cortex. In particular two aspects will be discussed. (1) What kind of parameters are forwarded to the cerebellar cortex? (2) How are these signals integrated within the cerebellar cortex?

[1]   Institute of Physiology, University of Munich, Pettenkoferstr. 12, 8000 Munich 2, FRG

Cerebellar Functions
ed. by Bloedel et al.
© Springer-Verlag Berlin Heidelberg 1984

2 Methods

2.1 Surgery

All the experiments were performed on adult cats, weighing 3 ± 0.5 kg. Under initial ether anesthesia, or in some cases under a short lasting barbiturate anesthesia (Thiopental, Hormonchemie, or Thiogenal, E. Merck), both femoral veins and one artery were catheterized. The external carotid arteries were tied. The animal, which was mounted in a stererotaxic headframe, was decerebrated at the intercollicular level. To avoid spontaneous or reflex movements, the animals were paralyzed by injections of Pancuronium (Organon) and artificially respired. Throughout the experiment arterial blood pressure, rectal temperature and expired CO_2 were monitored. Temperature and CO_2 were regulated to $37° \pm 1°C$ and 3-4 Vol % respectively. The cerebellar cortex was exposed at least two hr after decerebration. The dura was removed and the surface was covered with agar gel.

2.2 Natural Stimulation

The cat's left forepaw was passively moved around the wrist joint by an electronically controlled device. All the movements started from a low position (ϕ_L) and went up in the plantar-dorsal direction to a high position (ϕ_H) and back. The horizontal plane was defined as the zero position (see Fig. 1). The movements followed a time function, which was calculated in a minicomputer and stored on its memory (Nicolet MED-80 System). During data recording the movement function was scanned by the computer and fed to the electronic control device for positioning the paw.

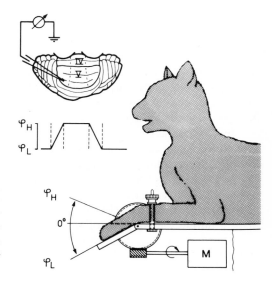

Fig. 1. Experimental design. The cat's forepaw was moved around the wrist joint. The movement always started from a low holding position ϕ_L and proceeded with a constant velocity to a high holding position ϕ_H. The upper part shows the anterior view of the cerebellum with ispilateral intermediate part of lobule Vc, from which unit activity was recorded. (After Rubia and Kolb, 1978)

2.3 Recording and Data Analysis

It is generally accepted that the sensory representation area of the cat's forepaw in the ipsilateral, intermediate cerebellar anterior lobe. By recording field potentials, the most significant responses to natural stimulation were obtained in sublobule Vc. In this area, single unit activity was recorded with glass micropipettes, filled with 3 mol/l NaCl, having a resistance of 2-3 $M\Omega$ at 170 Hz. The microelectrode was driven by a micromanipulator in steps of $2 \mu m$. The electrode was mounted so that recording tracks were perpendicular to the surface of the cerebellar cortex (18 deg lateral with respect to the sagittal plane). The recorded signals were band-pass-filtered and conventionally amplified by a factor of 1000. The signals were fed to a simple-voltage-level discriminator in order to obtain series of events. For the analysis of Purkinje cells two such discriminators as well as a logic circuit were used to reliably separate CS from SS activity (see Kolb, 1983). The computer was used on-line to construct Peristimulus-Time-Histograms (PSTH) with a binwidth of 5 ms; a data block of 1024 bins resulted in the 5.12 s timebase of the histograms. The binwidth was changed off-line to 40 ms by summing 8 bins.

In order to obtain an objective criterion whether the histograms showed time-locked responses or not, a statistical method derived by Weiss (1964) was used. Only those histograms are assumed to be responsive, which exceeded a significance level of 2σ.

The histograms obtained during linear ramp shaped movements have 4 characteristic sections: the time when the paw is at the low holding or at the high holding position (static sections) and the times during the upward or downward movement (dynamic sections). To characterize the unit activity, the first and second moment (i.e. linear and quadratic mean value) as well as the 95% confidence limits of the mean value were calculated from these characteristic sections of the histogram.

2.4 Unit Identification

Several criteria for unit identification have been reported (e.g., Thach, 1967; Eccles et al. 1971a, b). Units were identified as Purkinje cells either by the spontaneously occurring or by an evoked CS after electrical peripheral stimulation. For this purpose the superficial radial nerve was stimulated with square voltage-pulses of 0.5 ms duration and with an intensity of 10 times the threshold with respect to the occurrence of the field potentials within the cerebellar cortex.

Spike potentials from presumed MF appeared with a latency of 3-5 ms after electrical forelimb nerve stimulation and *before* the N_2 wave of the field potential. Furthermore, typical burst discharges with 2-6 spikes with frequencies of 600-800Hz were observed. The spikes were initially positive having an amplitude of about 5 mV. The unit could be kept isolated over an electrode displacement up to 100 μm.

Units, presumed to be GrC, showed a somewhat longer latency than MF, and discharged during the N_2-wave of the evoked field potential. Burst discharges also occured but less regularly than those of MF and with a larger variance of the frequency (300 to 1000 Hz). The spike amplitude was not greater than 2 mV and was very sensitive to small electrode movements. Generally, units could not be isolated over more than 5-10 μm.

3 Results

Out of a total of 902 cerebellar units identified according to the criteria mentioned above, there were 556 (61.5%) Purkinje cells, 163 (18%) mossy fibers and 183 (20.5%) granule cells.

Among the different types of movement functions, the linear ramp shaped function was mostly used (83%), since the different movement parameters can be best distinguished from each other. Non-linear ramp functions (quadratic) and sinusoidal functions were also used.

During ramp shaped movements those discharge patterns which exceeded a significance level of at least 2σ were classified into three different types. This has been qualitatively reported by Rubia and Kolb (1978) and quantitatively by Kolb (1981). *Type A* patterns were characterized by an increase of the unit activity only during the dynamic sections of the movements. The amount of increase was about the same during the upward and the downward movement. During the static sections of the movement no spikes or only insignificant discharges occurred (e.g. Fig. 6A). *Type B* patterns showed an increase of the unit activity preferentially during the upward movement and its following phase of high holding position (e.g. Fig. 2A, C). *Type C* patterns showed an opposite behavior to type B, i.e. an increase of unit activity preponderantly during the downward movement and its following phase of low holding position.

3.1 Responses to Static Parameters

The dependence of statistically significant unit activity on static parameters was tested in 25% of MF, 29% of GrC, 32% of CS and 41% of SS. Only those units, which were tested with at least three different sets of movement parameters, were considered. Information about the momentary position of the limb is transmitted in two different ways. (1) It can be directly coded by different tonic discharge rates, when the paw is at the low or high holding position respectively. (2) Without a change in tonic discharge, it can be indirectly coded by the phasic increase (or decrease) of unit activity, related to the momentary position during the dynamic phases of the movement. In Fig. 2A movements with an amplitude of 5 deg were applied within a range of -30° to +10°. The responses of two MF are illustrated with Peristimulus-Time-Histograms (PSTH, only highest and lowest starting positions), with a stackplot of all histograms (traces in the foreground are related to movements with negative starting positions) and with a graph of the unit discharge probability plotted against the parameter position. The MF responded to this type of ramp movement with an increase of unit discharge during the upward movement and with an increased tonic activity at the high holding position, whereas nearly no spikes occurred during the downward movement and at the low holding position. Furthermore, it can be seen qualitatively in the stackplot of Fig. 2A and quantitatively in the graph of the discharge probability, that the higher the high holding position, the higher the tonic discharge during this phase of movement. Other MF were found showing an opposite behaviour (Fig. 2B). These patterns are of type C, i.e. increased activity at the low holding position and during the downward

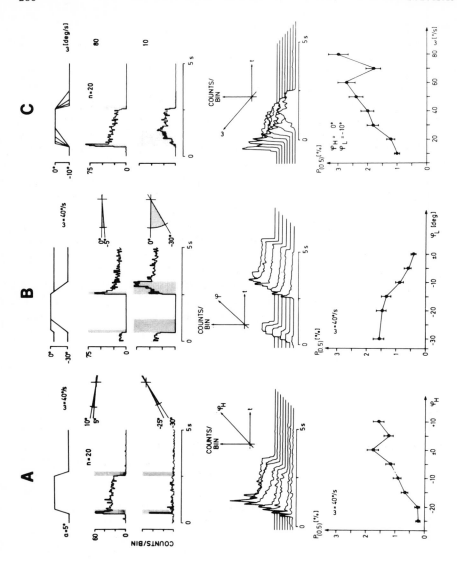

Fig. 2 A-C. Responses of two mossy fibers (one in **A** and **C**, the other in **B**) to the parameter position (**A** and **B**) and velocity (**C**). *Top line* mechanograms. *Below* two selected Peristimulus time histograms (PSTH). Middle part: Stackplots of all histograms obtained during different stimulations. *Bottom* Graph of the discharge probabilities of the unit against the tested parameter (ϕ_H in **A**, ϕ_L in **B** and ω in **C**). In these and all such following graphs the 95% confidence limits are included. For the PSTH here and in all subsequent figures: *Ordinate* counts/bin; *abscissa* time in s; dynamic sections on ramp movements are shaded and the number of sweeps are expressed by n. To the *right* of each PSTH is the actual movement amplitude or the tested velocity. Stackplot arrangements: PSTH obtained from the lowest starting positions in the foreground (**A**), in the background (**B**) and obtained during the lowest velocity in the foreground (**C**)

movement and no spikes during the upward movement and at the high holding position. In contrast to the MF of Fig. 2A, this example shows a negative correlation between starting position and tonic discharge probability, with the lower the starting
position the higher the unit discharge. At the MF input of the cerebellar cortex the
static parameters high and low holding positions are only separately transmitted. At
the neuronal level of GrC similar patterns were obtained, albeit more differentiated
with respect to higher derivatives of the movement function. On the other hand, at
this level (the first location of integration within the cerebellar cortex) patterns were
found, which possibly result from a convergence of synergistic as well as from antagonistic origins. Figure 3 shows the responses of two different GrC to ramp shaped
movements with a constant amplitude of 5 deg and a constant velocity of 40 deg/s,
applied in the ranges -20 deg to +20 deg (Fig. 3A) and -45 deg to +15 deg (Fig. 3B).
Both stackplots are arranged with the histograms obtained at more negative levels in
the foreground. The unit in Fig. 3A was of the B-type and showed response strengths,
which can be well related to both the high and low holding positions: the higher the
position the higher the discharge probability. Among all the units recorded and classified as MF, discharge patterns like these were never observed, since MF of type B
usually showed insignificant activity at the low holding position. The patterns of the
GrC in Fig. 3B are not homogeneous over the tested range. In the histograms obtained

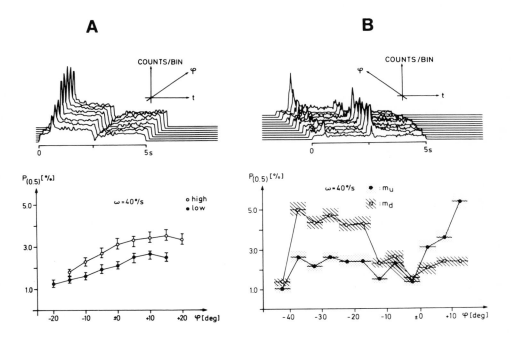

Fig. 3 A-B. Responses of two different granule cells illustrated by stackplots (arranged with histograms obtained from the lowest starting position in the foreground). Discharge probabilities of the
unit are calculated during the phases of high and low holding positions (**A**) and during the upward
(m_u) and downward (m_d) movement (**B**)

at positive starting positions (background of the stackplot), the discharge rate during the upward movement exceeds that during the downward movement (type B). The opposite behavior holds for movements starting from lower levels (foreground of the stackplots). Here the unit exhibits an increase of activity during the downward movement and its following phase of low holding position (type C). The alteration of discharge pattern as a function of the starting position may be interpreted as a convergence of unit activities of two different (possibly antagonistic) origins. Thus, the static information is transmitted, but only if it is associated with dynamic components, which we term the indirect coding of a static parameter.

It has been reported in several studies that the climbing fiber system is able to transmit information about natural peripheral stimulation (Eccles et al., 1972a, b, Leicht et al., 1973; Ishikawa et al., 1972a, b; Maekawa and Simpson, 1972; Simpson and Alley, 1974). Moreover, the climbing fiber system is capable of conveying information about static parameters via a tonic discharge (Kolb and Rubia, 1980). It should be emphasized that this group of olivary neurons is a minority, since the complex spike (CS) activity of the PC is primarily involved in dynamic processes. The mode of direct coding is observed in less than 3% of the units, whereas static information indirectly encoded was

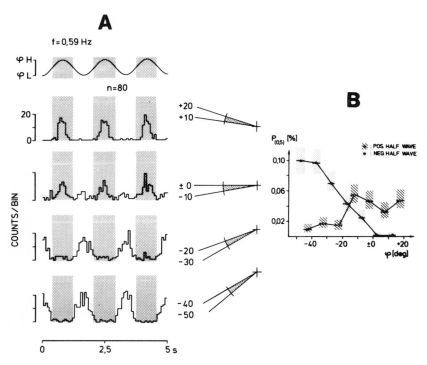

Fig. 4 A, B. Purkinje cell responding with the complex spike to sinusoidal movements with a frequency of 0.59 Hz. The sections of the positive halfwaves are shaded in the movement function as well as in the histograms (A). The unit's mean discharge probabilities are calculated within the positive and the negative halfwaves and are plotted against the tested position (B). (After Kolb and Rubia, 1980)

found more frequently. For these cases, sinusoidal movement functions seemed to be the appropriate stimulus, since the position stimulus is always associated with phase shifted dynamic stimuli. The responses of a PC discharging with the CS to sinusoidal movements is shown in Fig. 4. The frequency was 0.59 Hz with an amplitude of 10 deg. The movement was applied from different starting positions within the range -50 deg to +20 deg. The sections of the positive halfwaves of the sinusoidal function are marked. If one compares the responses to only the positive halfwave obtained at more positive starting positions, a positive correlation between the mean unit activity during the positive halfwave and the starting position can be recognized. A reciprocal behavior is true for the responses to the negative halfwave. In particular between -40 deg and +5 deg an accurate, linear relationship was found (see Fig. 4B). Thus, this change of the response patterns is not a shift in time, it is a shift according to the location within the tested range. These discharge patterns can be compared with those of the GrC in Fig. 3B. Depending on the starting position, both units show a reciprocal behavior with respect to the direction of the movement.

At the level of the PC discharging with SS, correlated responses to changes of static parameters over such a wide range as often observed on MF or GrC have not been found. This may be easily understood if one imagines the large scale of integration at this level; Figure 5 shows the responses of the SS of a PC to ramp shaped movements with an amplitude of 5 deg and a constant velocity of 40 deg/s, applied within the range -35

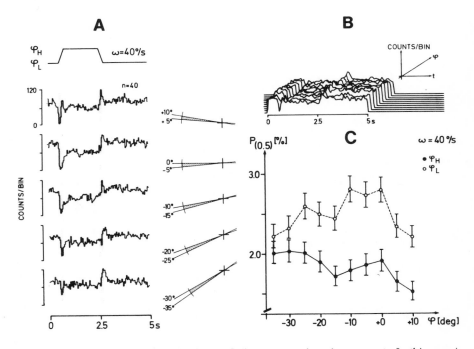

Fig. 5 A-C. Purkinje cell responding with Simple Spikes to ramp shaped movements. In this experiment the starting position was varied and the movement amplitude was always 5 deg. **A** PSTH. **B** Stackplots of all histograms; **C** The PC discharge probability, calculated during the phases of high and low holding positions

deg to 10 deg. The SS patterns obtained at the different levels were little affected by the absolute limb position. From the graph of the discharge probability versus low or high holding position (Fig. 5C), it can be assumed that a relationship exists only within certain small ranges. It has to be emphasized that this unit is the best sample of all the PC, where an analysis of the parameter position was performed.

3.2 Responses to Dynamic Parameters

In contrast to responses to static parameters, where both positive as well as negative correlations could be established, only positive correlations of the discharges of MF, GrC and the CS of PC to the parameter velocity were found. In 11% of MF, 39% of GrC, 28% of PC discharging with CS and 20% with SS the relationship between unit activity and movement velocity was studied.

The responses of a MF to the parameter velocity are presented in Fig. 2C. Ramp shaped movements were applied with 8 different velocities, with a constant amplitude of 10 deg and always starting from a position of -10 deg. The discharge probability increased by about a factor of 3 when the velocities were changed over about one decade. This is the maximal value we could find, which also holds for the climbing fibre system. One might expect that patterns without change in tonic discharges (patterns in which static information is not directly coded) would show a higher sensitivity to dynamic parameters. In Fig. 6 the responses of a GrC of type A to the same change of velocities

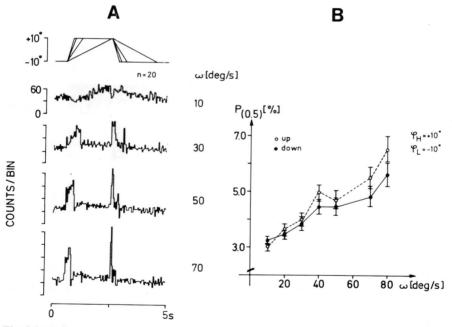

Fig. 6 A, B. Responses of a granule cell to ramp shaped movements with different velocites. **A** PSTH with the movement velocity to the right; **B** The granule cell's discharge probability, calculated during the upward and downward movement

(10 deg/s to 80 deg/s) as studied with the MF in Fig. 2C are shown. The discharge probability is 2.2 times higher during the upward movement with a velocity of 80 deg/s than with 10 deg/s. For the downward movement, the probability increase is 1.8. This is less than for the MF described above.

Purkinje cells discharging with CS are very sensitive to the parameter velocity. This has already been reported by Kolb and Rubia (1980). However, there was no single PC discharging with the SS, which showed statistically significant responses dependent on the velocity.

During ramp shaped movements, the acceleration signals cannot be accurately determined. Units often respond to these signals with short lasting peaks of increased frequency, which are evident in some previous figures (Fig. 2 and 6). In order to produce a gradual change in acceleration we usually applied ramp functions with quadratic increase and decrease in position, or sinusoidal movement functions with constant amplitude and logarithmic increasing and decreasing frequency. The latter function has the additional advantage, that during one presentation of the movement, continuously changing values of the acceleration occur. In Fig. 7A, such a movement function together with the CS responses of a PC is shown. The relative maxima of the averaged discharge rate of the unit lie approximately on a power function, which suggests that the activity was related preferentially to the derivatives of the movement function. This was tested by calculating the Pearson correlation coefficients between the histogram and the movement function or its derivatives. For the calculation (see Fig. 7B), the

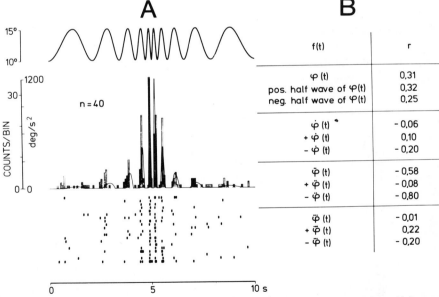

Fig. 7 A, B. A Purkinje cell discharging with the complex spike responding to a sinusoidal movement with a constant amplitude and logarithmic increasing and decreasing frequency. *Solid line* superimposed on the PSTH represents the absolute value of the negative acceleration; **B** Table of Pearson correlation coefficients *(r)* between PSTH in **A** and different functions [f(t)]. These are: Sinusoidal movement up to and including the third derivatives and their positive and negative values. (Kolb and Rubia, 1980)

complete function and their positive and negative values were separately used. The correlation coefficients range between +1 and -1. The best correlation was found between the averaged discharge rate and the negative acceleration, which is graphically superimposed on the histogram. Similar results were obtained by recording from MF, GrC, and the SS of the PC.

The results described so far are from single experiments and thus do not allow quantitative comparison. Therefore, we tried to compare the dynamic responses with the static responses by using scatter-plot techniques. Figure 8 shows plots of the different types of cerebellar units we recorded from. In order to have comparable results, only histograms were taken which showed statistically significant time-locked responses, which were obtained during ramp shaped movements with an amplitude of 30 deg, a starting position of -30 deg and a constant velocity of 40 deg/s. The data were calculated from a modified contrast formula and can cover values between +1 and -1. The dynamic response i.e. the contrast of the quadratic mean values of the activities during both dynamic sections of the movements, is plotted against the static contrast (see Kolb (1981) for more details). It can be seen (Fig. 8) that at levels with a low scale of integration (MF and GrC), both the static and dynamic responses occur. However, at the level of the PC, a level with a high degree of convergence, information about dynamic parameters is preferentially forwarded, especially that of the upward movement.

4 Discussion

4.1 Unit Identification

There is no doubt about the identification of Purkinje cells (PC). In agreement with Thach (1967, 1968, 1970a, b) and Eccles et al. (1971b) the best accepted criterion is

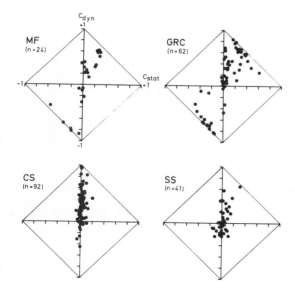

Fig. 8. Scatterplots of the different types of cerebellar units. Histograms, with statistically significant time locked responses, obtained during linear ramp shaped movements (ϕ_L = -30 deg, ϕ_H = 0 deg and ω = 40 deg/s). The dynamic contrast (i.e., the contrast between unit activity during the upward and that during the downward movement) is plotted against the static contrast (see text)

the appearance of both the mossy fiber-granule cell evoked SS and the climbing fiber-evoked CS. Even if no spontaneous CS occurs, cells can be identified as PC by eliciting CS using nerve-stimulation. As criteria for identfication of units as mossy fibers (MF) the spike size, the frequency of burst discharge, the unit isolation, and the short latency after peripheral nerve stimulation (Thach, 1967; Eccles et al., 1971a; Rubia and Kolb, 1978) are generally accepted. The crucial criterion, however, is the occurrence of a spike before the N_2 wave of the evoked field potential. It is possible that by using this criterion, only MF with the fastest conduction velocity are selected. Thus, many putative MF were rejected when this latter criterion was not fulfilled. This aspect has to be taken into account when the discharge patterns of MF are discussed. Units can be identified as granule cells (GrC) with considerable reliability by applying the criteria mentioned in the methods section, which are based on studies by Thach (1967) and Eccles et al. (1971a). However, a reliable identification can only be performed by a local parallel fiber stimulation, close to the place of recording, to evoke a Golgi cell inhibition. This test, which was originally induced by Eccles et al. (1966) is appropriate on GrC situated within the first GrC layer. We usually recorded down to a depth of 5 mm from the surface. Thus, with the exception of the first 700-800 μm of the recording track, this criterion was not testable.

4.2 Pattern Classification

All the discharge patterns presented in the form of PSTH, which exceeded a significance level of 2 δ, could be classified into one of 3 discharge types. This classification seemed to be very useful for an adequate description of the unit activity. The different types were first described qualitatively by Rubia and Kolb (1978) and have been carefully studied and quantified by Kolb (1981). From the specific shape of a histogram and consequently from its abstraction to a characteristic, well defined discharge type, conclusions about the pattern generating mechanism can be derived.

Although the different types were not restricted to a given location within the recorded sublobule, type A patterns were predominantly found within superficial parts of the cerebellar cortex. Since type A patterns are characterized by only phasic responses, it is likely that these patterns were generated by exteroceptors. For the MF system this agrees well with the findings of Ekerot and Larson (1972), who reported that the exteroceptive component of the cuneocerebellar tract terminates in the superficial zones of the cerebellar cortex. With respect to the climbing fiber system, distal cutaneous afferents ascending via the DF-SOCP and the DLF-SOCP terminate in the C_1 and C_3 zones of the intermediate part of the cerebellar anterior lobe (Rushmer et al., 1976; Ekerot et al. 1979).

The type B and C patterns showed mutually opposite behavior. The activity may be generated by the same types of receptors, which are antagonistically situated with respect to their specific functions. This aspect can already be deduced from the comparison of only single histogram of each type and particularly by the change of patterns obtained within the tested range (see Fig. 2A and B). According to the studies of Burgess et al. (1982), the parameter "joint position" appears to be signalled to an important degree by the level of activity in two populations of afferent fibers, each from antagonistic muscles or muscle groups. This was called an "opponent frequency code". This holds for other types of receptors, e.g. the slowly adapting mechanoreceptors described by Jänig (1970).

4.3 Information Transmission of Movement Parameters

A movement process changing joint position can be described as being composed of different parameters according to its time function and its derivatives. At the peripheral level, these stimuli are more or less selectively detected by cutaneous, articular, and muscle receptors. There are several studies reporting responses in the cerebellar cortex to adequate stimulation of cutaneous and muscle receptors (Eccles et al., 1972a, b, c, d; Leicht et al., 1973; Ishikawa et al. 1972a, b; Iosif et al., 1972). Less is known about information conveyed to the cerebellum from articular nerves. This is not surprising since in careful studies about the afferent activity of the articular nerve supplying the cat knee joint, it was assumed that the articular receptors are not capable of providing appreciable steady state position information (Clark and Burgess (1975), Clark (1975) and Grigg (1975)). It was concluded that for "position sense", muscle receptors are involved, whereas the central nervous system must be equipped to extract a reliable position signal from spindle discharge (Burgess et al., 1982). It is generally accepted that muscle spindle afferents convey the different movement parameters. This has been extensively studied by several groups (Grüsser and Thiele, 1968; Schäfer and Schäfer, 1969; Brown et al., 1969 and Matthews, 1972). By using ramp shaped lengthening of the cat soleus muscle in the absence of fusimotor activity, differences between the discharge of primary and secondary endings were obtained (Matthews, 1972). There is a greater sensitivity of primary endings to dynamic stimuli in comparison with that of secondary endings. In addition, as a consequence of the non-linear behavior of the primary endings, there is a greater sensitivity to small than to large stimuli. Such behavior is much less marked for the secondary endings (Matthews, 1972).

4.3.1 Responses at the Cerebellar Input Level

From the results presented in this study it can be stated that all parameters of a passive limb movement up to and including the second derivative are conveyed to the input of the cerebellar cortex. Tonic responses, directly related to limb positions, which were varied in a wide range are shown for MF in Fig. 2A and B in a few cases for the CS activity of PC (see Fig. 1, in Kolb and Rubia, 1980). These patterns are similar to tonic responses to passive limb movements of presumed MF applied in the awake monkey (Bauswein et al., 1984). In the present study, it can be seen that the high and low holding positions are transmitted separately via the MF input to the cerebellar cortex (Fig. 2A and B). There was either a positive correlation between unit activity and high holding position (type B, Fig. 2A) or a negative correlation between unit discharge and low holding position (type C, Fib. 2B). At this neuronal level we never found activity which signalled both static positions. This may result from the selection according to the latency criterion we used for the identification of MF. Thus, the recordings shown here are probably from high conduction velocity afferents originating in the primary endings of non-linearly behaving muscle spindles.

The parameter velocity was signalled by MF as well as CS of the PC usually showing a good positive correlation (see e.g. Fig. 2C).

4.3.2 Responses at the Granule Cell Level

At the level of granule cells (GrC) (the first location of integration within the cerebellar cortex) comparable patterns to those recorded from MF were also found. However, additional patterns were observed, which showed responses to both high and low holding positions. With these units a longer latency in comparison to that of MF is accepted, so secondary endings of muscle receptors have to be taken into account. Since these afferents do not show such a non-linear behavior as primary endings, the different patterns of Fig. 3A may be generated by this type of receptor afferent. Furthermore, patterns were obtained, which obviously result from a convergence of type B and C units (Fig. 3B). At the present stage of research it cannot be stated, whether this convergence takes place at the GrC-level or at precerebellar neuronal sites.

4.3.3 Responses at the Cerebellar Output Level

Comparable patterns of convergence also have to be considered in the climbing fiber system (Fig. 4A). However, this phenomenon has only been observed with sinusoidal movements, where static and dynamic parameters are not separated from each other. This aspect implies that the climbing fiber system is able to transmit information about static parameters, but preponderantly at those times when dynamic parameters are also conveyed. We term this the indirect mode of static information transmission. There are several studies dealing with the PC discharge during activation of different types of receptors in an extremity (Thach (1967), Konorski and Tarnecki (1970), Tarnecki and Konorski, 1970). With electrically controlled, passive movements, Rushmer et al. (1976) elicited climbing fiber responses to very small forepaw displacements of only 50 μm. The authors concluded that the climbing fiber acts as an "event marker", but from our own results with ramp shaped and sinusoidal movements (Kolb and Rubia, 1980), we have to expand this concept. In this sense, the climbing fiber system is not only an unspecific system for transmitting information about the occurrence of an event, it is also a system which precisely conveys specific information about the time course of passive movements. Therefore, the CS patterns reported by Rushmer et al. (1976) can be interpreted as an overlapping of velocity and acceleration responses. With respect to the SS activity, no clear dependence on the absolute limb position could be detected (see Fig. 5). The tonic SS discharge was not consistently correlated to the high or low holding position. This effect may result from the enormous convergence of integrated information onto a single PC. With these responses evoked by a passive movement our results agree with the findings mentioned above (Thach, 1967; Konorski and Tarnecki, 1970; Tarnecki and Konorski, 1970). Moreover, in the SS activity of the PC in Fig. 5, there is a difference in the tonic discharge during the phase of high and low holding position, and this difference is fairly constant over a wide range (see Fig. 5C). A time dependent adaptation process for signalling only relative displacements may be one important factor. With the applied type of ramp shaped movement, the limb position was changed by a displacement of 5 deg every 2.5 s, which was transmitted by this PC. The construction of all the histograms obtained at different starting positions took about 2000 s. Since most of the histograms do not differ significantly from each other, one may conclude that only short term variations are recognized by the SS. This may also be one of the reasons, why Armstrong et al. (1973) recorded no change in the discharge rate of 120 PS in response to changes in limb position. They used displacements of large amplitudes, and kept the extremity in each tested position for at least two min.

In the awake monkey, passive hand movements also elicited changes in the CS and SS activity (Bauswein et al., 1983, 1984). From a total of 149 PC recorded, tonic discharge in relation to hand position was never observed in the CS. However, one well documented cell discharges with different SS rates over a range of 55 deg. In contrast, tonic discharges of the SS were found when the monkey had to hold a handle against a mechanical stop (Thach, 1970b) or a constant load (Gilbert and Thach, 1977). However, in these experiments the hand position was associated with contraction of flexor and/or extensor muscles. Comparable results concerning the relation between somatosensory cortex activity and position and force have been recently reported by Jennings et al. (1983). In 89% of the neurons tested, the activity was related to both the limb position and the torque; very few neurons responded only to position or to torque. Furthermore, activity due to static parameters was also found in interpositus neurons of the awake cat (Burton and Onoda, 1978; Cody et al., 1981) and in neurons of the intact monkey (Thach, 1970a, 1978). The activity may supposedly be generated by MF collaterals.

Concerning the information transmission of the parameter position, one can conclude for the SS of the PC that the absolute value of limb positions is either transformed to another form of signal, which, for example, corresponds only to the relative position changes of the limb, or it has preferentially facilitative tasks, for example, setting the gain of the force on correcting movements.

The transmission of dynamic parameters by the climbing fiber system has been studied in detail (Kolb and Rubia, 1980) and can be seen in Fig. 7. No relation was found between SS activity and velocity. These findings agree with the results of our experiments with the intact monkey (Bauswein et al. 1984). Only a minority of PC, discharging with the SS, responded to passive movements (Harvey et al., 1977; Bauswein et al., 1984), but in these cases a specific relationship to this parameter could not be established. However, velocity related responses were obtained when active movements were performed (Mano and Yamamoto, 1980), or when interpositus neurons were recorded (Burton and Onoda, 1978; Cody et al. 1981). Considering only the SS activity as the large scale integrated MF input, one might interpret the disappearance of the specific velocity responses as the effect of the convergence onto one PC of velocity information from different sources. This information probably originates from functionally antagonistic muscles and can be recorded selectively at the cerebellar input. It is possibly integrated into a nonspecific pattern, which can be obtained at the level of PC during passive movements.

Furthermore, one must take into account that the responsiveness of the SS activity of a given PC may be altered by the climbing fiber input. This has been recently studied by Ebner and Bloedel (1981a, b, c). By means of generalized autocorrelation methods, the authors impressively showed an interdependence between the two types of spikes. This could be modified by the application of natural, peripheral stimulation, consisting of brief flexions of the forepaw. In further studies (Ebner et al., 1983; Bloedel et al., 1983) they showed the selective influence of the CS evoked by natural stimulation upon the SS of one single PC or up to three neighbouring PC (See Bloedel et al. this Vol.).

In a previous study (Rubia and Kolb, 1978) we divided PC into four different groups according to the relationship between CS and SS discharge during the movement. The first group (47%) was characterized by an increase of CS activity, which was associated with a decrease of SS activity and vice versa. Within the second group (22%) the averaged discharge rate of both types of spikes was either increased or decreased in a parallel fashion during the same phase of the movement. Since the CS activity is usually positively related to the velocity, the first group of PC should show negatively correlated SS activity, and the second group positively correlated SS activity. In fact, in seven PC such a trend with three positively and four negatively related SS activity was observed. However, these changes were so weak that they did not exceed the statistical significance level of 2σ. Whether these alterations result from information directed via the MF input, or from the effect of the climbing fiber activity, cannot be decided at the present stage of research. Absolute values of the different movement parameters are transmitted to the input of the cerebellar cortex, where they could be also verified. Since the CS patterns directly reflect the climbing fiber input, the complete output patterns (CS+ SS) of the cerebellar cortex contain specific information about movement parameters and to some extent their absolute values. In contrast, the SS patterns usually do not show information about specific parameters of a passive movement, but only relative changes. Therefore, the computation within the MF system is still unclear. Presumably the precisely transmitted movement parameters play a facilitatory role by cooperating with other parameters, such as force, this should be tested in future experiments using more sophisticated methods.

Acknowledgement. We are very grateful to Dr. Martin Galvan for improving the English. Furthermore we would like to thank Miss Luise Kargl for her helpful assistance during the experiments and for typing the manuscript. The study was supported by the Deutsche Forschungsgemeinschaft (Ru 177/12-9).

References

Armstrong DM, Cogdell B, Harvey RJ (1973) Firing patterns of Purkinje cells in the cat cerebellum for dfferent maintained positions of the limbs. Brain Res 50: 452-456

Bauswein E, Kolb FP, Leimbeck B, Rubia FJ (1983) Simple and complex spike activity of cerebellar Purkinje cells during active and passive movements. J Physiol 339: 379-394

Bauswein E, Kolb FP, Rubia FJ (1984) Cerebellar feedback signals of a passive hand movement in the awake monkey. Pflueger's Arch (submitted)

Bloedel JR, Ebner TJ, Yu QX (1983) Increased responsiveness of Purkinje cells associated with climbing fiber inputs to neighboring neurons. J Neurophysiol 50: 220-239

Brown MC, Goodwin GM, Matthews PBC (1969) After effects of fusimotor stimulation on the response of muscle spindle primary afferent endings. J Physiol 205: 677-694

Burgess PR, Wei JY, Clark FJ, Simon J (1982) Signaling of kinesthetic information by peripheral sensory receptors. Annu Rev Neurosci 5: 171-187

Burton JE, Onoda N (1978) Dependence of the activity of interpositus and red nucleus neurons on sensory input data generated by movement. Brain Res 152: 41-63

Clark FJ (1975) Information signaled by sensory fibers in medial articular nerve. J Neurophysiol 38: 1464-1472

Clark FJ, Burgess PR (1975) Slowly adapting receptors in cat knee joint: Can they signal joint angle? J Neurophysiol 38: 1448-1463

Cody FWJ, Moore RB, Richardson HC (1981) Patterns of activity evoked in cerebellar interpositus nuclear neurones by natural somatosensory stimuli in awake cats. J Physiol 317: 1-20

Ebner TJ, Bloedel JR (1981a) Temporal patterning in simple spike discharge of Purkinje cells and its relationship to climbing fiber activity. J Neurophysiol 45: 933-947

Ebner TJ, Bloedel JR (1981b) Correlation between activity of Purkinje cells and its modification by natural peripheral stimuli. J Neurphysiol 45: 948-961

Ebner TJ, Bloedel JR (1981c) Role of climbing fiber afferent input in determining responsiveness of Purkinje cells to mossy fiber inputs. J Neurophysiol 45: 962-971

Ebner TJ, Yu QX, Bloedel JR (1983) Increase of Purkinje cell gain associated with naturally activated climbing fiber input. J Neurophysiol 50: 205-219

Eccles JC, Llinás R, Sasaki K (1966) The mossy fibre-granule cell relay of the cerebellum and its inhibitory control by Golgi cells. Exp Brain Res 1: 82-101

Eccles JC, Faber DS, Murphy JT, Sabah NH, Táboříková H (1971a) Afferent volleys in limb nerves influencing impulse discharges in cerebellar cortex. I. In mossy fibers and granule cells. Exp Brain Res 13: 15-35

Eccles JC, Faber DS, Murphy JT, Sabah NH, Táboříková H (1971b) Afferent volleys in limb nerves influencing impulse discharges in cerebellar cortex. II. In Purkyně cells by mossy fibre input. Exp Brain Res 15: 484-497

Eccles JC, Sabah NH, Schmidt RF, Táboříková H (1972a) Cutaneous mechnoreceptors influencing impulse discharges in cerebellar cortex. I. In mossy fibres. Exp Brain Res 15: 245-260

Eccles JC, Sabah NH, Schmidt RF, Táboříková H (1972b) Cutaneous mechanoreceptors influencing impulse discharge in cerebellar cortex. II. In Purkyne cells by mossy fibre input. Exp Brain Res 15: 261-277

Eccles JC, Sabah NH, Schmidt RF, Táboříková H (1972c) Cutaneous mechanoreceptors influencing impulse discharge in cerebellar cortex. III. In Purkyne cells by climbing fibre input. Exp Brain Res 15: 484-497

Eccles JC, Sabah NH, Schmidt RF, Táboříková H (1972d) Integration by Purkinje cells of mossy and climbing fiber inputs from cutaneous mechanoreceptors. Exp Brain Res 15: 498-520

Ekerot CF, Larson B (1972) Differential termination of the exteroceptive and proprioceptive components of the cuneocerebellar tract. Brain Res 36: 420-424

Ekerot CF, Larson B, Oscarsson O (1979) Information carried by the spinocerebellar paths. In: Granit R, Pompeiano O (eds) Reflex control of posture and movement, vol 50. Elsevier/North Holland Biomedical Press Amsterdam, pp 79-90

Gilbert PFC, Thach WT (1977) Purkinje cell activity during motor learning. Brain Res 128: 309-328

Grigg P (1975) Mechanical factors influencing response of joint afferent neurons from the cat knee. J Neurophysiol 38: 1473-1484

Grüsser OJ, Thiele B (1968) Reaktion primärer und sekundärer Muskelspindelafferenzen auf sinusförmige mechanische Reizung. Pflueger's Arch 300: 161-184

Harvey RJ, Porter R, Rawson JA (1977) The natural discharges of Purkinje cells in paravermal regions V and VI of the monkey's cerebellum. J Physiol 271: 515-536

Iosif G, Pompeiano O, Strata P, Thoden U (1972) The effect of stimulation of spindle receptors and Golgi tendon organs on the cerebellar anterior lobe. II. Responses of Purkinje cells to sinusoidal stretch or contraction of hindlimb extensor muscle. Arch Ital Biol 110: 502-542

Ishikawa K, Kawaguchi S, Rowe MJ (1972a) Actions of afferent impulses from muscle receptors on cerebellar Purkinje cells. I. Responses to muscle vibration. Exp Brain Res 15: 177-193

Ishikawa K, Kawaguchi S, Rowe MJ (1972b) Actions of afferent impulses from muscle receptors on cerebellar Purkinje cells. II. Responses to muscle contraction, effects mediated via the climbing fibre pathway. Exp Brain Res 16: 104-114

Jänig W, Schmidt RF, Zimmermann M (1970) Single unit responses and the total afferent outflow from the cat's foot pad upon mechanical stimulation. Exp Brain Res 6: 100-115

Jennings A, Lamour Y, Solis H, Fromm C (1983) Somatosensory cortex activity related to position and force. J Neurophysiol 49: 1216-1229

Kolb FP (1981) Die Sensomotorik der Kleinhirnrinde. Experimentelle Ergebnisse und Funktions-modell. Inaugural-Diss, Tech Univ Munich

Kolb FP (1983) A simple method for reliable separation of cerebellar Purkinje cell complex and simple spikes. Pflueger's Arch 398: 341-343

Kolb FP, Rubia FJ (1980) Information about peripheral events conveyed to the cerebellum via the climbing fibre system in the decerebrate cat. Exp Brain Res 38: 363-373

Konorski J, Tarnecki R (1970) Purkinje cells in the cerebellum: Their responses to postural stimuli in cats. Proc Natl Acad Sci (Pol) 65: 892-897

Leicht R, Rowe MJ, Schmidt RF (1973) Cutaneous convergence on to the climbing fiber input to cerebellar Purkinje cells. J Physiol 228: 601-618

Mano NI, Yamamoto KI (1980) Simple-spike activity of cerebellar Purkinje cells related to visually guided wrist tracking movement in the monkey. J Neurophysiol 43: 713-728

Maekawa K, Simpson JI (1972) Climbing fiber activation of Purkinje cells in the flocculus by im-pulses transferred through the visceral pathway. Brain Res 39: 245-251

Matthews PBC (1972) Mammalian muscle receptors and their central actions. Arnold E (ed) LTD London 101-194

Pellionisz A, Llinás R (1980) Tensorial approach to the geometry of brain function: cerebellar co-ordination via a metric tensor. Neuroscience 5: 1125-1136

Pellionisz A, Llinás R (1982) Space-time representation in the brain. The cerebellum as a predic-tive space-time metric tensor. Neuroscience 7: 2949-2970

Rubia FJ, Kolb FP (1978) Responses of cerebellar units to a passive movement in the decerebrate cat. Exp Brain Res 31: 387-401

Rushmer DS, Roberts WJ, Augther GK (1976) Climbing fibre responses of cerebellar Purkinje cells to passive movement of the cat forepaw. Brain Res 106: 1-20

Schäfer SS, Schäfer S (1969) Die Eigenschaften einer primären Muskelspindelafferenz bei rampen-förmiger Dehnung und ihre mathematische Beschreibung. Pflueger's Arch 310: 206-228

Simpson JI, Alley KE (1974) Visual climbing fiber input to rabbit vestibulo-cerebellum: a source of direction-specific information. Brain Res 82: 302-308

Tarnecki R, Konorski J (1970) Patterns responses of Purkinje cells in cats to passive displacements of limbs, squeezing and touching. Acta Nbiol Exp 30:95-119

Thach WT (1967) Somatosensory receptive fields of single units in cat cerebellar cortex. J Neuro-physiol 30: 675-696

Thach WT (1968) Discharge of Purkinje cells and cerebellar nuclear neurons during rapidly alter-nating arm movements in the monkey. J Neurophysiol 31: 785-797

Thach WT (1970a) Discharge of cerebellar neurons related to two maintained postures and two prompt movements. I. Nuclear cell output. J Neurophysiol 33: 527-536

Thach WT (1970b) Discharge of cerebellar neurons related to two maintained postures and two prompt movements. II. Purkinje cell output and input. J Neurophysiol 33: 537-547

Thach WT (1978) Correlation of neural discharge with pattern and force of muscular activity, joint position, and direction of intended next movement in motor cortex and cerebellum. J Neuro-physiol 41: 654-676

Weiss TF (1964) A model for firing patterns of auditory nerve fibers. Tech Rep No 418 Cambridge, MA: Res Lab Electr, Mass Inst Technol

Constraints on Plasticity of Cerebellar Circuitry: Granule Cell-Purkinje Cell Synapses

D.E. HILLMAN and S. CHEN[1]

1 Introduction

The response of the nervous system to traumatic or attritional loss of specific cellular elements, as well as to failure of neurogenesis during development, has been addressed in a number of morphological (see reviews Cotman 1978, Lund 1978, Hillman and Chen 1984b) and physiological (Tsukahara 1981, Lynch et al. 1973) studies. Sprouting of remaining afferent axons from surrounding regions is regarded as the primary mechanism for restoring the number of connections (Liu and Chambers 1958, Westrum 1969, Raisman 1969, Raisman and Field 1973, Cotman and Nadler 1978, Lynch et al. 1975). This type of compensation has been reported in adult animals following partial destruction of afferents, developmental dysgenesis or early neuronal death. Some of these newly formed connections appear to be appropriate (Matthews et al. 1976b, Tsukahara 1981), while many others are aberrant (Westrum 1969, Llinas et al. 1973). The functional role of the latter afferents, if any, has not been determined. In general, the time course for this reorganization is prolonged (Matthews et al. 1976a) and apparently does not begin until 7-14 days after the injury.

A more rapid plasticity than that underlying sprouting was found when synapses formed between axons and dendrites which are in near apposition to each other (McWilliams and Lynch 1981, Chen and Hillman 1982a). Our studies show that this response is triggered in less than 24 hr following parallel fiber transections in the cerebellar cortex in adult animals (Chen and Hillman 1982a). Since parallel fibers normally establish over 90% of the connections on Purkinje cell spines, transections of these axons were expected to modify the ratio of parallel fiber-Purkinje cell connections. In fact within 12-30 hr following transections, all deafferented target sites on Purkinje cell spines were either: (1) occupied by remaining appositional parallel fibers, (2) pushed off by a new contact of a remaining parallel fiber (degenerating and normal bouton on the same postsynaptic site), or, (3) engulfed by glia surrounding the degenerating parallel fiber and the head of the spine. New synapses also appeared to form.

The takeover of deafferented synaptic sites was by axons lying near synapses or those axons that came into contact with dendritic shafts or spines as Bergmann glia became phagocytic. During this response, Bergmann glia processes partially withdrew from their envelopment of the dendritic shafts and spines allowing some parallel fibers

[1] Department of Physiology and Biophysics New York University Medical Center 550 First Avenue New York New York, 10016 USA

Cerebellar Functions
ed. by Bloedel et al.
© Springer-Verlag Berlin Heidelberg 1984

to move into physical contact with the Purkinje cell dendrites. These appositions may be the ones that take over old sites or form new synaptic sites similar to the process occurring during developmental synaptogenesis (Chen and Hillman 1982a). These two means of restoring the number of connections was seen within 12-24 h but was not obvious after 36 h. By 5 days, large reductions in afferent number was sufficient to cause changes in dendritic tree shape and the number of Purkinje cell spines (Chen and Hillman 1982a, b).

In the cerebellum, sprouting of remaining parallel fibers is not a significant consequence since these axons cannot branch effectively. Only short podial extensions were found (Chen and Hillman 1982a). This was because of their apparent lack of branching capability due to insufficient microtubules to recruit free ends needed to sustain an additional process (cf. Hillman 1979). Terminal growth of these axons around shallow lesions in folia was possible but was impeded by pial investment of the scar following transections through the molecular layer. In shallow transections of the folium, tightly packed parallel fibers deviated around the scar after 30 days.

The takeover of old postsynaptic sites, new synapse formation and podial extensions comprise mechanisms attempting to compensate for lost presynaptic sites. However, since the possibility for appositional contacts is also dependent on the number of degenerating parallel fibers (result of glial reaction described above), this response does not even begin to restore the number of synapses needed to match the reduction of afferents, and there is a marked decline in number of sites.

Thus, it is expected that other means of compensation must be taking place to restore and maintain the afferent input level to target neurons. This compensation is evident from a functional point of view since rather large deficits in the number of granule cells of the cerebellum has no readily detectable functional effect (e.g. heterozygous weaver mutants; Rakic and Sidman 1973) and massive reductions are necessary to alter function (e.g. homozygous weaver mutants; Rakic and Sidman 1973, Sotelo 1975 a, b).

2 Changes in the Size of Synaptic Sites

A most striking form of plasticity, recently reported, was the rapid enlargement of presynaptic boutons, postsynaptic spines and synaptic junctions of the parallel fiber-Purkinje cell connections following postnatal malnutrition (Chen and Hillman 1980, Hillman and Chen 1981a, b), parallel fiber lesions (Hillman and Chen 1984a) and neonatal chemical treatment (Yamano et al. 1983). The increased size of the postsynaptic spine heads was marked by a prominence of endoplasmic reticulum. The opposed afferent boutons gained synaptic vesicles in proportion to their increase in size (Chen and Hillman 1980, Hillman and Chen 1981c).

Most consistent was an enlargement in the synaptic contact area of membrane densities. This increase in size of the presynaptic and postsynaptic membrane specialization sites (PrSDs and PoSDs) occurred as equal-added, electron-dense area to most of the synaptic sites (cf. Fig. 1 for definition of terms). The time course of this synaptic plasticity appears to have been initiated within minutes to a few hours and may have

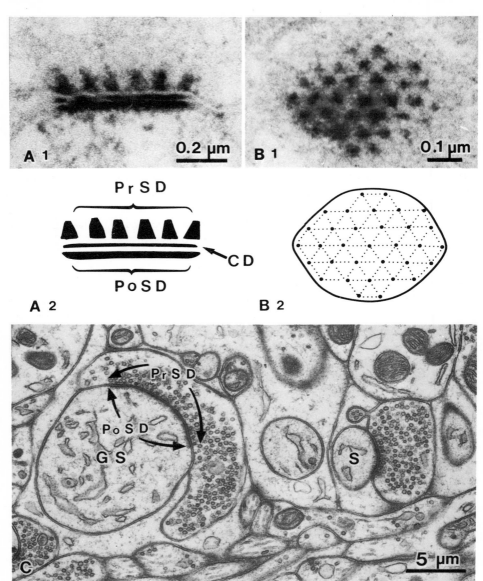

Fig. 1 A-C. The PrSDs and PoSDs of parallel fibers and Purkinje cells are dense membrane specialization (A, B, C). The PrSD and PoSD contact sites are directly opposed to each other and are the same size (note profile of synaptic site in **A1** and **2** and enface view in **B1** and **2**. In EPTA preparations **(A1, B1)**, the enface view shows that the grid composition of the PrSD consists of dense bodies arranged in regular rows **(B1, B2)** and that these densities are predominantly projecting from the inner surface presynaptic membrane. These bodies are round to pyramidal shaped and have been described as projections arranged in a lattice. In sagittal view, a plaque like area *(PoSD)* lines the inside of the postsynaptic membrane **(A1, A2)**. This density is directly opposed to the *PrSD*. An intermembrane density (cleft density, *CD*) is positioned between these two membrane specializations. The two interposed lines without stain are the lipid portions of each membrane (cont'd opposite)

been, for the most part, complete by 36 hr after lesioning the parallel fibers (Chen and Hillman 1982a). The enlargement in synaptic size was correlated to the deficit in the number of synaptic sites from parallel fibers on Purkinje cells (Hillman and Chen 1981b, 1984a).

Enlargement in the size of synaptic sites rather than a significant adding of synaptic sites from the remaining afferents appeared to be the principal means of compensation. This very clear and robust form of compensation may represent an intermediate step to sprouting in other systems and, in the cerebellum, appears to be an alternative to sprouting plasticity.

Other studies addressing the question of changes in area of individual synaptic sites have yielded tenuous results (cf. Hillman and Chen 1984b). Qualitative observations on the Reeler mutant demonstrated gigantic spines with a large contact area (Mariani et al. 1977). Persistence of PoSDs in the absence of afferents has been a consistent finding in a number of brain regions (Herndon 1968, Herndon et al. 1969, Hirano et al. 1972, Matthews et al. 1976a, Raisman et al. 1974, Smolen 1981, Sotelo 1968, 1973, 1975a, b, Taxi 1965, Westrum 1969, Wolff et al. 1979).

The persistence of PoSDs indicates that these sites were determined intrinsic to the neuron and suggest that the total contact area on each neuron might be constant (Chen and Hillman 1980, Hillman and Chen 1981b). Constancy in the amount of PoSD contact area most likely arises from the genome as a very specific control over the amount of macromolecules making up all of the PoSDs on each neuron. Thus, a quantitative study of the size of synapses in relation to the number of sites on each neuron was undertaken. The experimental paradigm was to use a set of perturbatons reducing the number of afferent parallel fiber synapses to Purkinje cells by varying amounts over a range from 0-100%. These sets established a frame of conditions under which the number of synapses and related size could be analyzed for determining if invariant parameters were present.

2.1 Constancy of Total Postsynaptic (PoSD) Contact Area: Reciprocal Relationship Between Number and Size of Synapses

The number and length of the combined PrSD-PoSD profiles of parallel fiber synapses on Purkinje cell spines have been determined in previous studies (Fig. 1c; Hillman and Chen 1981b, 1984a, b). The average values for profile length of the synaptic unit (PrSD-PoSD) were converted to average contact area based on the actual shape of the synaptic contact sites (Hillman and Chen 1981b, 1984a, b). This analysis demonstrated that the

---

In glutaraldehyde-osmium preparations (C), the PrSD-PoSD complex also appears as a dense region of these two membranes. Because the lipid portion of the membrane is also electron dense, this method does not define the components of the site as well as the EPTA method. Together with the synaptic vesicles this complex represents a synaptic site frequently referred to as active zones. Giant spine (GS) and normal sized-spine (S) were found following sectioning of parallel fibers.

Definition of terms: PrSD and PoSD contact area — Extracellular surface area overlying dense staining on respective pre- and postsynaptic membrane specializations.

Synaptic site or synapse — combined pre- and postsynaptic membrane specializations.

Vacant sites — PoSD without a facing PrSD

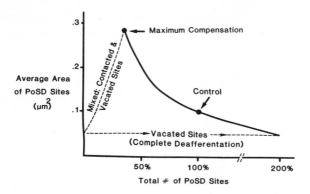

Fig. 2. Changes in the size of postsynaptic membrane specializations *(PoSDs)* over a range of reduction in afferent fibers from 0-100% (for data see Hillman and Chen 1984a). As the number of afferent synapses decreases, there is a reciprocal rise in the average size of sites until the number is reduced to about 65%. Reductions beyond this level began a drop in average size of sites until, at near total reductions, the size of vacant sites was 1/2 that for controls. A marked increase in the number of vacant sites over that of control synaptic sites was found. This corresponded to the doubling of the number of sites demonstrating that the total contact area on each Purkinje cell for these target specializations remained constant throughout the range of reduction between 0-100%

average area of synaptic contact between parallel fibers and Purkinje cells increased as a reciprocal (defined by X=1/Y where X is the number of synapses on each neuron and Y is the average area of the individual sites; cf. Hillman and Chen 1981b, 1984a, Fig. 2). The reciprocal relationship held for reductions in afferent number up to 65%. A reciprocal between area and number of sites demonstrates that total contact area is a constant over this range. (The average length of the synaptic profiles did not follow the reciprocal curve for number and length during this transition, cf. Hillman and Chen 1984a). A constant total contact area on each Purkinje cell was also apparent by calculating the product of the average area of PoSD sites and their number on each Purkinje cell over small ranges of reduction in the number of afferent synapse between 0-65% (Hillman and Chen 1981b, 1984a, cf. formula below).

$$\text{Constant total PoSD contact area} = \frac{\text{Number of sites}}{\text{Neuron}} \times \text{Average area of sites}$$

Each of these small groups, representing a level for reduction in the number of synapses, yielded a constant of about 5350 μm^2 (relative value; Hillman and Chen 1984a).

Afferent reductions slightly over 65% had a decrease in the average size of synaptic junctions and vacant PoSD sites appeared (Fig. 2). These vacant sites in spines were only one-half the size of the synapses on control spines, regardless if the number of synapses on each Purkinje cell was reduced by 65% or 100% (Hillman and Chen 1984a). This was not the case for partially vacant sites since the vacant area of these sites made up a large portion of the site (Hillman and Chen 1984a).

Analysis of the number of PoSDs on each Purkinje cell at maximum reduction of afferent parallel fibers revealed that the number of vacant PoSDs was double the number of contacted PoSD sites on control Purkinje cells (Hillman and Chen 1984a). Thus the total contact area of the PoSDs remained constant throughout the entire range of afferent reduction (0-100%). This indicates that there is a strong intrinsic factor which maintains a relatively consistent amount of PoSD macromolecules inserted into the plasma membrane on each Purkinje cell. Such molecules may include receptors (Kelly et al. 1976), ion channels (Landis and Reese 1974), site organizers (Carlin et al. 1981, Cartaud et al. 1981) as well as attachments sites (Cotman and Taylor, 1972, 1974) for linking with presynaptic structures.

2.2 Modifiability of Total Presynaptic (PrSD) Contact Area of Afferent Neurons

The response of remaining parallel fibers after partial loss is an obvious increase in total contact area of their presynaptic membrane specializations (PrSDs). The major finding supporting this was that the average contact area of presynaptic sites followed the reciprocal curve for a decrease in the number of sites for each target neuron (Fig. 3).

Interestingly, the total presynaptic grid area increased until the total contact area on each granule cell had attained an almost three-fold (200%) increase (Fig. 3). This upper limit occurred at about a 65% reduction in the number of spine synapses on Purkinje cells. At this level, the parallel fiber axons were not able to cover all of the PoSD contact area on the target Purkinje cells and thus vacant PoSDs sites began to appear. The potential for presynaptic sites to fill the available PoSD area is very strong since virtually no vacant sites were found until a 65% reduction in afferents was reached.

This increase in the total contact area of PrSDs was also indicated by the fact that number of grid densities increased for each granule cell. This occurred by adding dense projections to the lattice rows (cf. Fig. 1) of existing sites so that a round to slightly oval shape was maintained.

Thus two major parameters of synaptic size (individual and total PrSD contact area) varied in response to the reduction in the number of sites while one parameter (total PoSD contact area) remained constant. The interpretation of these parameters, with regard to their effect on organization and plasticity of circuitry, is embodied in a concept of CONSTRAINTS.

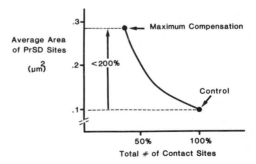

Fig. 3. Changes in the size of presynaptic specializations following the reduction in afferents. Note that a maximum average size of sites occurs when the reduction in afferents reaches 65%

3 Constraints on Plasticity of Synaptic Membrane Specializations

3.1 Total PoSD Contact Area on Each Purkinje Cell: An Invariant Parameter Representing a Primary Constraint to Size of Synapses

The difference in the response between the pre- and the postsynaptic membrane specializations (Fig. 4), namely the constancy of total PoSD contact area and a variability of total PrSD contact area, poses an interesting question regarding the properties of plasticity in the parallel fiber-Purkinje cell synapse. Such a predictability in the size of synapses according to change in the number of sites is suggestive of a constraining mechanism being involved. In other words, the net result of the reduction in the number of these spine sites is that a stabilizing factor represented by the constant total area of PoSD contact on each Purkinje cell forces a change in the average size of synaptic sites. Furthermore, since the parameter, average contact area of sites, is a mathematical function of the parameter, total PoSD contact area on each neuron, and since the total PoSD area is constant while the number of sites is readily varied, one can directly conclude that this constant serves as a highly specific constraint on the average size of sites (Fig. 5). Thus, the constant total amount of PoSD area on each Purkinje cell represents a fundamental parameter related to enlargement of synaptic sites in response to deafferentation but does not necessarily determine the individual sizes of synapses.

The underlying source of this constraining parameter is likely from invariant factors of molecules and macromolecular organization, originating as intrinsic factors (cf. Rakic 1974, Hillman 1979) that are defined by the genome (Hillman and Chen 1981b, 1984b). Such invariants play major roles in organization of organelles responsible for defining neuronal structure, synaptic connections as well as functional processes. Some obvious examples of invariants are seen as constraints from macromolecular structure of antigens and antibodies as well as enzymes involved in specificity of dynamic processes.

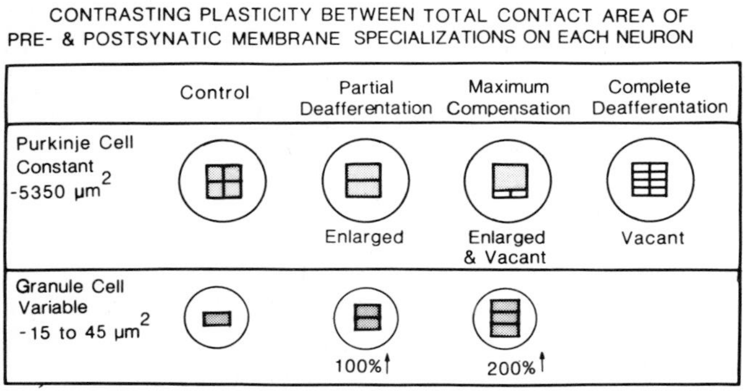

Fig. 4. Relative distribution of total synaptic area and synaptic sizes on target and afferent neurons in response to different degrees of reduction in number of afferent synapses. Note constancy in total contact area of the target and a plasticity in the total area of axonal contacts on afferent neurons. The individual synapses or vacant sites adjust accordingly

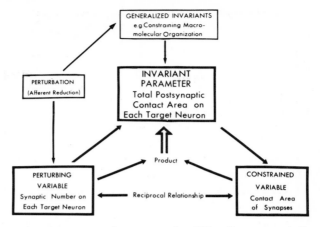

Fig. 5. Relationships between an invariant parameter and two types of variables. One represents the strength of the perturbation (Perturbing Variable) and the other is a variable that is constrained by an invariant (Constrained Variable). The invariant parameter in the example is believed to be closely associated with genetic coding in macromolecules which are the true constraining factors on this dynamic response in plasticity (Generalized Invariant). Various strengths of different types of perturbations (Frame of Conditions), directed at a local area of structural organization, cause a reciprocal response between parameters representing the strength of the perturbation and the variable parameter that is constrained by the invariant factor. The result is that the size of each site enlarges as a reciprocal to the number of sites. The product of the these two variables is invariant through the frame of conditions. The example shown results from a series of levels for reduction in the number of synapses on each target neuron and the effect of the constraining macromolecular organization on the average area of individual synaptic sites

3.1.1 Constraint on the Size of Individual Synapses

The previously described relationship between the invariant in total PoSD contact area and the variability of individual size of synapses are the result of constraints acting during reactive and developmental synaptogenesis. Total PoSD contact area on Purkinje cells of the cerebellum qualifies as an invariant based on the lack of a significant change over the range of perturbations to the number of these sites between 0 and 100% (Hillman and Chen 1981b, 1984a). In addition to the constraint over the individual size of sites, this invariant also had a constraining relationship over the total PrSD contact area of granule cells.

3.1.2 Constraint Over Total PrSD Contact Area

Total area of presynaptic membrane specializations (PrSDs) is variable over a large range of afferent reduction (0-65%). This factor is physically related to the afferent neuron; yet, it responds to the reduction of afferents equal to the individual size of PoSD sites. Thus, it must also be constrained according to the increase in sizes of individual

RELATIONSHIPS BETWEEN CONSTANTS AND VARIABLES
WITHIN A FRAME OF CONDITIONS

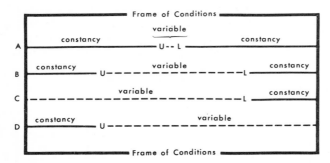

Fig. 6 A-D. Relationship between constants, variables, and frame of conditions defined by a series of perturbations yielding a defined variable range. In **A**, a parameter has two levels of constants, upper and lower values *(U, L)* separated by a variable range of inherent and experimental variations which is very small. The difference between the upper and lower values is significantly small and the parameter can be considered to be a "primary invariant parameter". In **B, C**, and **D**, there is a broad range of conditions where a parameter is variable. In some cases, there is a range of conditions where the variable becomes constant. This may occur at either the upper or the lower level of constancy or at both the upper or lower levels. The importance of these parameters lies in their transitions from variables to constants. This point of change represents a "limitation on the variability" and is a "secondary invariant" since its influence is added to that from the primary type

PoSD sites (Figs. 1, 3, 4, 5, 7). This strongly suggests that the PrSD area must be bound by interactive factors to the amount of PoSD contact area. In this way synaptic connectivity can be adjusted over a large range in response to deficits in the number of afferent neurons (Figures 7 & 8). This parameter is the second essential component to compensation of afferent input to the Purkinje cell.

3.2 Limitations of Variability: Secondary Constraints on Size and Number of Synapses

Secondary constraints occur as maximum and minimum limits of variability (Fig. 6). In the cerebellum, these were limits to which the series of increasing strengths of specific perturbations on the number of synapses could drive the variable, area of individual synaptic sites, through the constraining effect of constancy in total PoSD contact area. A graphic illustration in Fig. 6 shows the relationship between the primary invariant, constancy in total contact area, to the secondary invariant, limit of variability. A parameter represented as A in Fig. 6 is constant throughout a set of defined perturbations (Frame of Conditions) with the exception of a small variability representing inherent and experimental variations. This variability is bound by upper and lower values (U and L) representing two constant levels. Since the variable range is significantly small compared to the overall alteration produced by the series of perturbations (0-100%), this parameter represents the primary invariant previously described.

In contrast, B, C and D have a broad range of conditions where a parameter is variable. These are cases where there is a transition from the variable to a constant value over a relatively wide range within the set of perturbations (Frame of Conditions). This transition can occur at both or either of the upper and lower levels of the variable range. The important aspect of these parameters lies in this transition point acting as a limitation for variabilities. This represents a second type of invariant having a constraining action. Such a transition site is seen in the size of synaptic sites shown in Figs. 2, 3 and 7. The underlying source of these limits is much more complicated than the first type of invariant described but is also likely an expression of factors related to molecular and macromolecular properties while their influence as an invariant is masked over a certain range.

3.2.1 Maximum Limit on Total PrSD Contact Area

One obvious limit is in the maximum amount of total PrSD contact area which can be gained by each afferent granule cell (Figs. 3, 4, 7). This level is reached when the total PrSD area reaches 200% of control values. At this level, PoSD contact sites become vacant and the afferent number reduced by about 65%. The capacity for compensation by parallel fiber-Purkinje cell connections is defined by this limit (Fig. 7).

3.2.2 Maximum Number of PrSD Sites on Each Afferent Neuron

Another constraint appears to be the maximum number of PrSD sites that can occur on each afferent axon. This maximum limit is indicated by studies in the cerebellum (Hillman and Chen 1981b), the optic system (Schneider 1973, 1981) and the superior cervical ganglia (Ostberg et al. 1976). In the cerebellum, the number of sites was limited to 150 for each parallel fiber (Hillman and Chen 1981b, Table 1, column F) in a malnutrition study in the rat. Quantitative analysis of synapses in superior cervical ganglia

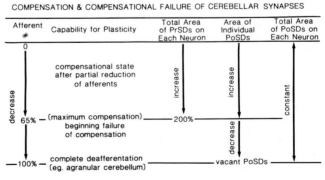

Fig. 7. Capability for plasticity of both granule cell afferents and Purkinje cells as target neurons following 0-100% reduction in the number of afferent synapses. The total area of PoSDs on each target neuron remains constant while total area of PrSDs on afferent neurons increased proportional to the degree of afferent reduction. The average contact area of synaptic sites increased up to about 65% reduction in the number of afferents. Beyond this point the afferent neurons failed to cover all of the constant PoSD area, and vacant PoSD sites appeared. At this level further compensation failed

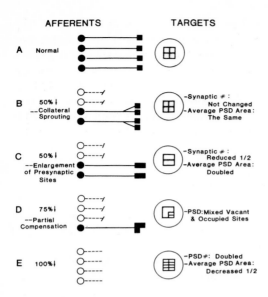

Fig. 8 A-E. Relationship between afferents and target neurons following various levels of reduction in the number of afferent sources. In the cerebellum sprouting is not prominent **(B)**. However, enlargement of target synaptic sites occurred but the total target area on each neuron remained constant. Because the number of afferent sites was reduced, the afferent responded to cover the available target area up to 65%. The area doubled at 50% reduction in number of synaptic sites **(C)**. Above 65% some of the target area became vacant occurring as small vacant sites and as partially covered large postsynaptic sites **(D)**. Complete reduction in afferents resulted in a doubling of the number of target sites that were only one-half the size of controls **(E)**

following axotomy demonstrated that there is a maximum limit to the number of synaptic sites on each axon (Ostberg et al. 1976). Schneider, working on the optic system, found that there was a limit to the length of the axonal arbor and presumed a corresponding limit on the number of synaptic contacts. He indicated that the axonal arbor was smaller if the competition for sites was high, suggesting possible limits on size rather than size being a constant throughout life.

3.2.3 Maximum Number of Synaptic Sites on Each Target Neuron

Studies on the compressed optic tectum suggest that there is a maximum number of sites on each target neuron (Murray, Sharma and Edwards 1982). When the number of afferent fibers to one colliculus was doubled by removal of the contralateral one, the number of sites on targets did not increase. This result was contradicted by Marotte (1981) on the same system, showing up to a 100% increase in the number of synaptic sites when the normal complement of optic nerve axons was allowed to regenerate to a bilaterally halved tectum. Recently, Smolen (1983) demonstrated that there was a maximum limit to the number of sites on neurons of the superior cervical ganglion in the adult rat, while a higher synaptic density was found in adolescent animals.

Results from our studies on the cerebellum indicate that a maximum limit on the number of synaptic sites is present but the source may be the minimum size of contacted sites. A minimum limit on the size of contacted sites (described below) and the constancy of total PoSD contact area could produce a constraint on the number of sites. A maximum number of synaptic sites could be the result of a maximum limit on the number of spines. However, this is unlikely because, when sites become vacant, spine number doubled (Hillman and Chen 1984a). This latter conclusion is further exemplified by the fact that the number of vacant PoSD sites appears constrained by minimum size of these sites (see below).

3.2.4 Minimum Size for Vacant PoSDs Sites on Spines

Our results show that the average area of virtually all vacant PoSD sites on spines is about 1/2 that for contacted sites in control animals (Hillman and Chen 1984a). The minimum size of PoSD vacant spine sites is consistent whether perturbations are produced in the adult following normal development of circuitry or in agranular cerebella produced by mutations, X-irradiation, viruses or chemicals all resulting in abnormal development (Hillman and Chen 1981). However, these small sizes are not characteristic of vacant PoSDs on dendritic shafts or somas (Pinching 1969, Somogyi et al. 1982, Sotelo 1978). This would suggest that factors of spines allow minimum limits to be met while those of dendrites do not.

When all excitatory afferents are removed, the number of vacant PoSD sites is maximal. This is believed to be due to a limit on minimum size of vacant sites and the constancy in total contact area of PoSDs.

3.2.5 Minimum Size of Synapses

A number of findings indicate that there might be a minimum size of PoSD-contacted sites. Recent studies showed that number of synapses on targets was maximally limited when the ratio of afferent neurons to the number of targets was doubled (Murray et al. 1982). A maximum number of synaptic sites may not be due to a limit on the actual number of sites but rather to a minimum size for each synapse. When the number of afferent neurons is normal, an optimum minimal size of contacted sites is maintained. Adding afferents apparently does not change the size or number of synaptic sites on the target (Murray et al. 1982). Thus since the total contact area is constant, the total number of synapses on each target neuron could be further constrained by a minimal size limit of synapses. We hypothesize that there is a minimum size for functional sites; however, the optimum operational size is somewhat larger than this minimum.

The source of this minimum size limit for contacted sites may be set by limits on the size of each presynaptic grid structure rather than by the postsynaptic membrane specializations. Commonly the smallest sites on spines are composed of seven dense projections. This lattice structure occurs as projections arranged in three rows of two-three-two (see Fig. 1 B_2). The area of this PrSD is equal to about the smallest synaptic site. Early developing synapses have dense sites which are smaller than seven dense projections. These small putative PrSD sites do not have particles associated with membranes as found in freeze-fractured specimens of mature synapses (Landis 1983). This suggests that dense projections may not develop at very small sites.

3.2.6 Minmum Total PrSD Area Limiting Cell Survival

A minimum total contact area for presynaptic membrane specializations is not well defined but is suggested by retrograde cell degeneration. For example in mutant mice, Staggerer and Nervous, a lack of PoSD targets results in granule cell death (Sotelo and Changeux 1974, Sotelo 1979, Sotelo and Triller 1979). It has been postulated that once a certain minimum target area is reached, the afferent neuron may not have sufficient target interactions to sustain its functional integrity and as a result undergoes neuronal death (Bleier 1969, Udin and Schneider 1981, Lewis and Cotman 1980, Cowan 1973, Aguaya et al. 1976).

4 Maintaining Efficacy of Synapses: Macromolecular Reorganization of PoSDs and Increase in PrSD Area

One of the major considerations regards the purpose of the response in the size of synapses. The obvious implication is that efficacy is being maintained by the constancy in total contact area of the target when afferent connections are lost. The findings described above suggest that the level of total contact area by the afferent parallel fibers can increase until a certain limit is met. Possible mechanisms for this process are that the PoSDs increase in area by incorporation of macromolecules from old sites or newly synthesized molecules which arrive from a pool and insert in remaining PoSD sites. The change in the size of PoSD sites could occur within a normal turnover of macromolecules occurring between a cytoplasmic pool and the plasma membrane (Hillman and Chen 1984b). In this way, the total PoSD contact area is maintained and also the presynaptic neurons are stimulated to increase the amount of PrSD contact area to cover the PoSD sites. In addition, there is both an increase in the number of synaptic vesicles and an enlargement of the PrSD contact area to cover the available target area (Figs. 1, 3). These apparent changes occur very rapidly, allowing the neuron to compensate almost immediately (min to h) following the deafferentation.

These changes in pre- and postsynaptic structure strongly suggest that the efficacy of synapses is maintained. Efficacy of synapses may be represented on the presynaptic side of the synapse as an increase in the number of calcium channels and the number of synaptic vesicles as well as sites for their release. On the postsynaptic neuron, the number of receptor sites and related sodium channels are likely being maintained and represented by the PoSD.

5 Adaptation in Circuitry Through Modification of Relative Synaptic Sizes

Evidence from deafferentation studies shows that total postsynaptic contact area is conserved and total presynaptic specializations of the remaining afferent axons can increase (within certain limits) to cover the conserved PoSD contact area. Therefore, the individual size of sites is tightly linked to the number of afferent synapses on each neuron. This leaves almost no margin for adaptation in the size of synapses unless the number of sites is changed. One exception is that the relative size of synapses from different afferents on the target neuron can change. This modulation would be a small shift of the PoSD macromolecules between differents synapses (Fig. 9) while each afferent source gains or loses some of its PrSD structures (dense projections).

The resulting change in the relative area of contact from one afferent source neuron to another may represent the circuitry component of learning. Shifts in the relative size of sites could be the fixation process for ingraining learned information into memory. This status could be maintained until disruption by further neuronal loss allowing relearning, or it might continually be reorganizing as other connections are optimized for the learned state.

Change in the relative size of synapses may be represented by varied sizes of PoSD sites following deafferentation (Chen and Hillman 1982a, Hillman and Chen 1981c, 1984a) or deficits of afferent neurons due to developmental malnutrition (Hillman and Chen 1981b). An intriguing observation is that the distribution of synaptic sizes increases as the number of afferents is decreased. This could be interpreted as a greater number of synapses having a smaller difference in synaptic sizes because there are more synapses, between which the differences can be divided. In contrast, smaller total number of synapses are expected to have larger differences since there are fewer sites for distributing these differences. The proposed small shift in size of sites is difficult to measure since there may not be a change in average size of sites (Fig. 9, compare B and C).

SUBTLE PLASTICITY

--Remolding of Individual Synaptic
Sizes Without Rewiring The Circuitry

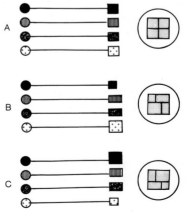

Fig. 9 A-C. The hypothetical effect of relative shifts in the size of synapses on targets among different source afferents **(A, B)**. Note that the influence of each afferent neuron can be changed between sources by taking over area from other sites or giving up some of the area of their contact sites. In **A**, the set of newly developed synaptic junctions are all in equal size. As the developmental molding of the circuit occurs the relative area shifts between sites without making or breaking connections. Finally in **C**, the remodelling of the relative synaptic sizes is depicted following effects on circuits in other parts of the nervous system. Note the average area does not change

6 Conclusions

A major recent finding in the cerebellum is that total contact area of postsynaptic membrane specializations is invariant when the number of excitatory afferents to Purkinje cell spines was altered between 0-100%. In contrast, the total contact area of afferent axons readily increases to fill the conserved area of target sites as the number of afferents decreases. The resulting effect was a rapid change in the size of synapses between parallel fibers and Purkinje cells as a primary means of restoring a constant afferent contact area on target sites of deafferented Purkinje cells. Restoring the number of afferent sites by synapse formation from opposed and possibly terminal growth of the axon may also occur to some degree.

The compensation in total area of contact by the parallel fiber-Purkinje cell synapses had limits. The total contact area which could be gained by each afferent neuron was about 200%. At this compensatory level (about 65% reduction in the number of sites), PoSDs began to be vacated of afferent contacts. Therefore, the limit for compensation was reached and the Purkinje cell no longer sustained a complete input. Other limits were found on the size and number of synapses as well as vacant sites.

From an analysis of a number of parameters, it is evident that changes in the individual size of synapses was reciprocal to the reduction in number of afferent connections and changed as a result of the constraint from the constancy in "total contact area for excitatory synapses on each target neuron". This invariant parameter of total PoSD contact area was established by demonstrating a reciprocal relationship between the number of these synaptic sites and the average size of synapses occurring over a wide range for modification in the number of synapses. Furthermore, this "constraint" from the postsynaptic neuron also had a control over "total synaptic contact area of afferent neurons" allowing the remaining parallel fibers to cover the vacated portion of the total postsynaptic contact area with presynaptic grid densities. However, secondary constraints from limits on the variable, "total presynaptic contact area", placed a restriction on the range of afferent reductions over which compensatory plasticity in synapse size could take place. The functional implication of the compensation is that the efficacy of the input to the Purkinje cell is maintained over a specific compensatory range but fails once the limit is met. The underlying source of the constraints involved in this plasticity is suggested to be from macromolecular organization and is closely controlled through the genome.

References

Aguaya AT, Peyronnard JM, Terry LC, Romine JS, Bray GM (1976) Neonatal neuronal loss in rat superior cervical ganglia: retrograde effects on developing preganglionic axons and Schwann cells. J Neurocytol 5: 137-155

Bleier R (1969) Retrograde transsynaptic cellular degeneration in mammillary and ventral tegmental nuclei following limbic decortication in rabbits of various ages. Brain Res 15: 365-393

Carlin RK, Grab DJ, Siekevietz P (1981) Function of calmodulin in postsynaptic densities. III. Calmodulin-binding protein of the postsynaptic density. J Cell Biol 89: 449-455

Cartaud J, Sobel A, Rousselet A, Devaux PF, Changeux JP (1981) Consequences of alkaline treatment for the ultrastructure of the acetylcholine receptor-rich membranes from Torpedo marmorata electric organ. J Cell Biol 90: 418-429

Chen S, Hillman DE (1980) Giant spines and enlarged synapses induced in Purkinje cells by malnutrition. Brain Res 187: 487-493

Chen S, Hillman DE (1982a) Plasticity of the parallel fiber-Purkinje cell synapse by spine takeover and new synapse formation in the adult rat. Brain Res 240: 205-220

Chen S, Hillman DE (1982b) Marked reorganization of Purkinje cell dendrites and spines to adult rat following vacating of synapses due to deafferentation. Brain Res 245: 131-135

Cotman CW (1978) Neuronal plasticity. Raven Press, New York

Cotman CW, Nadler JV (1978) Reactive synaptogenesis in the hippocampus. In: Cotman CW (ed) Neuronal plasticity. Raven Press, New York, pp 229-260

Cotman CW, Taylor D (1972) Isolation and structural studies on synaptic complexes from rat brain. J Cell Biol 55: 696

Cotman CW, Taylor D (1974) Localization and characterization of concanavalin. A receptor in the synaptic cleft. J Cell Biol 62: 236-242

Cowan WM (1973) Neuronal death as a regulative mechanism in the control of cell number in the nervous system. In: Rockstein MC, Sussman ML (ed) Development and aging in the nervous system. Academic Press, London New York, pp 19-41

Herndon RM (1968) Thiophen induced granule cell necrosis in the rat cerebellum: An electron microscopic study. Exp Brain Res 6: 49-68

Herndon RM, Margolis G, Kilham L (1969) Virus-induced cerebellar malformation. An electron microscope study. J Neuropathol Exp Neurol 28: 164

Hillman DE (1979) Neuronal shape parameters and substructures as a basis of neuronal form. In: Schmidt FO, Worden FW (eds) The neurosciences: fourth study program. MIT Press, Cambridge, pp 477-498

Hillman DE, Chen S (1981a) Vulnerability of cerebellar development in malnutrition. I. Quantitation of layer volume and neuron numbers. Neuroscience 6: 1249-1262

Hillman DE, Chen S (1981b) Vulnerability of cerebellar development in malnutrition. II. Intrinsic determination of total synaptic areas on Purkinje cell spines. Neuroscience 6: 1263-1275

Hillman DE, Chen S (1981c) Plasticity of synaptic size with constancy of total synaptic contact area on Purkinje cells in the cerebellum. In: Vidrio FA, Galina MA (ed) Symp proc XI Int Congr Anat. Alan Liss, New York, pp 229-245

Hillman DE, Chen S (1984a) Reciprocal relationship between size of postsynaptic densities and their number: Constancy in contact area. Brain Res (in press)

Hillman DE, Chen S (1984b) Plasticity in the size of pre- and postsynaptic membrane specializations. In: Cotman C (ed) Synaptic plasticity and remodelling. Guilford Press, New York

Hirano A, Dembitzer HM, Jones M (1972) An electron microscope study of cycasin-induced cerebellar alteration. J Neuropathol Exp Neurol 31: 113-125

Kelly P, Cotman CW, Gentry C, Nicolson GL (1976) Distribution and mobility of lectin receptors on synaptic membranes of identified neurons in the central nervous system. J Cell Biol 71: 487-496

Landis D (1983) Formation of synaptic junctions during postnatal development in cerebellar cortex. Soc Neurosci Abst 9: 1176

Landis DM, Reese TS (1974) Differences in membrane structure between excitatory and inhibitory synapses in the cerebellar cortex. J Comp Neurol 155: 93-126

Lewis E, Cotman CW (1980) Factors specifying the development of synaptic number in the rat dentate gyrus: Effects of partial target loss. Brain Res 191: 35-52

Liu CN, Chambers WW (1958) Intraspinal sprouting of dorsal root axons. Arch Neurol Psychiat 79: 46-61

Llinas R, Hillman DE, Precht W (1973) Neuronal circuit reorganization in mammalian agranular cerebellar cortex. J Neurobiol 4: 69-94

Lund RD (1978) Development and plasticity of the brain. Oxford Univ Press, New York

Lynch G, Deadwyler S, Cotman CW (1973) Post-lesion axonal growth produces permanent functional connections. Science 180: 1364-1366

Lynch G, Rose G, Gall C, Cotman CW (1975) The response of the dentate gyrus to partial deafferentation. In: Santini M (ed) Golgi centennial symposium proceedings. Raven Press, New
York, pp 505-517

Mariani J, Crepel F, Mikoshiba K, Changeux JP, Sotelo C (1977) Anatomical physiological and biochemical studies of the cerebellum from Reeler mutant mouse. Philos Trans R Soc London Ser
B 281: 1-28

Marotte LR (1981) Density of optic terminals in half tecta of goldfish with compressed retinotectal
projections. Neuroscience 6 (4): 679-702

Matthews DA, Cotman CW, Lynch GS (1976a) A quantitative ultrastructural analysis of synaptic
changes in the rat dentate gyrus following entorhinal lesions. I. Magnitude and time course of
degeneration. Brain Res 115: 1-21

Matthews DA, Cotman C, Lynch G (1976b) A quantitative ultrastructural analysis of synaptic
changes in the rat dentate gyrus following entorhinal lesions. II. Re-acquisition of morphologically normal synaptic contacts. Brain Res 115: 23-41

McWilliams JR, Lynch G (1981) Sprouting in the hippocampus is accompanied by an increase in
coated vesicles. Brain Res 211: 158-164

Murray M, Sharma S, Edwards MA (1982) Target regulation of synaptic number in the compressed
retinocortical projection of the goldfish. J Comp Neurol 209: 374-385

Ostberg A-JC, Raisman G, Field PM, Iversen LL, Zigmond RE (1976) A quantitative comparison of
the formation of synapses in the rat superior cervical sympathetic ganglion by its own and by
foreign nerve fibers. Brain Res 107: 445-470

Pinching AJ (1969) Persistence of postsynaptic membrane thickenings after degeneration of olfactory
nerves. Brain Res 16: 277-281

Raisman G (1969) Neuronal plasticity in the septal nuclei of the adult rat. Brain Res 14: 25-48

Raisman G, Field PM (1973) A quantitative investigation of the development of collateral reinnervation after partial deafferentation of the septal nuclei. Brain Res 50: 241-264

Raisman G, Field PM, Ostberg AJC, Iversen LL, Zigmond RE (1974) A quantitative ultrastructural
and biochemical analysis of the process of reinnervation of superior cervical ganglion in the adult
rat. Brain Res 71: 1-16

Rakic P (1974) Intrinsic and extrinsic factors influencing the shape of neurons and their assembly
into neuronal circuits. In: Seeman P, Brown GM (eds) Frontiers in neurology and neuroscience
research. Univ Toronto, pp 112-132

Rakic P, Sidman RL (1973) Organization of cerebellar cortex secondary to deficit of granule cells
in Weaver mutant mice. J Comp Neurol 152: 133-162

Schneider GE (1973) Early lesions of superior colliculus: Factors affecting the formation of abnormal relational projections. Brain Behav Evol 8: 73-109

Schneider GE (1981) Early lesions and abnormal neuronal connections. TINS July 187-192

Smolen AJ (1981) Postnatal development of ganglionic neurons in the absence of preganglionic input. – Morphological observations in synapse formation. Dev Brain Res 1: 49-58

Smolen AJ (1983) Retrograde transneuronal regulation of the afferent innervation to the rat superior
cervical sympathetic ganglion. J Neurocytol 12: 27-45

Somogyi J, Hamori J, Silakov VL (1982) Free postsynaptic sites in the lateral geniculate nucleus of
adult cats following chronic decortication. Cell Tiss Res 225: 437-442

Sotelo C (1968) Permanence of postsynaptic specialization in the frog sympathetic ganglion cells
after denervation. Exp Brain Res 6: 294-305

Sotelo C (1973) Permanence and fate of paramembranous synaptic specializations in "mutants"
and experimental animals. Brain Res 62: 345-351

Sotelo C (1975a) Synaptic remodeling in mutants and experimental animals. In: Vital-Durand F,
Jeannerod M (eds) Aspects of neural plasticity, vol 43, pp 167-190

Sotelo C (1975b) Anatomical, physiological and biochemical studies of the cerebellum from mutant
mice. II. Morphological study of cerebellar cortical neurons and circuits in the Weaver mouse.
Brain Res 94: 9-44

Sotelo C (1978) Purkinje cell ontogeny: Formation and maintenance of spines. In Corner MA,
Baker RE, Van DE, Pol NE, Swaab DF, Uyling HBW (eds) Progress in brain research: maturation of the nervous system, vol 48, pp 149-168

Sotelo C (1979) Synaptic stabilization – comparative studies on the cerebellum of staggerer and nervous mutant mice. In: Meisami E, Brazier MAB (eds) Neural growth and differentiation. Raven Press, New York

Sotelo C, Changeux JP (1974) Transsynaptic degeneration 'en cascade' in the cerebellar cortex of staggerer mutant mice. Brain Res 67: 519-526

Sotelo C, Triller A (1979) Fate of presynaptic afferents to Purkinje cells in the adult nervous mutant mouse: A model to study presynaptic stabilization. Brain Res 175: 11-36

Taxi J (1965) Contribution a l'etude des connexions des neurons moterus du system nerveux autonmome. Ann Sci Natl Zool (Paris) 7: 413-674

Tsukahara N (1981) Sprouting and the neuronal basis of learning. TINS (Sept): 234-237

Udin SB, Schneider GE (1981) Compressed retinotectal projection in hamsters: Fewer ganglion cells project to tectum after neonatal tectal lesion. Exp Brain Res 43: 261-269

Westrum LE (1969) Electron microscopy of degeneration in the lateral olfactory tract and plexiform layer of the prepyriform cortex of the rat. Z Zellforsch 98: 157-287

Wolff J, Joo F, Dames EW, Feher O (1979) Induction and maintenance of free postsynaptic membrane thickenings in the adult superior cervical ganglion. J Neurocytol 8: 549-563

Yamano T, Shimada M, Ohno M, Utsunomiya T, Oya N (1983) Synaptic changes in Purkinje cell dendritic spine of mouse cerebellum after neonatal administration of cytosine arabinoside. Acta Neurophysiol 60: 19-23

Comparison Between the Developmental Calendars of the Cerebral and Cerebellar Cortices in a Precocial and an Altricial Rodent

A. SCHÜZ and F.M. HEIN[1]

Changes in the structure of the brain which occur after birth are interesting because they might be, and in part have proven to be, subject to environmental influences. This is true, for instance, for the development of dendritic spines and synapses in the cerebral cortex of mice and rats (f. ex. Cragg 1967, Fifková 1970, Valverde 1971, Winkelmann et al. 1977). However, in precocial animals such as the guinea-pig the majority of spines and synapses in the cerebral cortex develop before birth (Schüz 1981). This makes us hesitant to connect these changes to processes of learning.

Another very striking postnatal change concerns the cerebellum. In rats and mice, humanes etc. the migration of granular cells from the external to the internal granular layer (Fig. 1a) and the connection between parallel fibers and Purkinje cells occur mainly after birth. Here again, learning processes may be suspected to mold the development. In the guinea-pig, however, already at birth most of the granular cells have migrated downwards (Fig. 1b). The external granular layer has become as thin as in a mouse of about two weeks of age. The different cell types have reached already a high degree of maturity as can be seen from Fig. 2: the parallel fibers are well developed, the soma of the Purkinje cells is already smooth, their dendrites extend over the whole thickness of the molecular layer and are densely covered with spines. The inner granular layer is full of mature granular cells showing the typical claws. The Golgi cells, too, have their adult shape. The stellate and basket cells are also well developed. The only striking pecularity on stellate and basket cells compared to the adult seems to be a higher number of long, spinelike appendices on their dendrites and sometimes also on the soma.

Thus, in the cerebellum, too, a developmental calendar seems to be ruling which is not affected by the event of birth happening earlier or late in different species. Consistent results have been found in birds (Saetersdal 1956) and in rats with prolonged gestation time (Zagon 1975).

The decrease in the thickness of the external granular layer is shown for mice and guinea-pigs on a plot that also shows the increase in the number of spines in the cerebral cortex (Fig. 3). In the precocial as well as in the altricial animal the differentiation of the granular layer in the cerebellum is roughly synchronous with the increase in spines in the cerebral cortex, and both processes seem to be completed at about the same time. In the case of the cerebral cortex we gained the impression that the rather explosive development of spines and synapses on pyramidal cells inaugurates the critical period of learning. This anatomical change immediately precedes the first exploration of the world which in the case of rats and mice happens when they begin to leave the

---

[1] Max-Planck-Institut für biologische Kybernetik, Tübingen, FRG

Cerebellar Functions
ed. by Bloedel et al.
© Springer-Verlag Berlin Heidelberg 1984

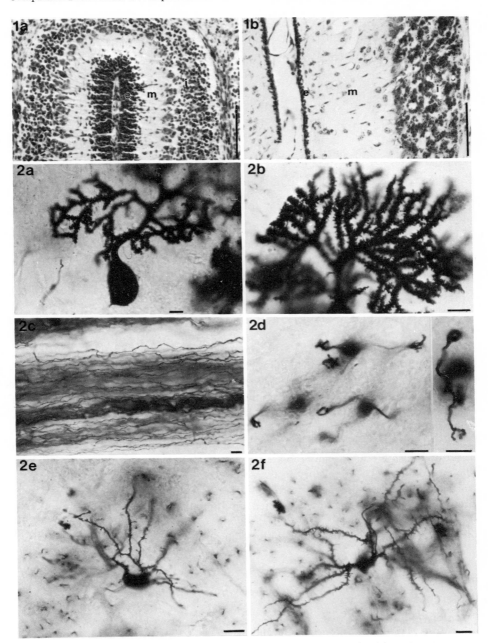

Fig. 1 a-b. Nissl preparation of the cerebellar cortex of an 8-day old mouse (a), and of a newborn guinea-pig (b). *e* external granular layer; *i* internal granular layer; *m* molecular layer. *Bar* 100 μm

Fig. 2 a-f. Stage of development of the different cell types in the cerebellum of the newborn guinea-pig: **a** and **b** Purkinje cells; **c** parallel fibers; **d** granular cells; **e** stellate cell; **f** basket cell. Golgi preparations. *Bar:* 10 μm

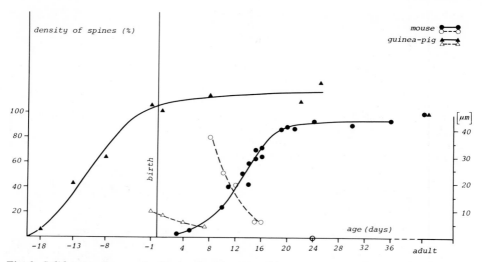

Fig. 3. *Solid curves* increase in the density of spines *(left scale)* along dendrites of pyramidal cells in the cerebral cortex of mice and guinea-pigs. The values for the mouse are taken from Valverde (1971). *Broken curves* decrease in the thickness of the external granular layer *(right scale)* in the cerebellum of the two species

nest, but right after birth in the case of the guinea-pig. We have not yet investigated synapse formation in the cerebellum of the guinea-pig, but for the cerebellum of the mouse it is known (Larramendi 1969) that the synapses between parallel fibers and Purkinje cells are made during the diminution of the external granular layer. The increase in synaptic density in the molecular layer has leveled out even before the disappearance of the external granular layer. If this is also true for the guinea-pig, we may suspect that not only in the cerebral cortex but also in the cerebellum, a learning machine is set up which is ready to incorporate information when the animal begins to discover the environment. The parallelity in the development of the cerebral and the cerebellar cortices could mean that motor learning in the cerebellum as envisaged by Marr (1968) and Albus (1971) is intimately connected with the other kind of learning.

Acknowledgement. We are very grateful to Prof. V. Braitenberg for helpful discussions.

References

Albus J S (1971) A theory of cerebellar function. Math Biosci 10: 25

Cragg B G (1967) Changes in the visual cortex on first exposure of rats to light. Nature (London) 215: 251-253

Fifkova E (1970) The effect of monocular deprivation on the synaptic contacts of the visual cortex. J Neurobiol 1: 285-294

Larramendi L M H (1969) Analysis of synaptogenesis in the cerebellum of the mouse. In: Llinás R (ed) Neurobiology of cerebellar evolution and development. 1st Int Symp Inst Biomed Res, Am Med Assoc/Educ Res Found

Marr D (1968) A theory of cerebellar cortex. J Physiol 202: 437

Saetersdal T A S (1956) On the ontogenesis of the avian cerebellum, part 2. Measurements of the cortical layers. Univ Bergen Arbok Naturvit Rekke 3: 1-53

Schüz A (1981) Pränatale Reifung und postnatale Veränderungen im Cortex des Meerschweinchens: Mikroskopische Auswertung eines natürlichen Deprivationsexperimentes. (English summary). J Hirnforsch 22: 93-127

Valverde F (1971) Rate and extent of recovery from dark rearing in the visual cortex of the mouse. Brain Res 33: 1-11

Winkelmann E, Brauer K, Klütz K (1977) Untersuchungen zur Spinedichte von Lamina-V-Pyramidenzellen im visuellen Cortex von Laborratten nach langdauernder Dunkelaufzucht. J Hirnforsch 18: 21-28

Zagon I S (1975) Prolonged gestation and cerebellar development in the rat. Exp Neurol 46: 69-77

Three Types of Large Nerve Cells in the Granular Layer of the Human Cerebellar Cortex

E. Braak and H. Braak[1]

Morphological classification of nerve cell types is generally done in Golgi preparations. Golgi-impregnated neurons are completely filled with precipitates of silver chromate rendering examination of cytoplasmic details impossible. With a new technique most of the precipitate is dissolved and the remainder is converted to small particles stable enough to withstand various counterstaining procedures. Lipofuscin or other cytoplasmic components can now be stained by suitable techniques.

Most of the nerve cell types in the human brain show a highly characteristic pattern of pigmentation. The size, shape, affinity to aldehydefuchsin, and the pattern of distribution of the lipofuscin granules can serve as excellent criteria for classifying nerve cells (Fig. 1). This can readily be demonstrated by means of the new technique which enables one to perceive simultaneously the pattern of pigmentation of individual nerve cells through transparent Golgi impregnations of their cell bodies and processes.

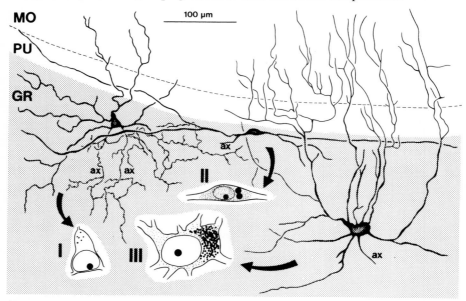

Fig. 1. Three different types of large nerve cells in the granular layer of cerebellum. For further information see text

[1]   Frankfurt (Main), FRG

Cerebellar Functions
ed. by Bloedel et al.
© Springer-Verlag Berlin Heidelberg 1984

Golgi preparations reveal the existence of three types of large nerve cells within the granular layer (GR) of the human cerebellar cortex. Type I cells (I) correspond to the well known Golgi cells. They have a rounded or polygonal cell body with only a few dendrites that radiate in all directions. The axon (ax) ramifies profusely close to the parent soma. Cells of this type are most frequently encountered among the large neurons within the granular layer. Type I neurons contain only a few small lipofuscin pigment granules. Type II cells (II) have a fusiform or triangular cell body with a few rather extended dendrites that rarely ramify. Cells of this type are either devoid of lipofuscin or contain a few large lipofuscin granules stained intensely by aldehydefuchsin. Type III cells (III) are multipolar neurons with a fair number of dendrites originating from any point of the soma. The dendrites extend into the lower two third of the molecular layer (MO). Here and within the Purkinje cell layer (PU) they repeatedly branch off forming a dense dendritic arborization. Most cells of this type are evenly distributed throughout the entire granular layer. Type III cells are filled with tightly packed lipofuscin granules. The various cerebellar folia show differences in the packing density and pattern of distribution of the type III cells.

The pattern of pigmentation is characteristic for each of the three types of large nerve cells. They can therefore be distinguished not only in Golgi preparations but also in simple combined pigment-Nissl preparations.

References

Braak E, Braak H (1983) On three types of large nerve cells in the granular layer of the human cerebellar cortex. Anat Embryol 166: 67-86

Local Circuit Neurons in the Cerebellar Dentate Nucleus of Man

H. BRAAK and E. BRAAK[1]

Golgi preparations reveal the existence of two classes of nerve cells in the human dentate nucleus. Relatively large projection cells (P) predominate. Small local circuit neurons (I) are scattered throughout the nuclear gray. By means of the newly developed de-impregnation technique the pattern of lipofuscin pigmentation of both cell types can be studied (Fig. 1).

The projection cells store a considerable amount of finely granulated and faintly stained pigment, whereas the local circuit neurons contain only a few large and intensely stained lipofuscin granules. The local circuit neurons give off a few smoothly contoured

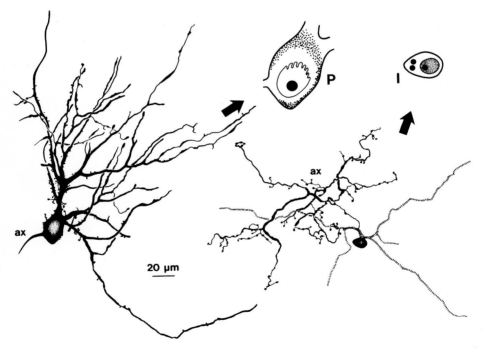

Fig. 1. Large projection cells *(P)* and small local circuit neurons *(I)*. Different patterns of lipofuscin pigmentation

[1]   Frankfurt (Main), FRG

Cerebellar Functions
ed. by Bloedel et al.
© Springer-Verlag Berlin Heidelberg 1984

and rather extended dendrites. The axon (ax) arises either from the cell body or a dendrite by way of a cone-shaped initial portion. A thin thread-like segment follows. Further distally, the caliber of the axon increases abruptly. This thick portion branches several times at short intervals giving off fine processes with bead-like enlargements. Occasionally, a second axon is generated.

The pattern of pigmentation is characteristic for the two classes of nerve cells in the dentate nucleus. Both classes can therefore be distinguished not only in Golgi preparations but also in pigment-Nissl preparations thus rendering quantitative evaluations possible.

References

Braak H, Braak E (1983) Morphological studies of local circuit neurons in the cerebellar dentate nucleus of man. Human Neurobiol 2:49-57

Brain Stem Afferents Bilaterally Branching to the Cat Cerebellar Hemispheres

A. ROSINA and L. PROVINI[1]

It was recently observed (Rosina and Provini 1981) that basilar pontine nuclei (PN) projections to the cat cerebellar hemisphere are more bilateral than previously described. Subsequent work on animals with chronic mid-sagittal section of the cerebellum has shown that this bilaterality can be accounted for by divergent axon collaterals of individual PN neurons, given off at intracerebellar level (Rosina et al. 1980).

However in these experimental conditions it was not possible to evaluate whether those bilateral collaterals only stem from PN neurons whose axon recrosses within the cerebellum (after having crossed within the pons) as the original observations by Rosina and Provini (1981) had suggested, or whether a crossed component is also present.

By using the double-fluorescent retrograde tracing (Kuypers et al. 1980) in a sequential way, an experimental paradigm was designed which allows to recognize the crossed or recrossed components of this interhemispheric transcommissural system, and to evaluate their relative incidence.

If a fluorescent tracer (Fast blue, FB) is injected into the hemisphere of an intact cerebellum it will be retrogradely transported by all classes of PN neurons which project to the cerebellar hemisphere (i.e., neurons A, B, C, D and C', D' of Fig. 1). If a spectrally different fluorescent tracer (Nuclear yellow, NY) is injected into the other hemisphere after cerebellar midsagittal section, it will be retrogradely transported only by those PN neurons whose axon reaches the NY-injected hemisphere via the ipsilateral brachium pontis (i.e., neurons A', B' and C, D of Fig. 1). In fact retrograde transport of the tracer by the intracerebellar axonal branches, either crossed or recrossed, will be prevented.

Thus only the PN neurons whose intracerebellar branches have taken up the FB tracer, first injected (i.e., neurons C and D of Fig. 1) will be double-labeled. As a result

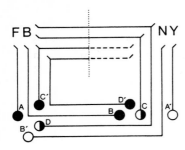

Fig. 1. Schematic representation of the different kinds of projections from pontine nuclei to the cerebellar hemisphere. See text for further explanation

[1]   Istituto di Fisiologia dei Centri Nervosi, CNR, Via Mario Bianco, 9, 20131 Milano, Italy

only one half of the neurons whose axons branch within the cerebellum and link the two cerebellar hemispheres will be double-labeled (i.e., neurons C, D and not C', D' of Fig. 1). Moreover the double-labeled neurons found in the PN ipsilateral to the FB-injected hemisphere (i.e., neurons D) will represent the recrossed component of the system, while double-labeled neurons found in the PN contralateral to the FB-injected hemispere (i.e., neurons C) will represent the crossed component of the system.

This same experimental design allows us to evaluate the crossed or recrossed components of any precerebellar neuronal set projecting bilaterally to the hemispheres by intracerebellar axonal branching.

The above described paradigm, applied in six experiments on young cats, in which the tracers were injected into crus I or II of the cerebellar hemisphere (for details of the method see Rosina and Provini 1983) gave in brief the following results.

The double-labeled PN neurons, projecting bilaterally to crus I or II by means of intracerebellar axonal branching, account for 5 to 10% of the entire population of PN neurons projecting to the injected cerebellar areas. Among them the double-labeled neurons found in the PN ipsilateral to the FB tracer injection (recrossing neurons, D in Fig. 1) greatly outnumber the double-labeled neurons found on the opposite side (crossing neurons, C in Fib. 1) by an average ratio of 9 to 1. The pontocerebellar system connecting the two hemispheres is therefore mainly composed of PN neurons whose axons cross the midline twice, as originally suggested by Rosina and collaborators (1980). Within the PN nuclei the caudal parts of ventral paramedian and peduncular nuclei are the largest contributors to the system, while no double-labeled neurons were observed in the dorso-lateral nuclei.

A few double-labeled neurons bilaterally branching to the two cerebellar hemispheres were seen in the nucleus reticularis tegmenti pontis (NRTP), in the perihypoglossal complex (PH) and in the medullary paramedian reticular formation (MPRF), where the presence of neurons with intracerebellar axonal branching had already been observed (Provini and Rosina 1980, Rosina and Provini 1980, and unpublished material). In these bilaterally branching systems, however, crossed and recrossed components are equally represented.

The mossy fiber interhemispheric systems described here have some interesting functional implications. The pontine component the PN where bilaterally projecting neurons are located relay information mainly from the parietal, premotor and visual association areas (Baker et al. 1976, Brodal 1983, Rosina and Provini 1981). Thus it does not seem too farfetched to suggest that the PN component plays a role in the coordination of forelimb movements (cf. Brinkman 1981) and in the execution of manual tasks requiring visual guidance (cf. Myers et al. 1962, Ron and Robinson 1973, Mower et al. 1980). As to the component originating in NRTP, PH and MPRF it is well known (Precht 1977) that these precerebellar stations mediate visual and oculomotor informations to the cerebellum. These informations could be utilized by the cerebellar hemisphere in the control of saccades and of smooth movements of the eyes, as well as in the visual control of more complex manipulative tasks, as already suggested (Ron and Robinson 1973).

References

Baker J, Gibson A, Glickstein M, Stein J (1976) Visual cells in the pontine nuclei of the cat. J Physiol 255: 415-433

Brinkman C (1981) Lesions in supplementary motor area interfere with a monkey's performance of a bimanual coordination task. Neuroscience 27: 267-270

Brodal P (1983) Principles of organization of the corticopontocerebellar projection to crus II in the cat with particular reference to the parietal cortical areas. Neuroscience 10: 621-638

Kuypers HGJM, Bentivoglio M, Catsman-Berrevoets CE, Bharos AT (1980) Double retrograde neuronal labeling through divergent axon collaterals, using two fluorescent tracers with the same excitation wavelength which label different features of the cell. Exp Brain Res 40: 383-392

Mower G, Gibson A, Robinson F, Stein J, Glickstein M (1980) Visual pontocerebellar projections in the cat. J Neurophysiol 43: 355-366

Myers RE, Sperry RW, McCurdy NM (1962) Neural mechanisms in visual guidance of limb movement. AMA Arch Neurol 7: 195-202

Precht W (1977) The functional synaptology of brainstem oculomotor pathways. In: Baker R, Berthoz A (eds) Control of gaze by brain stem neurons. Developments in neuroscience, vol I. Elsevier/Amsterdam, pp 131-152

Provini L, Rosina A (1980) La proiezione cerebellare del complesso periipoglossale. Boll Soc Ital Biol Sper 56 (18bis): 239

Ron S, Robinson DA (1973) Eye movements evoked by cerebellar stimulation in the alert monkey. J Neurophysiol 36: 1004-1022

Rosina A, Provini L (1980) Mossy fibre branching from precerebellar reticular nuclei. Neurosci Lett S5: S442

Rosina A, Provini L (1981) Pontine projection to crus I and crus II of the cat cerebellum. A horseradish peroxidase study. Neuroscience 6: 2613-2624

Rosina A, Provini L (1983) Somatotopy of climbing fiber branching to the cerebellar cortex in cat. Brain Res 289: 45-63

Rosina A, Provini L, Bentivoglio M, Kuypers HGJM (1980) Ponto-neocerebellar axonal branching as revealed by double fluorescent retrograde labeling technique. Brain Res 195: 461-466

Subject Index

aberrant cerebellofugal projections 165
aberrant fiber connections 165
ablation of the cerebellum (see: cerebellectomy)
acceleration signal 291
3-acetylpyridine 230, 234, 238, 275
adaptation 9, 120f, 138, 142, 313
    of long latency EMG responses 138
    of long loop responses 9
    of OKAN 121, 142
    of synapse size 313
    of VOR (see: vestibulo-ocular reflex,
    adaptation of)
alcohol 137
aldehydfuchsin 322
alpha motoneuron 42
altricial rodent 318
amphibia 104
ankle strategy 54ff
ankle synergy 55
ankle torque 63
anterior lobe 126, 131, 136, 196, 284, 293
    and ataxia of stance and gait 131
    atrophy of 136
    lesion of spinocerebellar part 131
ape 194
archicerebellum 86, 128
Arnold-Chiari malformation 141
aspartate 263
associative memory 208
asthenia 128
ataxia 129ff, 164, 276
    and inferior olive 276
atrophy 131, 135f, 148f, 160
autocorrelation 296
autocorrelogram 260

balance condition 52
Bang-Bang timing model 209
barbiturates 236, 278
    and Gaba action 278
basal ganglia 36, 48
basal ganglia and trajectory control 48
basket cell 170, 232, 236, 269, 272, 318
bear 194
Behrmann projection 189

bidirectional pattern of discharge 40
body schema 82
boutons 301
brainstem nuclei 36
brain trauma 164
build-up of force 129
burst-tonic neurons 113

cerebellar hemispheres
    and ataxia 130
    and build-up of force 129
    and dysdiadochokinesis 129
    and dysmetria 129
    lesion of (see also: cerebellum, lesion of)
    128, 134
    and timing of movements 129
    and tremor 129, 130
cerebellar input 294
cerebellar learning (see also: motor learning)
    172
cerebellar lesion (see: cerebellum, lesion of)
cerebellar lesions and oculomotor deficit 122
cerebellar models and sensorimotor theory 208
cerebellar nuclei 16, 40, 119, 164, 196
cerebellar nuclei, cooling of 16, 142
cerebellar symptoms 83
cerebellar tensor ellipsoid 221
cerebellar vermis 142
cerebellectomy (see also cerebellar hemispherec-
    tomy 80, 140, 164, 239)
    and cerebellofugal projections 165
    and optokinetic nystagmus 140
    and smooth pursuit 140
cerebello-pontine angle tumors 141f
cerebello-prefrontal projection 82
cerebello-rubral fibers 164
cerebellum
    and clearing 206
    and dynamic loops 207
    and early antagonist response 27
    and Hebb-Synapse 209
    and intention-execution comparator 207
    lesion of 14, 16, 122, 131, 137

cerebellum
    and motor memory 209
    and motor set 14
    and phasic control 206
    and prediction 27ff
    and read out 209
    and shaping of PC dynamism 209
    and synergy models 208
    and tensor network theory 211ff
cerebro-cerebellar interactions 77
cervical myelopathy 137
chorea 137
clearing (see: cerebellum and clearing)
climbing fiber 87, 110, 115, 156, 170, 171,
    173, 174, 177, 220, 230, 256, 265f, 268,
    275, 278, 288, 293, 295
    and calcium currents 174
    collaterals 266
    and metric tensor 220ff
    retrograde labeling with [^{3}H]-D-asp 265
climbing fiber system (see: climbing fiber)
compensation of vestibular lesion 172
complex spike 100, 205, 233, 236, 260, 268,
    269, 275, 284, 293
    and calcium currents 236
conditioned movement 72
conflict stimulation 112ff
conjugate drift of the eyes 239
conjunctive hypothesis 256
constraints on plasticity 306
continuous movements 3, 4
control systems approach 210
cooling 16, 27, 46, 142, 235, 278, 280
    of cerebellar nuclei 16, 46, 142
coordination vectors 181
covariant assembly 212ff
covariant embedding procedure 213, 216
crosscorrelation analysis 254
cryocoagulation 275
CS (see: complex spike)
cuneocerebellar tract 293

dead beat effect 67
decerebrate rigidity 280
Deiters neurons 231, 237, 240, 241
    and inferior olive inactivation 237
dendritic spines 318
dentate nucleus 14, 32, 40, 70, 80, 129, 324
    lesion of 130
    and lipofuscin 324
    and projection neurons 324
    and small circuit neurons 324
deoxyglucose uptake 238, 239, 275
    and lesion of inferior olive 238
developmental calendar 318

discontinuous movements 3
distributed system 177
dorsal cap 87, 239
dorsal cerebellar vermis (see: posterior vermis)
dorso-lateral nuclei 327
double-fluorescent retrograde tracing 326
double labeling 165
downbeat nystagmus 143
dyadic product 219, 222
dynamic loop 207
dynamic parameters 290
dysarthria 138, 142, 148ff
dysdiadochokinesis 129
dysmetria 82, 129
dysprosody 138

early antagonist response 25, 27
efference copy 32, 88
Eigenvalue 217, 220, 221, 222
Eigenvector 217, 220, 221, 222
electric fish 168
electrocoagulation 275
extensor rigidity 128
external granular layer 318
exteroceptors 293
eye position 114
eye velocity 88, 114, 118

fast blue (FB) 326
fast eye movements 114
fastigial nuclei 139, 237
fastigio-reticulo-spinal pathway 280
field potential analysis 73ff
finger-nose test 130
flocculectomy 86, 90, 104, 115, 116, 118,
    140, 141
    and cancellation of VOR 141
    and OKN 141
    and smooth pursuit 141
flocculo-nodular lobe (see also: flocculus) 178
flocculus 86, 89, 93, 94, 101, 109ff, 114, 119,
    141ff, 178, 241
    and comparison monkey/rabbit 119
    and gaze paretic nystagmus 142
    lesion of 101, 142
    and smooth pursuit 109ff, 141
forelimb motor cortex 70
Friedreich's ataxia (see: Friedreich's disease)
Friedreich's disease 134, 136f, 148f, 159,
    160
frontal cortex 49
frontal eye fields 48
functional compensation 164
fundamental tensor 218

GABA 48, 236
gain change 250, 252, 256, 257
gain change hypothesis 250, 252, 257
gain of stretch reflexes 34
gait width 164
gamma motoneurons 42, 45
gaze-paretic nystagmus 90, 142, 143
gaze velocity Purkinje cell 88, 95, 115, 118,
    142
gigantic spine 303
giraffe 194
globus pallidus 48
Golgi cell 170, 232, 236, 293, 318
Golgi preparation 322
granular layer
    Type I cells 323
    Type II cells 323
    Type III cells 323
granule cells 114, 179, 284, 295
gravitational forces 57f
guinea pig 188

^{3}H-D-aspartate 263
hand movements
    visually initiated 73
harmaline 130, 173, 175, 234, 238, 280
harmaline intoxication 130
head velocity 88
Hebb-postulate 209 (see also: Hebb-Synapse)
Hebb-Synapse 206
heel-shin test 130
hemicerebellectomy (see: cerebellar hemispherec-
    tomy)
heriditary late cerebellar atrophy 135
hip strategy 54
hip synergy 55
Hodgkin-Huxley model 205
horizontal optokinetic eye nystagmus 100
horizontal semicircular canal 112
hypermetria 82, 164
hyporeflexia 128
hypotonia 128, 276
    and inferior olive 276

image slip (see also: retinal slip) 88, 118
image slip velocity (see also: retinal slip) 114,
    115, 120
inactivation period 256
inferior olive 87, 96, 166, 172, 175, 221, 230,
    235ff, 240f, 260, 275f, 280
    and ataxia 276
    and calcium currents 176
    cooling of 235
    and deoxyglucose uptake 238f
    and electronic coupling 177

    and eye drift 239
    and eye movements 172
    and harmaline tremor 238
    and hypotonia 276
    lesion of 172, 236, 238, 241, 276
    and Marr-Albus-Hypothesia (see also: in-
        ferior olive and motor learning) 172
    and motor learning 172, 240, 242
    and oscillatory behavior 176
    and postural activity 238
    and rebound excitation 176
    role of 172f, 240, 278
    stimulation of 172
    and symptomatology of cerebellectomy
    239
    and tonic inhibitory effect 278
    and VOR 172, 241
inhibition 272
inhibitory mechanism 32
instruction 24
intent 24
intention 130, 216
intention-execution comparator 207
intention vector 216, 217
interaction of climbing fiber and parallel fiber
    input 207
intermediate cerebellum 126
internal granular layer 318
interneuron 278
interpositus nucleus 32, 40, 70, 80, 164, 237,
    296
I.O. (see: inferior olive)
isoelevation 190
isoelevation map 190

joint position 293

Kennard principle 164
kinaesthetic discrimination 82
kinetic tremor 13

labyrinthectomy 112, 116
Lagrangian formalism 62
late cortical cerebellar atrophy 131
lateral cerebellar hemisphere (see: cerebellar
    hemispheres)
lateral cerebellar nuclei (see: cerebellar nuclei)
lateral geniculate body 165
lateral inhibition model 205, 223
lateral vestibular nuclei 275
learning (see: motor learning)
lesion of inferior olive (see: inferior olive, lesion
    of)
lesion of the spinocerebellum (see also cerebellum,
    lesion of) 131

lesion of the vestibulocerebellum (see also: cerebellum, lesion of) 133
lipofuchsin 322, 324
local circuit neurons 324
locomotor behavior 164
long latency EMG responses (see: long loop
  responses)
long-loop reflex (see: long loop responses)
long loop responses 7, 10, 12, 16f, 19, 135,
  137
  and cerebellar dysfunction 16ff, 135
  chorea 137
  and motor set 7
  and perturbation of movement 7
  and sensorimotor cortex 10, 17
lower vermis atrophy 141
Lugaro cell 170

M1 135
M2 135
M3 135
macromolecules and postsynaptic contact area
  312
manatee 188
Marr-Albus-Hypothesis 172, 247, 268
mechanical waves 198
medullary paramedian reticular formation
  (MPRF) 327
Mercator-Sanson projection 188
metric tensor 218, 220
microtubules 301
migration of granular cells 318
molecular layer 170, 318
monkey 119, 296
Moore-Penrose generalized inverse 219
mossy fiber 86, 87, 88, 110, 114, 178, 179,
  181, 284, 293
  and eye position 114
  and eye velocity 114
  and fast eye movements 114
  identification of 293
  and retinal slip 114
  role of 181
  and vestibular nerve input 114
movement apraxia 49
movement parameters, representation in cerebellar cortex 282ff
movement stability 36
movement trajectories 36, 46, 52
  stability of 46
multi-joint movements 1f
multiple sclerosis and -long latency
  EMG responses 137
multisensory-multimotor general sensorimotor
  theory 224

muscle responses 24
muscle spindle afferents 294
muscle synergy 53
myoclonic encephalopathy 143

neocerebellar dysfunction 19
neocerebellum 12, 19, 70, 128 (see also: cerebellar hemispheres)
nodulus, lesions of 89
non-linear oscillators 260
non-orthogonal coordinate axes 212
non-programmed discontinuous movements 16
non-programmed movements and cerebellar dysfunction 16
NOT (see: nucleus of the optic tract)
NRTP (see: nucleus reticularis tegmenti pontis)
nuclear yellow 165, 326
nucleus of the optic tract 91, 97
nucleus prepositus hypoglossi (PH) 92, 97, 99,
  101, 119 (see also: perihypoglossal complex)
nucleus reticularis tegmenti pontis (NRTP) 87,
  88, 91, 97, 99, 101, 327
nucleus vestibularis (see: vestibular nuclei)

ocular pursuit (see: smooth pursuit)
ocular symptoms of cerebellum diseases 86ff,
  109ff, 139ff
OKAN (see: optokinetic afternystagmus)
OKN (see: optokinetic nystagmus)
olivo-ponto-cerebellar atrophy 135, 148, 149,
  160
omni-directional pause cell 48
opponent frequency code 294
opsoclonus 143
optic tectum 310
optokinetic afternystagmus (OKAN) 89, 97,
  111, 113ff
optokinetic nystagmus (OKN) 88f, 109ff,
  115f, 141
optokinetic reflex (see: optokinetic nystagmus)
oscillatory behavior 176

palatal myorrhythmia 130
paleocerebellum 128
paraflocculectomy 140
paraflocculus 101
parallel fiber 87, 170, 178, 179, 181, 232, 268,
  300, 318
  transection of 300
paramedian pontine reticular formation 113
parietal cortex 48f, 327
parietal lobe (see: parietal cortex)
Parkinson's disease 59, 137, 149
  and long latency EMG responses 137
pars reticulata 48

pattern recognition 208
pause cell 48
P-cells (see: Purteinje cell)
peduncular nuclei 327
perihypoglossal complex (see also: nucleus pre-
     positus hypoglossi) 113, 137
perturbation of movement 7, 25
phasic control 206
physiological tremor 45
plastic changes
     and climbing fiber activation 171f
     of VOR (see also: vestibulo-ocular reflex)
     120f
plasticity 87, 230, 240, 300
plateau potentials 269ff
pons 119
pontine nuclei 32, 99, 165, 326
porpoise 188, 194
position sense 294
posterior lobe 70, 126
posterior vermis 139, 142
     adaptation of saccadic pulse 142
     lesion of 142
     saccadic dysmetria 142
postsynaptic contact area 301ff
postsynaptic density 301
postural body balance 9
postural movements 52
posture 52
posturography 131
potassium conductance
     176
precentral cortex
     neurons of 12
     and trajectory control 10
precocial animals 318
prediction 25
prefrontal cortex 70ff
premotor cortex 20, 70, 327
premovement potentials 80
prepositus hypoglossi (see: nucleus prepositus
     hypoglossi)
preprogrammed response 26
presynaptic contact area 301ff
presynaptic density 301
pretectum 91, 97, 99, 101
primary endings 294
primary fibers 119
primary vestibular fiber 110
primary vestibular neurons 112
primate 88
probing 168
programmed movements 3, 4
projection cells 324
pseudobulbar palsy 148, 149
Pt (see: pretectum)

Purkinje cell 86ff, 114ff, 170ff, 186ff, 205ff,
     230ff, 247ff, 260ff, 269ff, 275ff, 278f, 280,
     284ff, 300ff, 318ff, 323
     and gaze velocity 95, 115, 118
     identification of 292
     and optokinetic nystagmus 114, 117f
     and smooth pursuit 88, 95, 115, 118, 147
     and vestibulo-ocular reflex 115
Purkinje cell dynamism, shaping of 206
Purkinje cell ensembles 177, 230
pursuit system 100, 104 (see also: smooth pur-
     suit)
pyramidal tract 71

rabbit 103, 115, 116, 119
ramp shared movement 285
Ramsey-Hunt-Syndrome 130
rat 90, 164ff, 274
reaction time 76
read-out 206
rebound excitation 176
rebound nystagmus 143
reciprocal delay 60
recrossing neurons 327
recruitment of cerebro-cerebellar interactions
     77
red nucleus 164, 165
Reeler mutant 303
retinal ganglion cell 102
retinal slip 87, 91, 97, 99, 100
Riemannian metric tensor 219
Riemannian spaces 218
robots and brain theory 202

saccade (see also: fast eye movements) 327
saccadic dysmetria 142
saccadic eye movement 48
saccadic eye movements and
     substantia nigra pars reticulata neurons 48
sagittal stripes 258
sagittal zone 196, 258
secondary endings 294
segmental stretch reflex 28, 30, 45, 135
selforganization 208
sensorimotor cortex 17, 165
sensorimotor theory 208
sensorimotor transformation 213ff
sensory metric transformation 213
sensory reception 213
sensory vector 216
Shy-Drager syndrome 149
simple spikes 88, 93, 100, 114ff, 189ff, 234ff,
     248, 275, 278
single joint movements 1, 2, 12

sinusoidal movement function 289
slowly adapting mechanoreceptors 294
slow pursuit tracking 48
smooth movements 327
smooth pursuit 88, 100, 104, 109, 111ff, 140
somatosensory cortex 296
spasticity 159
spatial orientation 82
speech 138
     and cerebellar hemispheres 138
     and cerebellar lateralization 139
     superior vermis 138
spinal tumors 137
spindle afferent 41, 45
spine, gigantic 303
spines 301, 303
spinocerebellum 126
sprouting 300, 301, 303, 310
square wave jerks 143
stability of movement trajectory 46
stance 14, 52, 131
     in cerebellar patients 14
static parameters 285
stellate cell 170, 269, 272, 318
step tracking task 3
strategy 53
striate cortex 76
substantia nigra 48
superficial thalamo-cortical projections 73
superior colliculus 48
superior paravermal segment of the left hemi-
     sphere 139
superior vermis 138
support surface 52, 55
suspensory strategy 54
sway trajectories 56
switching mechanism 80
synaptic site size 301
synergics 53
synergy generators 60

temporal lookahead module 223
tensor 177
tensor analysis 218
tensor ellipsoid 218
tensorial brain theory 201
tensorial network theory 177, 182, 211
tensor theory 215
thalamic zone 165
thalamo-cortical projection
     deep 73
     superficial 73
thalamus, VA-VL region of 70
time constant 110
timing of force 129

timing hypothesis 186
timing of movement and cerebellum (see also:
     timing hypothesis) 12
time-sharing 206
tonic hypothesis (see also: tonic theory) 280
tonic inhibitory effect 278
tonic theory 230 (see also: tonic hypothesis)
toxic agents and cerebellum 135
training 31
trajectories (see: movement trajectories)
trajectory control 1, 14
     and cerebellar lesion 14
tremor 40, 44, 129, 130
     dentate nucleus 40
trophic theory of climbing fiber function 230
true blue 165
type I cell 323
type II cell 323
type III cell 323
type I neurons 113
type II neurons 113
type A pattern 285
type B pattern 285
type C pattern 285

ungulate 188
unidirectional pattern 40
urethane anesthesia 237, 278

velocity profile 2, 3
velocity signal 290
velocity storage 89, 92, 96, 102, 104, 111, 118,
     119, 141
velocity storage integrator 141
velocity-to-position integrator 90
ventral paramedian nuclei 327
vermis 194, 136 (see also: posterior vermis)
     lesion of 136
vestibular commissure 99
vestibular compensation and climbing fiber 172
vestibular nerve 112, 114
vestibular neurons 96
vestibular nuclei 86, 97, 99, 101ff, 110, 113,
     119, 128
     projection to 128
     and smooth pursuit 113, 119, 128
vestibular stimulation 93, 94, 113,
     in darkness 114
vestibular nystagmus (see: vestibulo-ocular re-
     flex)
vestibulocerebellum 86, 139
     and oculomotor functions 139
     and postural ataxia 133
vestibulo-collic compensation 212f

vestibulo-ocular mechanism (see: vestibulo-ocu-
    lar reflex)
vestibulo-ocular reflex (VOR)   86ff, 109, 112,
    115f, 118, 121, 140, 223, 241, 242, 247,
    257, 268
    adaptation of   87f, 121, 242, 247, 257, 268
    cancellation of   141
    and inferior olive   242
    suppression of   112, 115f, 118, 327 (see also:
    cancellation of)
    and tensor theory   223
vestibulo-spinal pathway   280
viscoelastic forces   58
vision   208
visual association areas   327

visual cortex   89
visually initiated hand movements   73
visual streak   112
visual-vestibular interaction   90, 95, 109
VN (see: vestibular nuclei)
VOR (see: vestibulo-ocular reflex)

walking   52
weaver mutants   301
white mouse   188

y-group   119

zona incerta   165

Studies
of
Brain
Function

Coordinating Editor:
V. Braitenberg

Editors: H.B. Barlow,
T.H. Bullock, E. Florey,
O.-J. Grüsser, A. Peters

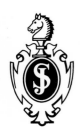

Springer-Verlag
Berlin
Heidelberg
New York
Tokyo

Volume 12
M. Heisenberg, R. Wolf

Vision in Drosophila

Genetics of Microbehavior
1984. 112 figures. Approx. 200 pages. ISBN 3-540-13685-1
In preparation

Volume 11
G.A. Orban

Neuronal Operations in the Visual Cortex

1984. 188 figures. XV, 367 pages. ISBN 3-540-11919-1

Volume 10
U. Bässler

Neural Basis of Elementary Behavior in Stick Insects

Translated from the German by C.M.Z. Strausfeld
1983. 124 figures. XI, 169 pages. ISBN 3-540-11918-3

Volume 9
E. Zrenner

Neurophysiological Aspects of Color Vision in Primates

Comparative Studies on Simian Retinal Ganglion Cells and the Human Visual System
1983. 71 figures. XVI, 218 pages. ISBN 3-540-11653-2

Volume 8
J. Hyvärinen

The Parietal Cortex of Monkey and Man

1982. 85 figures. XI, 202 pages. ISBN 3-540-11652-4

Volume 7
G. Palm

Neural Assemblies

An Alternative Approach to Artificial Intelligence
1982. 147 figures. VIII, 244 pages. ISBN 3-540-11366-5

Studies of Brain Function

Coordinating Editor:
V. Braitenberg

Editors: H.B. Barlow,
T.H. Bullock, E. Florey,
O.-J. Grüsser, A. Peters

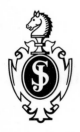

Springer-Verlag
Berlin
Heidelberg
New York
Tokyo

Volume 6
M. Abeles

Local Cortical Circuits

An Electrophysiological Study
1982. 31 figures. VIII, 102 pages. ISBN 3-540-11034-8

Volume 5
H. Collewijn

The Oculomotor System of the Rabbit and Its Plasticity

1981. 128 figures. IX, 240 pages. ISBN 3-540-10678-2

Volume 4
H. Braak

Architectonics of the Human Telencephalic Cortex

1980. 43 figures, 1 table. X, 147 pages. ISBN 3-540-10312-0

Volume 3
J.T. Enright

The Timing of Sleep and Wakefulness

On the Substructure and Dynamics of the Circadian Pacemakers Underlying the Wake-Sleep Cycle
With a Foreword by E. Flory and an Appendix by
J. Thorson
1980. 103 figures, 2 tables. XVIII, 263 pages
ISBN 3-540-09667-1

Volume 2
W. Precht

Neuronal Operations in the Vestibular System

1978. 105 figures, 3 tables. VIII, 226 pages
ISBN 3-540-08549-1

Volume 1
W. Heiligenberg

Principles of Electrolocation and Jamming Avoidance in Electric Fish

A Neuroethological Approach
1977. 58 figures, 1 table. XI, 85 pages. ISBN 3-540-08367-7